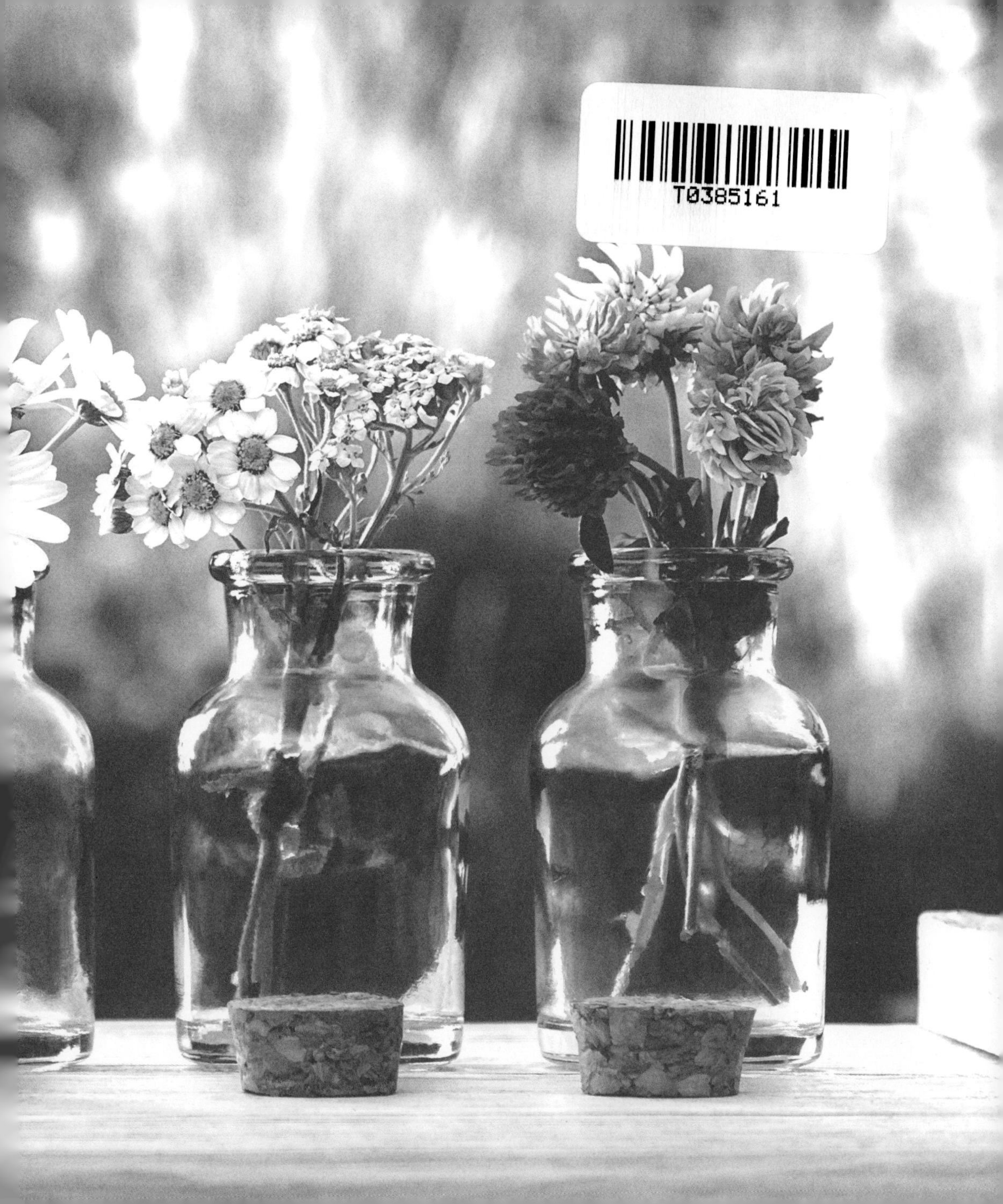
T0385161

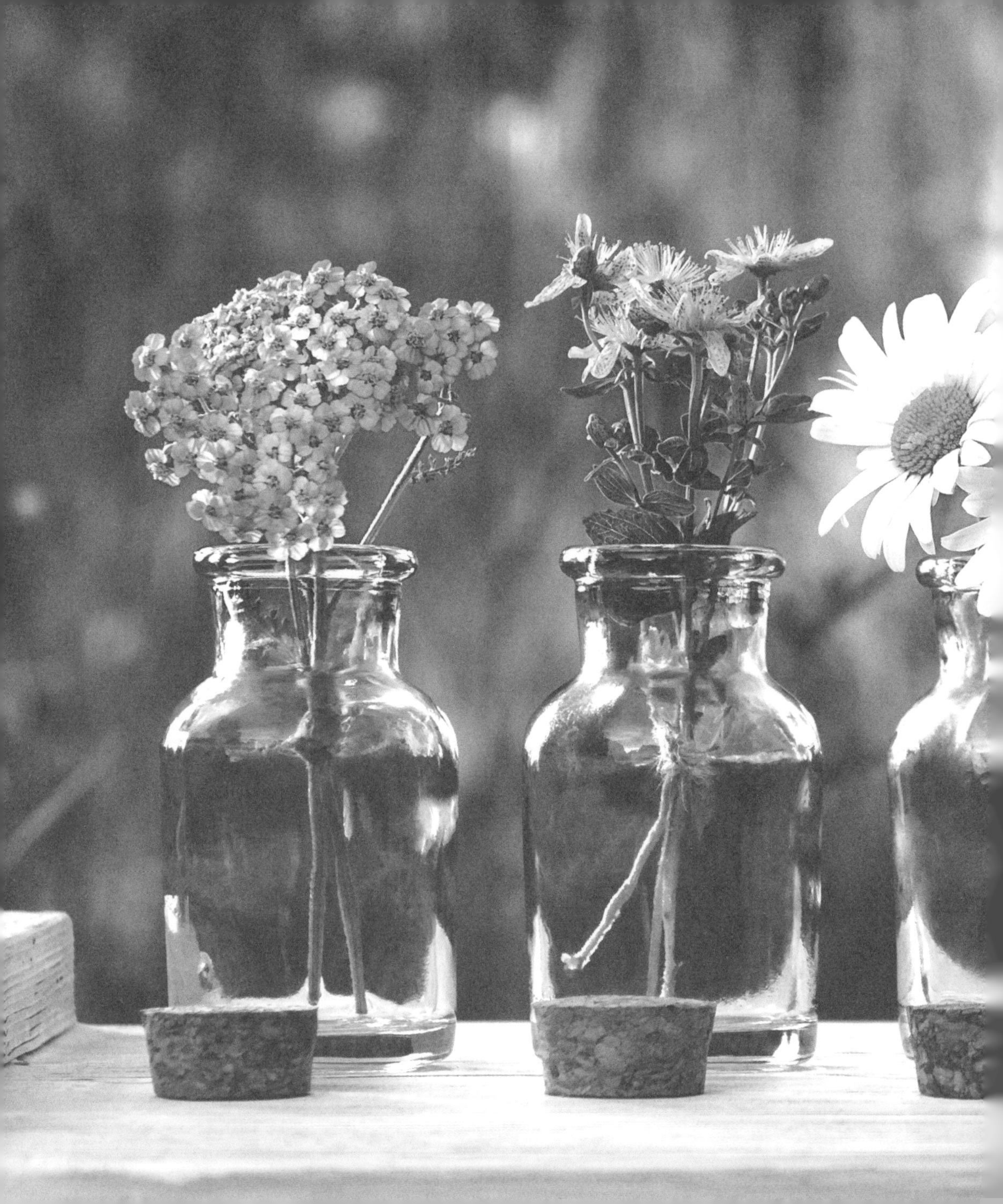

THE GARDEN APOTHECARY

THE GARDEN APOTHECARY

An Hachette UK Company
www.hachette.co.uk

Summersdale Publishers Ltd
Part of Octopus Publishing Group Limited
Carmelite House
50 Victoria Embankment
LONDON
EC4Y 0DZ
UK

www.summersdale.com

Printed and bound in China

ISBN: 978-1-78783-979-3

THE GARDEN APOTHECARY

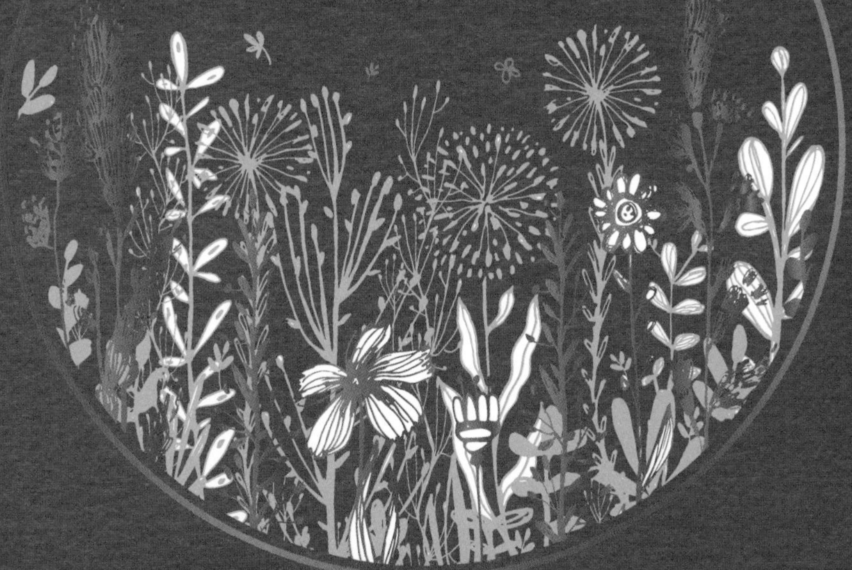

RECIPES, REMEDIES AND RITUALS

CHRISTINE IVERSON

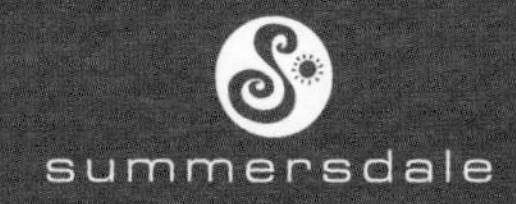

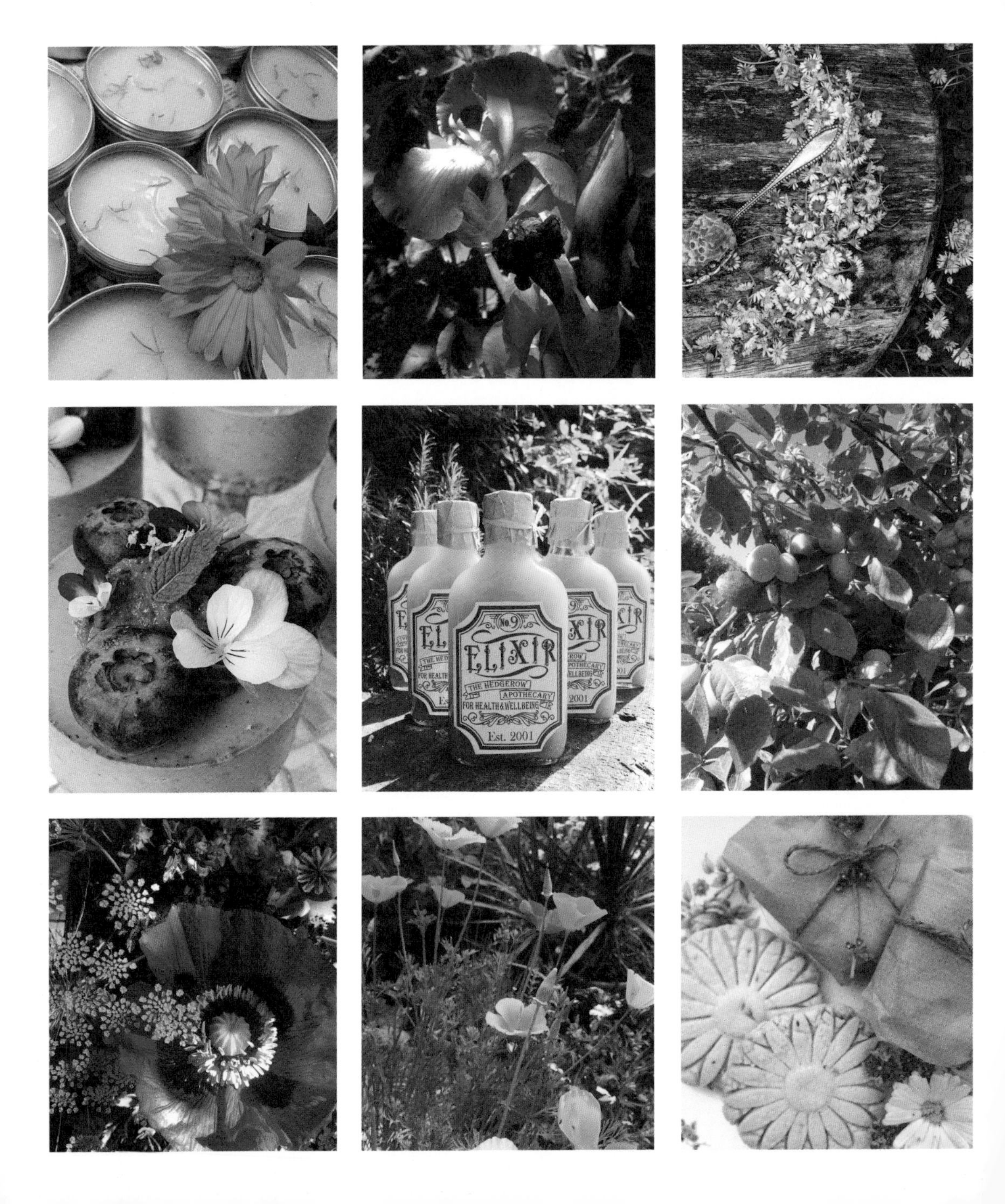
No.9
ELIXIR
THE HEDGEROW
APOTHECARY
FOR HEALTH&WELLBEING
Est. 2001

CONTENTS

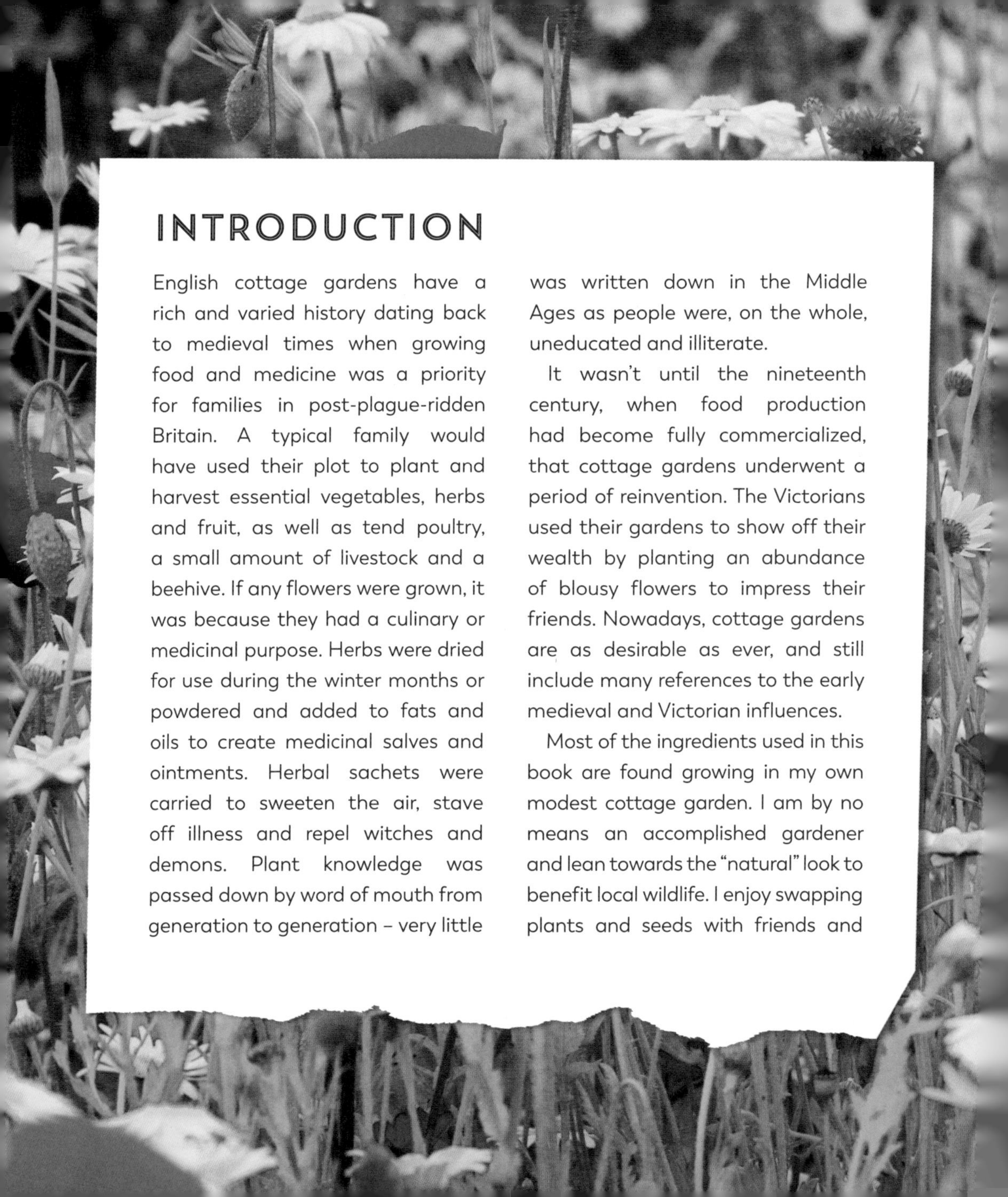

INTRODUCTION

English cottage gardens have a rich and varied history dating back to medieval times when growing food and medicine was a priority for families in post-plague-ridden Britain. A typical family would have used their plot to plant and harvest essential vegetables, herbs and fruit, as well as tend poultry, a small amount of livestock and a beehive. If any flowers were grown, it was because they had a culinary or medicinal purpose. Herbs were dried for use during the winter months or powdered and added to fats and oils to create medicinal salves and ointments. Herbal sachets were carried to sweeten the air, stave off illness and repel witches and demons. Plant knowledge was passed down by word of mouth from generation to generation – very little was written down in the Middle Ages as people were, on the whole, uneducated and illiterate.

It wasn't until the nineteenth century, when food production had become fully commercialized, that cottage gardens underwent a period of reinvention. The Victorians used their gardens to show off their wealth by planting an abundance of blousy flowers to impress their friends. Nowadays, cottage gardens are as desirable as ever, and still include many references to the early medieval and Victorian influences.

Most of the ingredients used in this book are found growing in my own modest cottage garden. I am by no means an accomplished gardener and lean towards the "natural" look to benefit local wildlife. I enjoy swapping plants and seeds with friends and

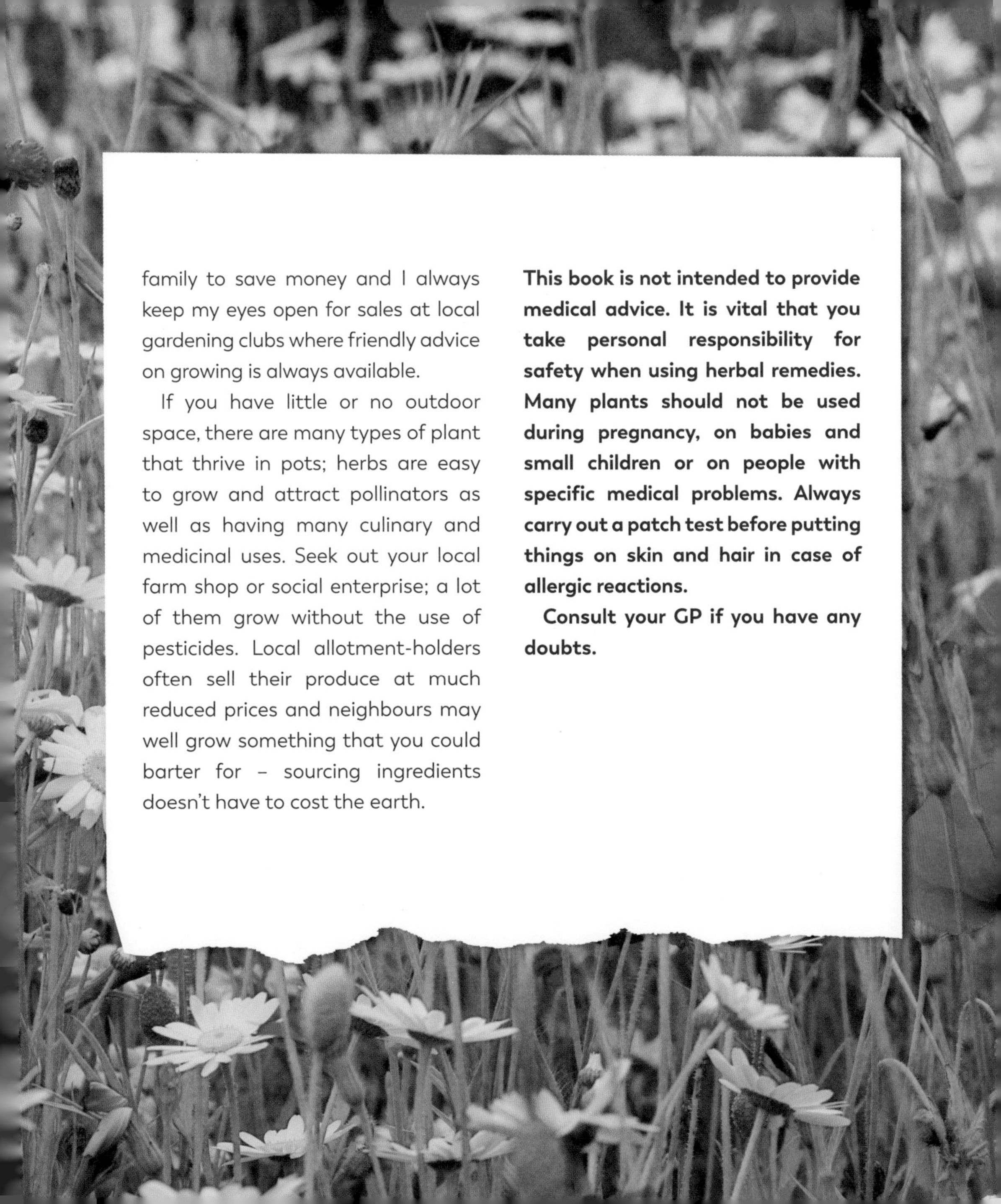

family to save money and I always keep my eyes open for sales at local gardening clubs where friendly advice on growing is always available.

If you have little or no outdoor space, there are many types of plant that thrive in pots; herbs are easy to grow and attract pollinators as well as having many culinary and medicinal uses. Seek out your local farm shop or social enterprise; a lot of them grow without the use of pesticides. Local allotment-holders often sell their produce at much reduced prices and neighbours may well grow something that you could barter for – sourcing ingredients doesn't have to cost the earth.

This book is not intended to provide medical advice. It is vital that you take personal responsibility for safety when using herbal remedies. Many plants should not be used during pregnancy, on babies and small children or on people with specific medical problems. Always carry out a patch test before putting things on skin and hair in case of allergic reactions.

Consult your GP if you have any doubts.

NOTE FROM THE AUTHOR

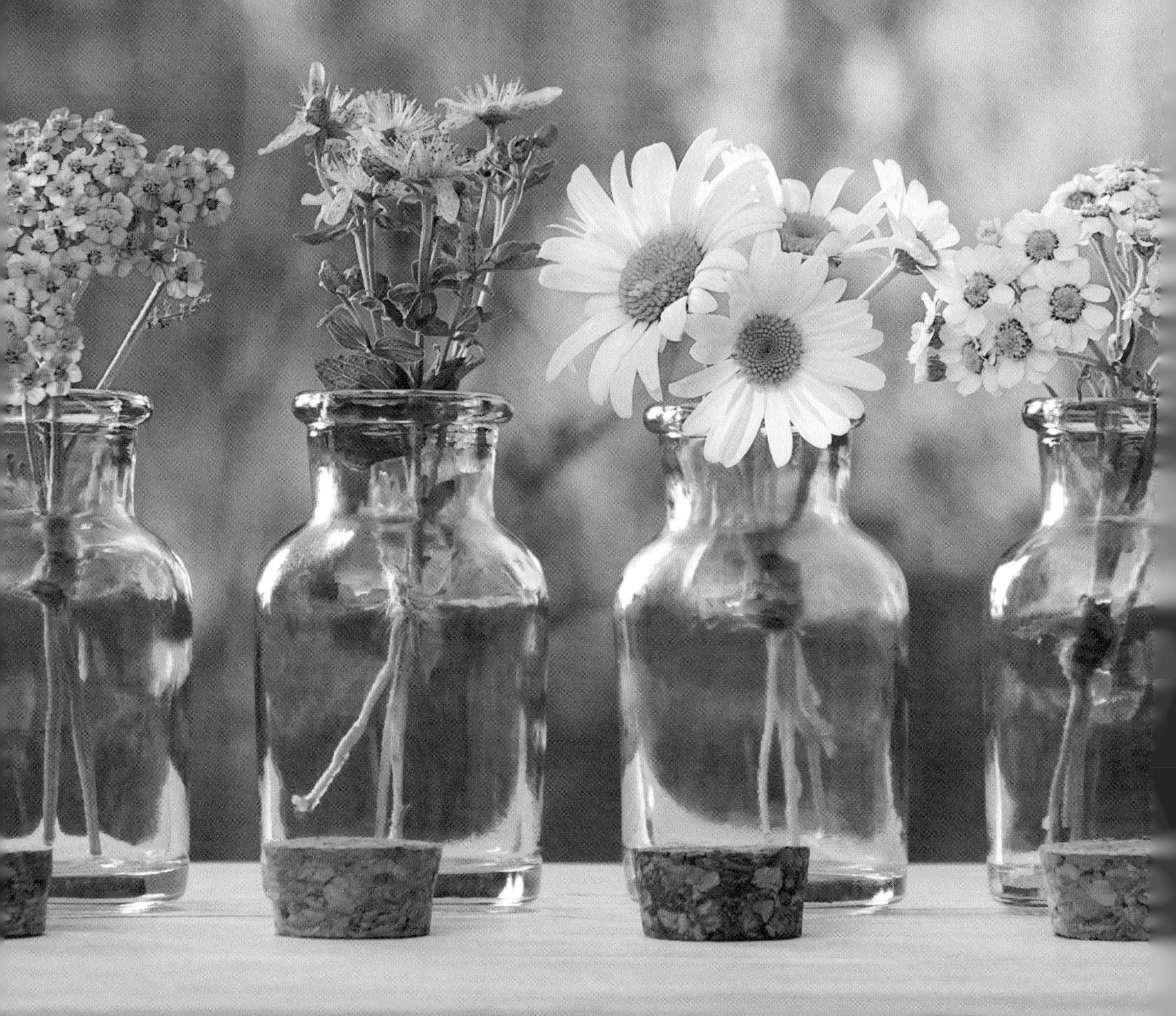

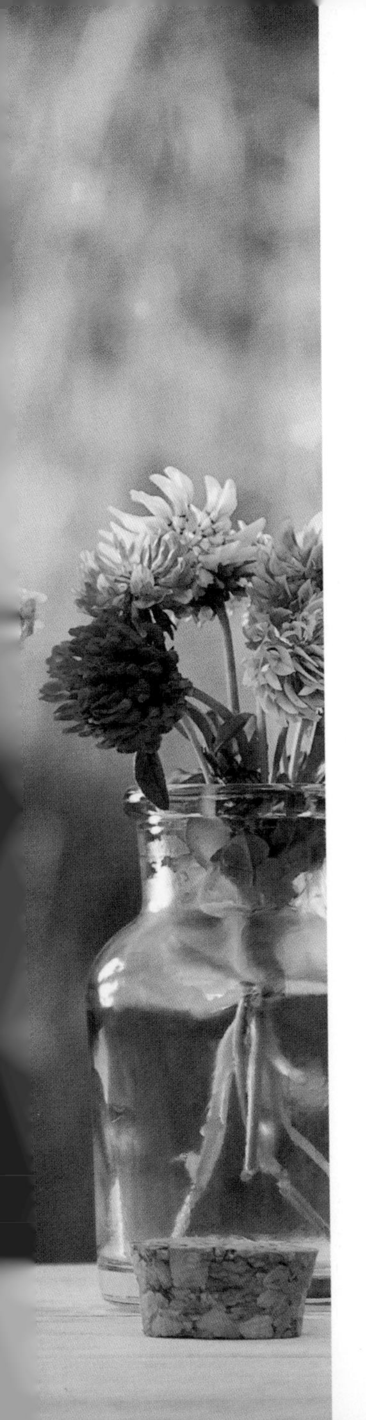

In 2020 our world changed significantly; access to open countryside was restricted, hedgerows and fields were off limits and we were "locked down" in our own homes for many months. Like a lot of people I found that gardening was hugely beneficial for my well-being, especially after some tricky and stressful times at work. This time certainly made me appreciate my little green patch.

With two nieces in the nursing profession I wanted to make them something natural to calm their poor skin. Constant hand washing was taking its toll and they were really suffering with dry and inflamed hands, which no amount of chemical-laden hand cream would soothe. Unable to venture out into the hedgerows I wandered into my own back garden for inspiration and discovered calendula. Healing Hand Balm (see page 54) was born!

Creating your own simple remedies needn't be daunting; it's just like following a cake recipe but with less familiar ingredients. Start with something simple and you'll soon find the confidence to be a little more daring – but be warned: it's very addictive!

THE GREAT HERBALISTS

I have used many references from the writings of one of the most famous English apothecaries (chemists) Nicholas Culpeper. He upset his medical colleagues by writing *The English Physician* in English instead of the preferred Latin. Culpeper wanted his teachings of medical and pharmaceutical knowledge to be available to everyone. I have also frequently referenced Pliny the Elder, who interestingly is believed to have died when Mount Vesuvius erupted in Pompeii in AD 79. Pliny, a commander in the Roman army, naturalist and author, famously wrote the 37-book *Naturalis Historia*, described as "an encyclopaedia of all contemporary knowledge – animal, vegetable and mineral", giving a wonderful insight into beliefs and practices in the first century.

PREPARING FLOWERS AND HERBS

It's important to prepare fresh botanicals before infusing them into carrier oils; excess moisture in the plants can turn the oil rancid rendering it useless. You don't need equipment like dehydrators to prepare your herbs and flowers. I use a piece of chicken wire fashioned into a frame for drying flower heads and petals. Herbs and flowers don't have to be absolutely dry but do need to be "wilted" for a couple of hours to remove some of the moisture. Lay petals and leaves onto kitchen paper overnight – whole flower heads will take a bit longer. Bunches of woody herbs can be hung up in cool airy places like outhouses or garden sheds, but avoid the cooking smells and smoke of the kitchen.

HERBS

Herbs are at their best before they begin to flower. Harvest them mid-morning on a dry day before the sun has burned away the flowers' essential oils.

- Remove any old, dead or diseased leaves – there's no need to wash them if you grow without the use of pesticides – give them a gentle shake to remove any insects.
- Tie the herbs into loose bundles with natural twine, hang upside down and put a brown paper bag over them to catch leaves as they dry.
- Keep them away from direct sunlight and leave for at least two weeks or until the leaves are crunchy. It's important that your herbs are completely dry or they could be spoiled by mould growth – check on them regularly and discard any that smell musty or have fluffy mould growing on them.
- Crumble the herbs with your fingers and store in an airtight container, where they will keep for about a year. I've found that rubbing the dried herbs through a colander effectively removes any woody stalks and crumbles the leaves up finely as well.

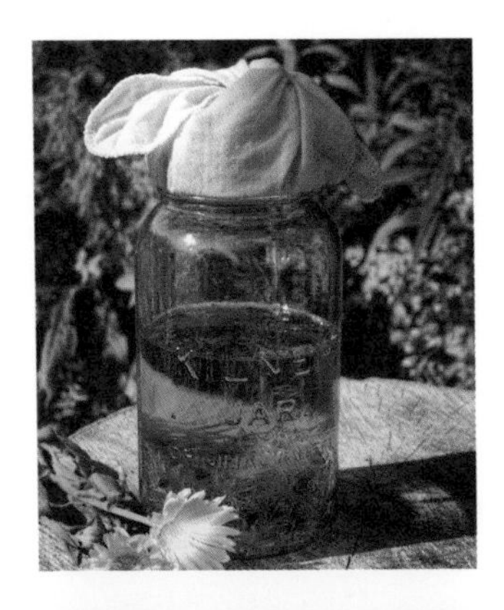

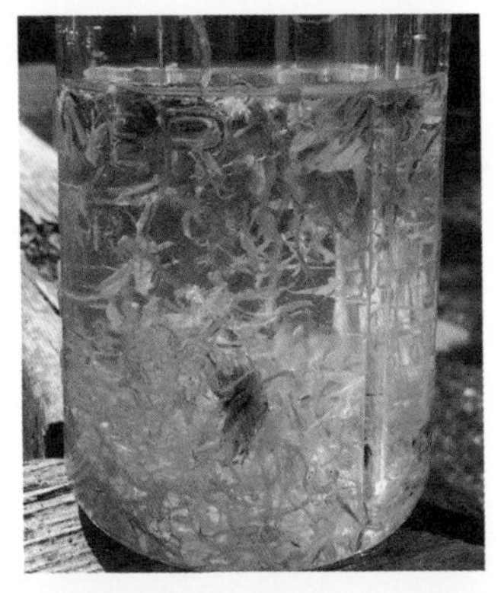

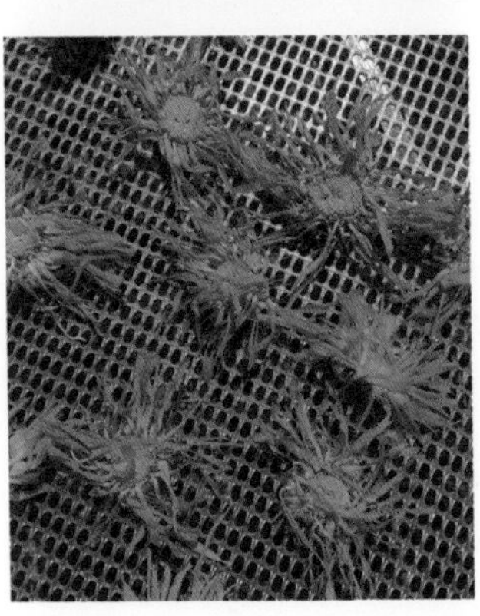

FLOWER HEADS AND PETALS

Harvest flower heads and petals mid-morning on a dry day when the flowers are looking their best. Avoid drying in direct sunlight as this can destroy the very health-giving properties that you wish to harness in your remedies. All you need for the drying process is a flat surface that allows air to circulate freely; chicken wire is perfect for this. Alternatively, hang up some muslin to create a flat hammock, or even use an old wire shelf from the oven. I place my chicken wire tray under the shade of a big old apple tree in the garden on a dry day, although if it's windy you might lose a few flowers. Remember to bring them back inside before nightfall otherwise the flowers will get damp with the morning dew.

- Lay baking paper over the wire of your drying surface, to prevent smaller petals falling through the gaps.
- Spread petals across the surface in a single layer, trying not to overlap them. They will dry quite quickly.
- Place flower heads far enough apart so they don't touch – these will take a while longer. They will shrivel and become crumbly as they dry. Place in a cool, airy place away from direct sunlight and turn them over occasionally.
- When they feel crunchy and crumble easily, store in an airtight container, label and date. Depending on the drying environment and type of flower they can take anything from two to four weeks to dry completely. Flower heads and petals will keep for up to a year.

CHOOSING THE RIGHT CARRIER OIL

There are a wide variety of plant-based carrier oils available on the market, all with different beneficial properties for you to choose from. These are used in homemade infused oils, lotions, massage oils and balms; they also "carry" essential oils that need to be diluted before going onto the skin. You can use many of the oils that you have in your kitchen larder or there are a huge variety of sellers online; try and find one that is reputable and stocks good quality oils – remember this product will be absorbed into your skin and into your bloodstream.

Many oils are pressed from nuts, seeds and kernels. If you have any allergies make sure you research thoroughly before using them, and always do a patch test first.

TYPE OF OIL	PROPERTIES	HAIR/SCALP		SKIN	
		Oily	Dry	Oily	Dry
Almond	Moisturizing Antioxidant High in vitamin E Natural SPF Nourishing	✓	✓	✓	✓
Apricot Kernel	Easily absorbed Antioxidant Anti-ageing Antiseptic High in vitamin A	X	✓	X	✓
Avocado	Soothing Hydrating Natural SPF Antioxidant Anti-inflammatory	X	✓	✓	✓

TYPE OF OIL	PROPERTIES	HAIR/SCALP		SKIN	
		Oily	Dry	Oily	Dry
Coconut	Easily available Antioxidant Anti-inflammatory Anti-microbial Anti-ageing Promotes hair growth	X	✓	X	✓
Grapeseed	High in vitamin E Easily absorbed Antibacterial Antioxidant Anti-dandruff	✓	✓	✓	✓
Jojoba	Antiseptic Hypoallergenic Hydrating Anti-inflammatory Anti-fungal Anti-acne Healing	✓	✓	✓	✓
Olive	Easily available Skin brightening Antioxidant Anti-ageing Collagen boosting Cleansing	X	✓	✓	✓
Peach Kernel	Easily absorbed High in vitamin E Hypoallergenic Good for older skin	X	✓	X	✓
Sunflower	Easily available Anti-inflammatory Moisturizing Easily absorbed	✓	✓	✓	✓

HOW TO MAKE INFUSED CARRIER OILS

Creating infused carrier oils is a lovely way to harness the properties of your garden flowers and herbs and turn them into the wonderful lotions, balms and salves contained in this book. I particularly love to make calendula infused carrier oil – not only does it become the most beautiful golden orange colour, it has wonderful skin healing benefits, too.

SUN METHOD

Healers and apothecaries have used this traditional method for hundreds of years and although it takes time and relies heavily on the appearance of the sun this is definitely my preferred way. I just love to see jars of different coloured botanical oils working their magic and infusing on my south-facing windowsill.

INGREDIENTS

Herbs or flowers, these can be dried or fresh

Carrier oil of your choice

Equipment needed

Glass jar

Muslin square

String or elastic band

METHOD

Fill the jar halfway with your plant material.

Cover with your chosen carrier oil shaking to burst any bubbles. Ensure that all plant material is completely covered – anything sticking out could go mouldy.

Top with the muslin and secure with string or an elastic band.

Place on a sunny windowsill for at least 2 weeks until the oil has taken on some colour and scent.

Strain the oil through the muslin, squeezing to extract all the oil. Compost the plant material left behind.

Label and date – you might think that you'll remember which oil it is, but believe me you won't!

Keep in a cool dark place and use within a year.

QUICK INFUSION METHOD

In the winter months this technique enables you to infuse carrier oil without the help of the sun. This method is a lot quicker than the sun method, but may not extract as many beneficial oils as the traditional method. Be careful not to fry your plant material by heating the oil too much.

INGREDIENTS

Herbs or flowers, these can be dried or freshly wilted

Carrier oil of your choice

Equipment needed

Heatproof bowl

Saucepan

Boiling water

METHOD

Put the plant material and carrier oil into your heatproof bowl suspended over the pan of boiling water; ensure the water doesn't touch the bottom of the bowl.

Simmer gently, without a lid, for 2 hours checking the water level in the pan regularly.

Allow to cool, strain, label and date.

Keep in a cool dark place and use within a year.

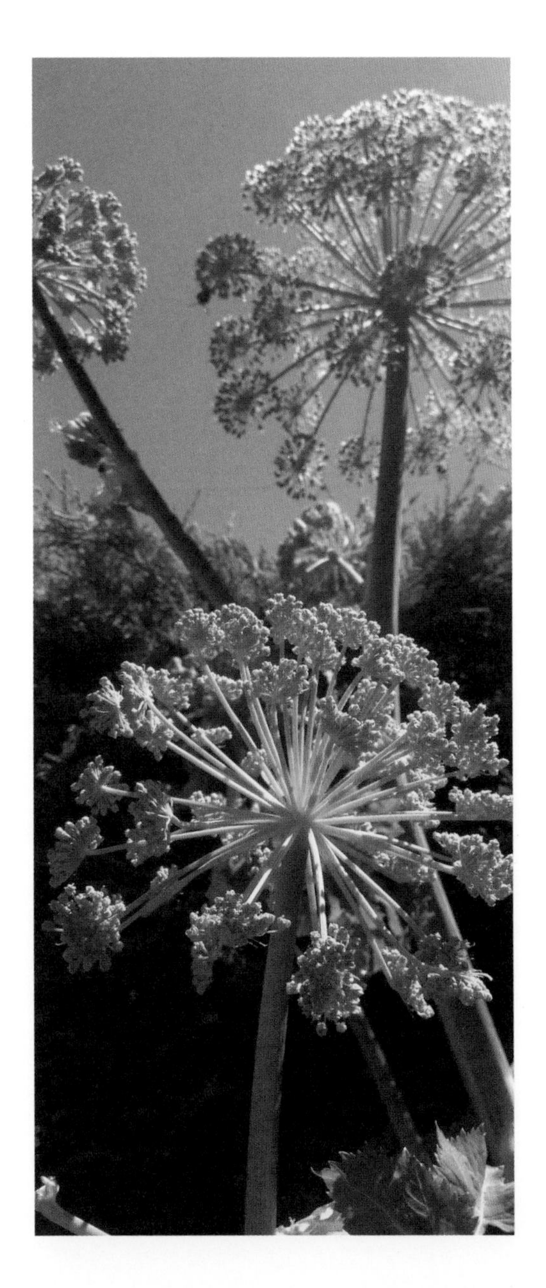

STERILIZING JARS AND BOTTLES

It's good practice to sterilize all your jars and bottles before use. This will extend the shelf life of your product by removing bacteria and germs.

Wash jars and bottles in hot soapy water and rinse.

Lay the jars in an oven preheated to 140°C (285°F) for 10–15 minutes until dry.

Soak the lids in boiling water in a bowl, dry thoroughly with kitchen paper before use.

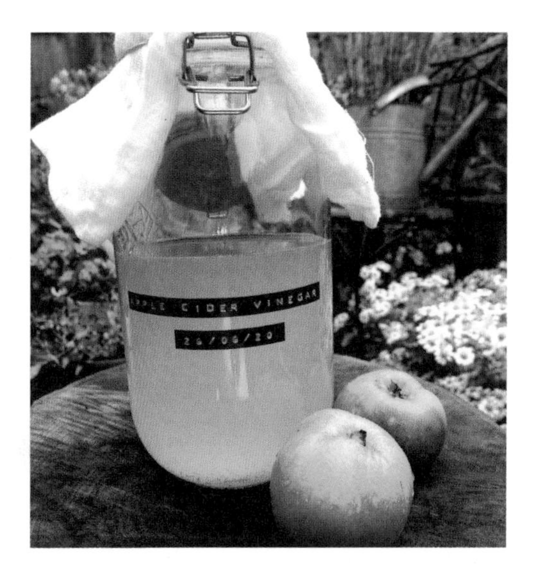

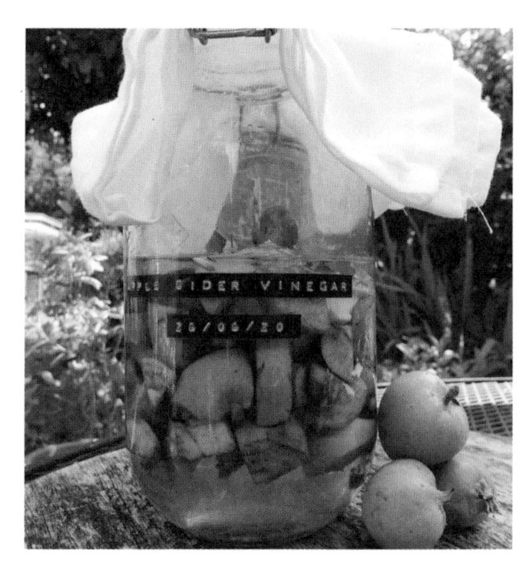

SETTING POINT FOR JAM: You'll need this when making the jams included in some of the recipes. Before beginning your jam-making put a couple of small plates in the freezer. To test for setting point, take the pan off the heat and place a small blob onto one of the cold plates. Let it stand for a minute, then push the blob with your finger and you should see it wrinkle. If the jam is still liquid, pop it on to boil for another 5 minutes and test again.

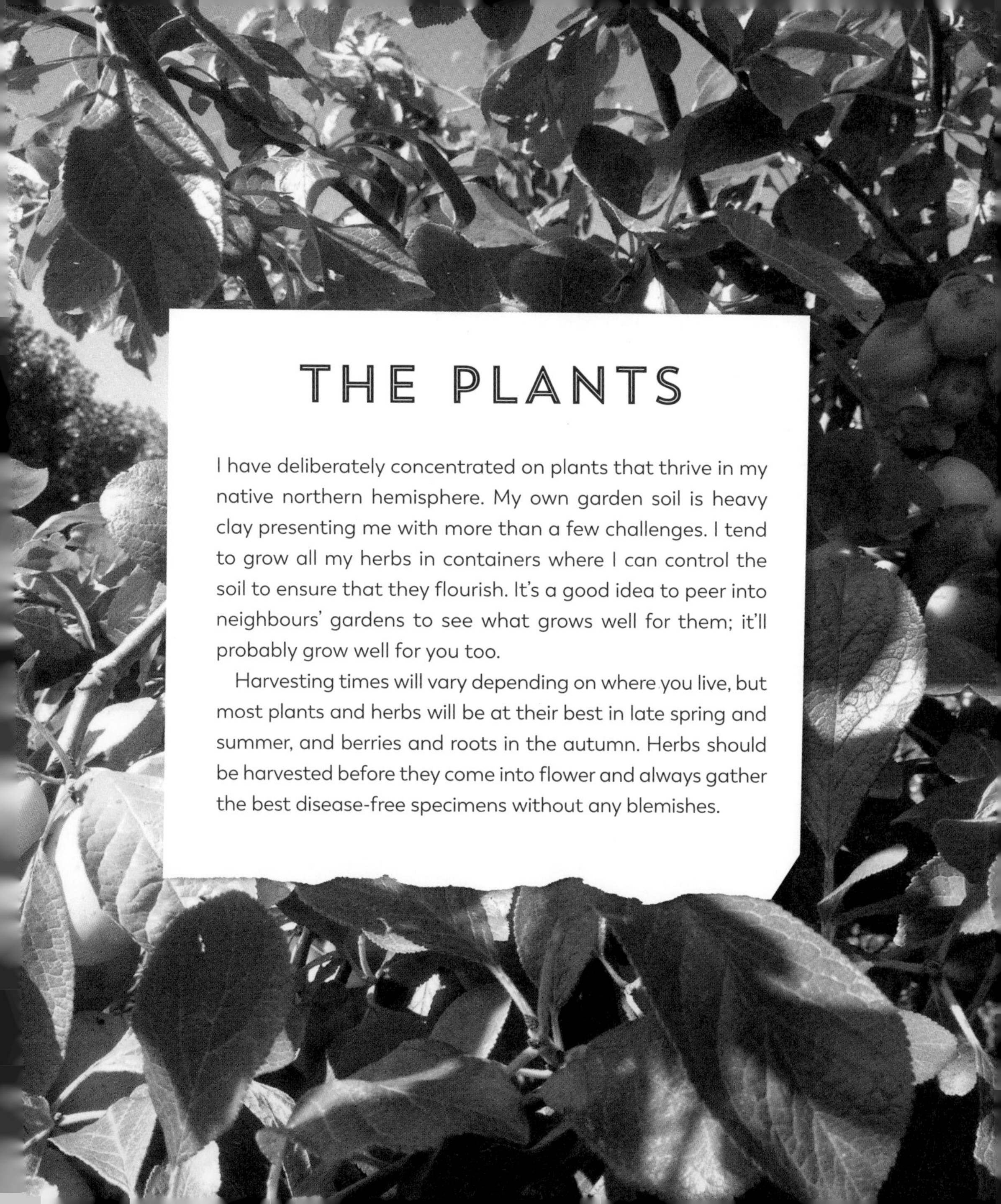

THE PLANTS

I have deliberately concentrated on plants that thrive in my native northern hemisphere. My own garden soil is heavy clay presenting me with more than a few challenges. I tend to grow all my herbs in containers where I can control the soil to ensure that they flourish. It's a good idea to peer into neighbours' gardens to see what grows well for them; it'll probably grow well for you too.

Harvesting times will vary depending on where you live, but most plants and herbs will be at their best in late spring and summer, and berries and roots in the autumn. Herbs should be harvested before they come into flower and always gather the best disease-free specimens without any blemishes.

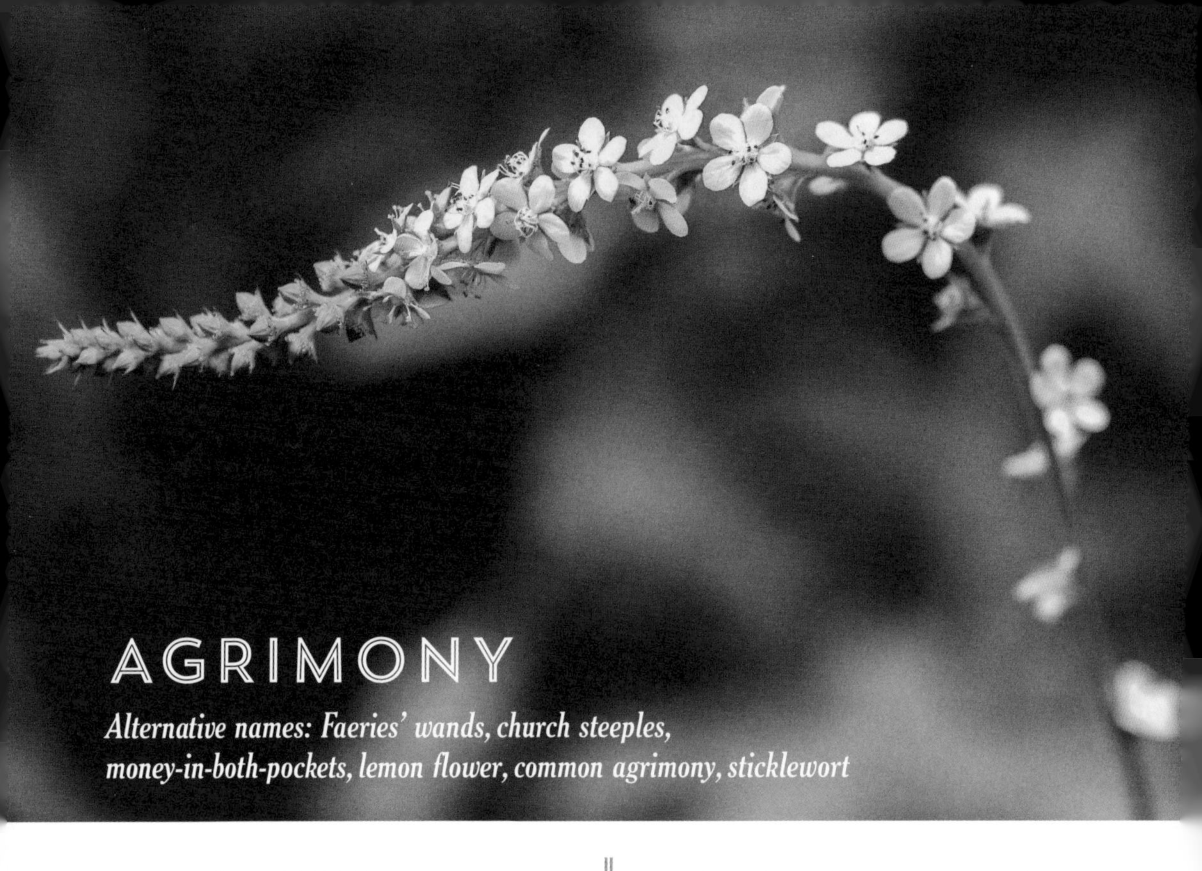

AGRIMONY

Alternative names: Faeries' wands, church steeples, money-in-both-pockets, lemon flower, common agrimony, sticklewort

HOW TO IDENTIFY: Tall hairy spikes carry five-petalled apricot-scented yellow flowers and serrated leaves.

HISTORY: Native to the UK, the name agrimony comes from the Greek word *argemone* meaning "plants that heal the eyes". The fruits of agrimony have been found in Neolithic excavations, although unfortunately their use at that time is unknown.

The Roman author and naturalist Pliny the Elder considered agrimony "an herbe of princely authority", using it to treat liver and kidney problems.

Dr Edward Bach of flower remedies fame chose agrimony as one of his 38 flower essences to be used by those who put on a "brave face" while actually harbouring inner turmoil.

FOLKLORE: With its wand-like flower-covered spikes, agrimony was used to ward off hexes and block curses, returning them back to their sender.

During a witch trial in Scotland in 1716, Ferquhar Ferguson admitted to using agrimony to cure someone who was "elf shot", which has been explained in Anglo Saxon texts as being injured by invisible arrows. Unsurprising then that agrimony would be carried about the person to create a "psychic shield" as protection against witches, elves and evil influences. It was also sometimes used as a tool to seek out witches.

Flowers that resemble holy objects were believed to have the ability to protect against evil spirits; one folk name for agrimony is "church steeples" explaining why it was regarded as so powerful.

FOLK MEDICINE: This native plant has long been used on medieval battlefields to staunch blood flow as well as a treatment for warts and snakebites. Agrimony seeds and leaves were made into a solution for healing wounds known as *eau d'arquebusade* or "musket shot water".

The Physicians of Myddfai were a group of thirteenth-century doctors, practising in Wales, their cure for mastitis recommends:

"Take agrimony, betony and vervain and pound well, then mix with strong old ale, strain well, and set some milk on the fire; when this boils add the liquor thereto and make a posset [spicy, hot milk drink] thereof, giving it to the woman to drink warm. Let her do this frequently and she will be cured."

And from Culpeper:

"It openeth and cleanseth the liver, helpeth the jaundice, and is very beneficial to the bowels, healing all inward wounds, bruises, hurts, and other distemper... is good against the biting and stinging of serpents, and helps them that have foul, troubled or bloody water, and causes them to make clear water speedily."

In medieval England, agrimony was placed underneath the pillow to cure insomnia, the patient staying asleep the whole time that it was there. An ancient rhyme of unknown origin explains:

"If it be leyd under a mann's head,
He shall sleepyn as he were dead;
He shall never drede ne wakyn
Till fro under hi heed it be takyn."

OTHER COMMON USES: Flowers gathered in late summer produce a pale yellow natural dye; autumn flowers can be used for a deeper yellow colour.

BEDROOM POTPOURRI

The fragrant honey scent of agrimony flowers is retained even when dried; the soporific properties of all the other flowers in this remedy make a calming potpourri to keep on your bedside table. Orris root, with a scent itself that has been compared to Parma violets, has the ability to enhance other scents. This recipe makes enough to fill a medium-sized bowl.

INGREDIENTS

25g dried agrimony flowers

25g dried rose petals

25g dried camomile flowers

25g dried meadowsweet

25g dried lavender

25g dried lemon balm

3 tbsp orris root

3 drops lavender essential oil

3 drops rose essential oil

METHOD

Mix the dried flowers and orris root together thoroughly in a bowl.

Add the oils and mix again.

Place a handful of the potpourri in an open bowl beside your bed, keeping the rest in a sealed container for later use. Alternatively, tuck into a draw-string pouch and place under your pillow.

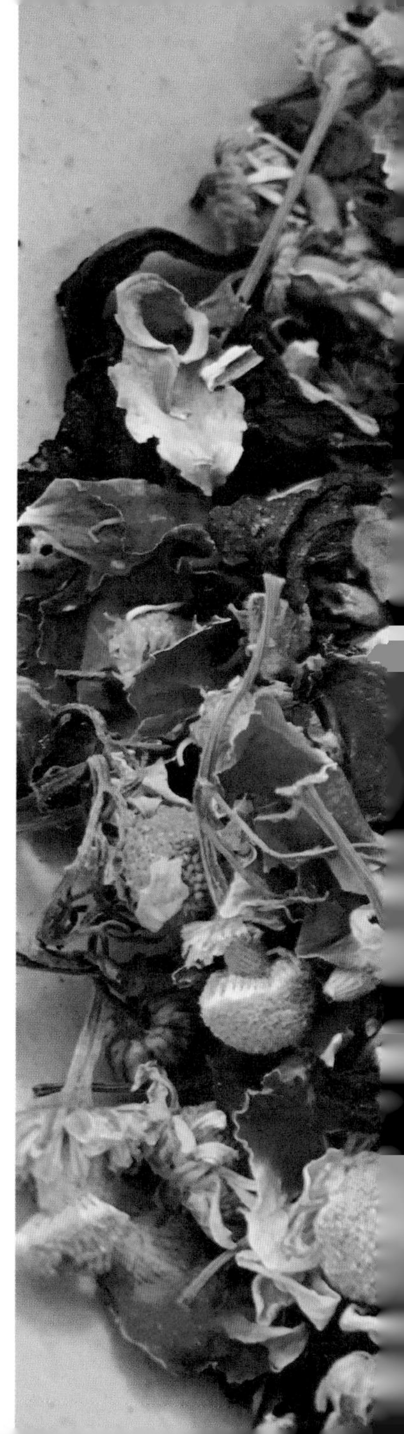

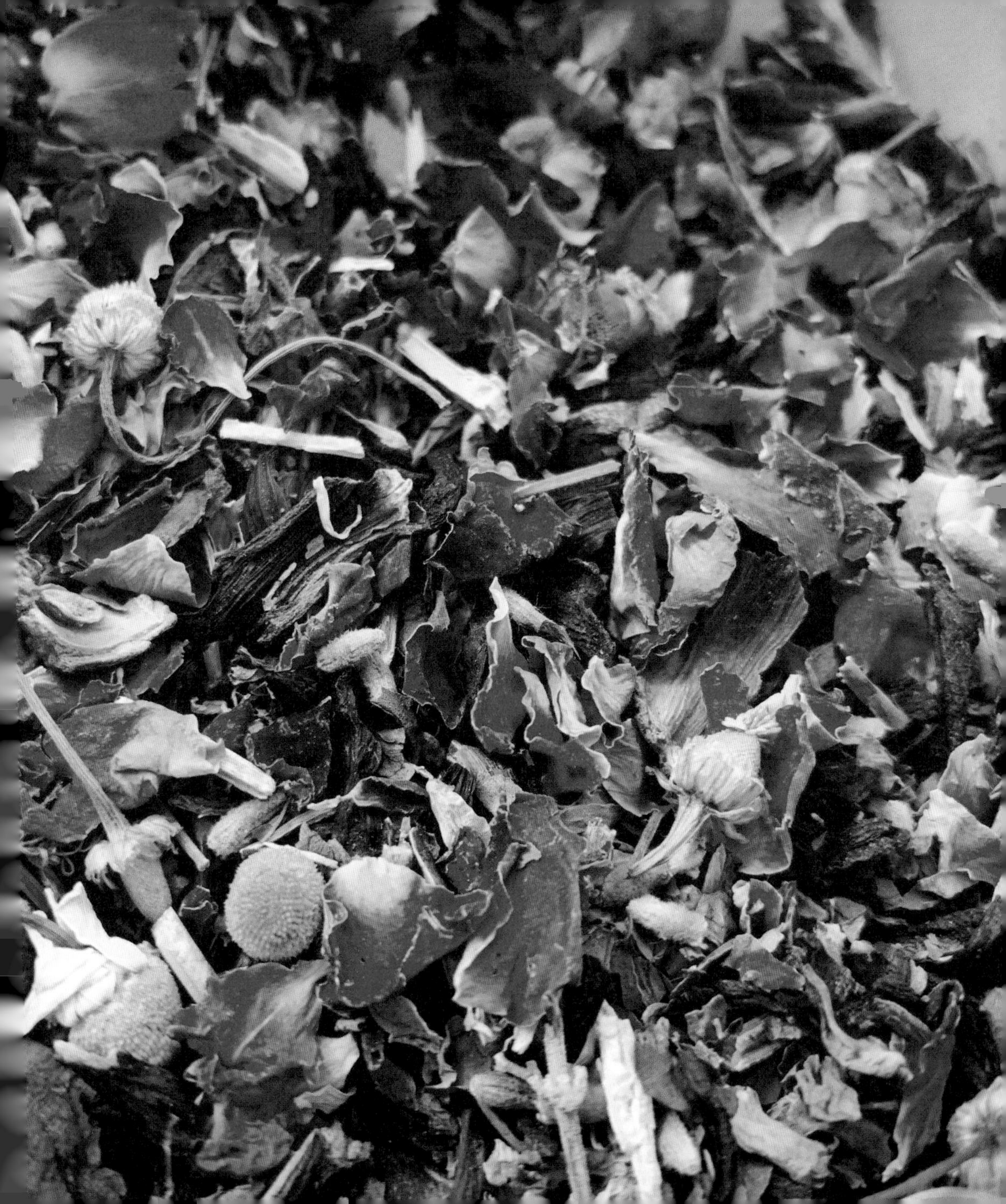

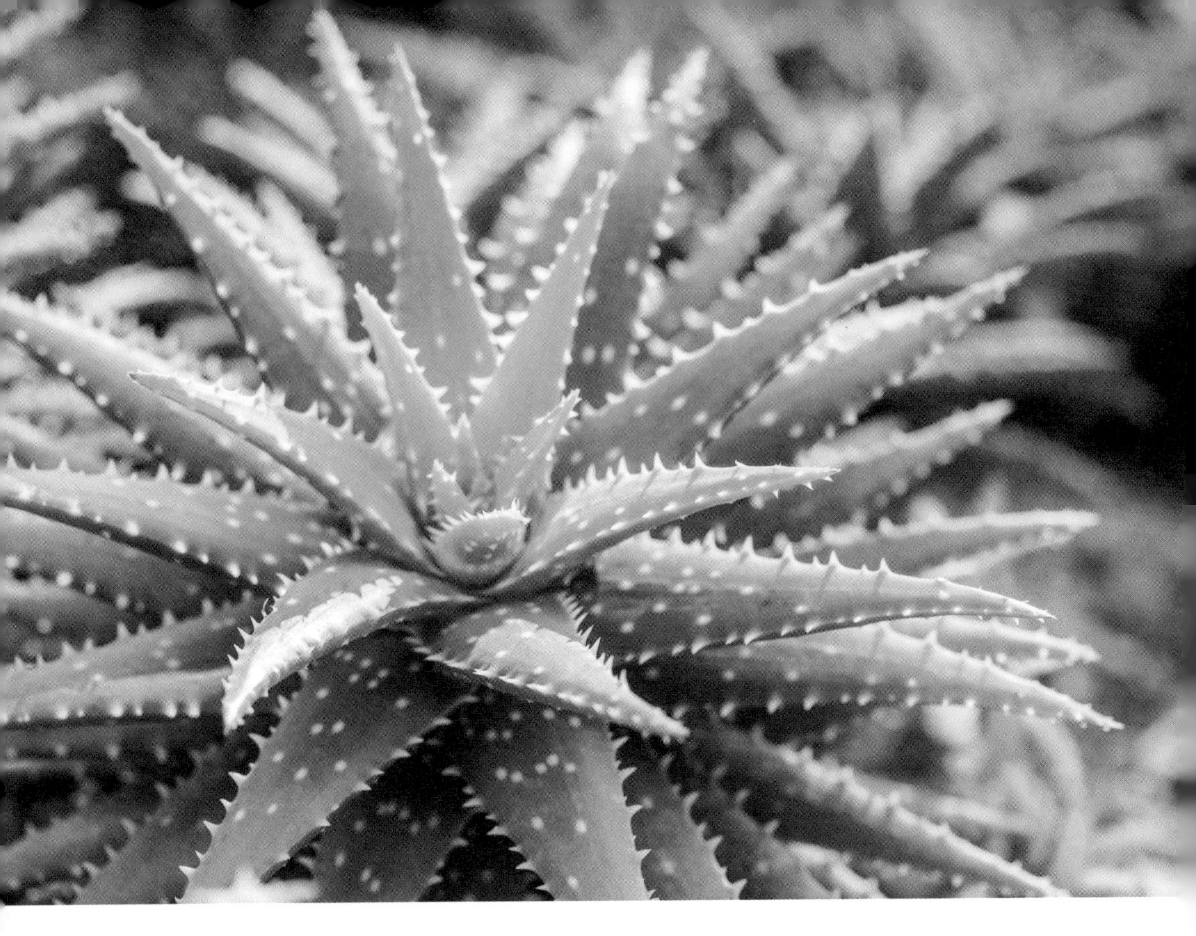

ALOE VERA

Alternative names: Burn plant, first-aid plant, medicine plant

HOW TO IDENTIFY: Although not native to the UK, aloe vera can successfully grow on windowsills and in greenhouses. Aloe vera is a member of the succulent family, with thick fleshy upright pointed leaves with little "teeth" along their edges.

HISTORY: Thousands of years ago, Cleopatra and Nefertiti are both known to have used the nourishing juice of aloe vera in their beauty routines. Aloe vera was also used in the embalming process for its antibacterial and anti-fungal properties.

The fifteenth-century explorer Christopher Columbus grew aloe plants on board his ships to use medicinally as a wound healer. Sixteenth-century Native American tribes applied aloe to their skin and their wooden cooking and working implements to prevent insect infestation.

During World War Two, aloe juice provided by botanical gardens was used effectively to heal radiation burns caused by X-rays.

FOLKLORE: In South American culture, aloe leaves are strung up around the house to ward off evil spirits, keep members of the household safe from accidents and ensure good luck.

Pilgrims to Mecca hang aloe over the doorways of their homes as a protective measure and to symbolize that they are going on a pilgrimage.

FOLK MEDICINE: The Roman author Pliny the Elder recommended that aloe juice was used to cure the sores of leprosy and to reduce perspiration. The Knights Templar drank aloe juice with palm wine and hemp, which they called the "Elixir of Jerusalem" believing that it would add years to their lives.

Also known as "first-aid plant" and "medicine plant" this gives us a clue to the respect that was given to this wonderful healing plant. Culpeper advises:

"Aloes made into a powder, and strewed upon new bloody wounds, stops the blood and heals them; it likewise closes up old ulcers, particularly those about the private parts and fundament [bowel]: boiled with wine and honey it heals rifts and haemorrhoids...removes obstructions of the viscera, kills worms in the stomach and intestines..."

OTHER COMMON USES: An aloe leaf can be cut and rubbed on minor burns to give instant relief and speed up healing. Aloe is very skin friendly and is used in cosmetics and in sun creams. I'm sure many of you had bitter aloes painted on your fingernails as a child to deter biting – I certainly did.

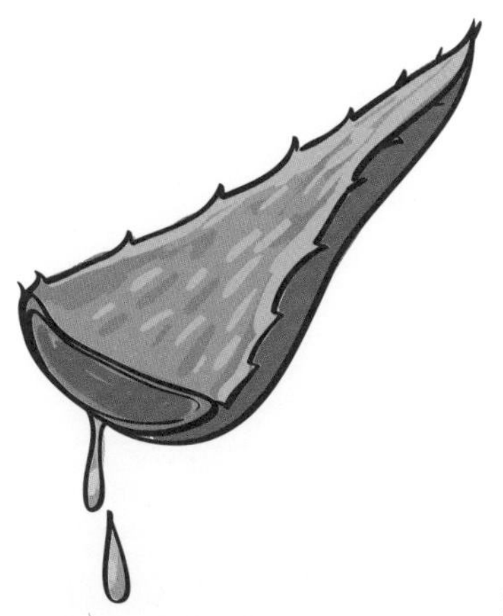

ALOE VERA AFTER-SUN SOOTHER

Needless to say it's healthier not to let your skin get sunburned, however if you do get caught out this kitchen recipe will help to soothe the burn. Aloe is anti-inflammatory, anti-viral, anti-fungal and antibacterial, and will gently relieve, cool and rehydrate sun-damaged skin. Coconut oil moisturizes the skin and relieves the itchiness of sunburn. Lavender essential oil is a great burn healer, reduces inflammation and relieves pain.

Extracting aloe gel from the plant is pretty straightforward. Cut a large leaf from the plant and remove the green outer-leaf casing. Put the clear slippery gel into a food processor and blitz until it turns to liquid. Alternatively, organic aloe vera gel is easily available on the high street and online if you don't have access to a plant.

Makes about 50ml

INGREDIENTS

4 tbsp aloe vera gel

2 tbsp extra virgin coconut oil

4 drops lavender essential oil

Equipment needed

A clean, sterilized jar

METHOD

In a clean bowl, combine all the ingredients thoroughly.

Spoon into the jar and refrigerate.

Gently apply a compress of a cold wet towel over the burned area to cool the skin before applying the gel.

The coconut oil in the after-sun gel will have set in the fridge, give it a stir to loosen it before applying gently to the skin.

Use within a month.

This lotion should only be used for mild cases of sunburn, please seek medical advice for more severe cases.

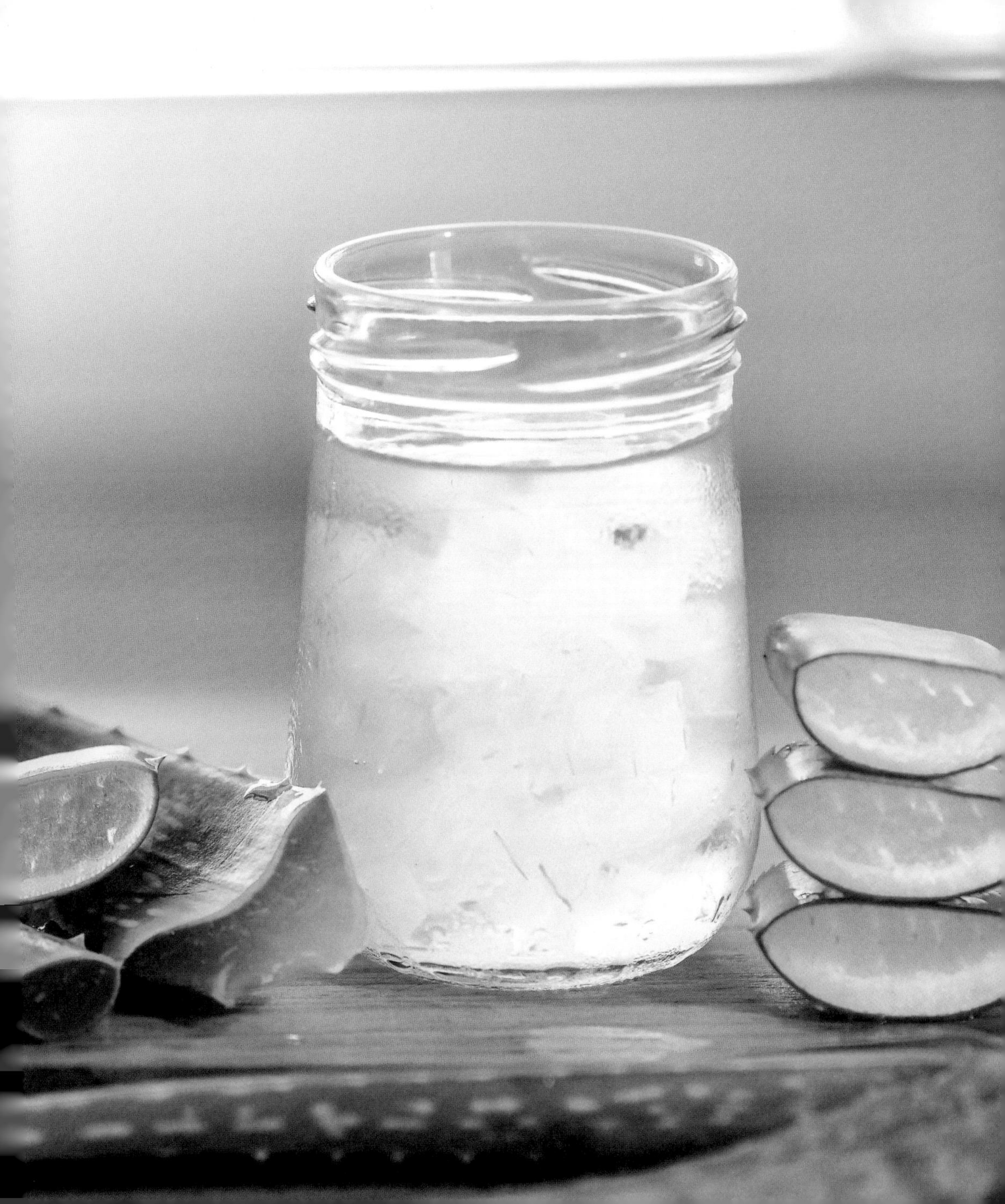

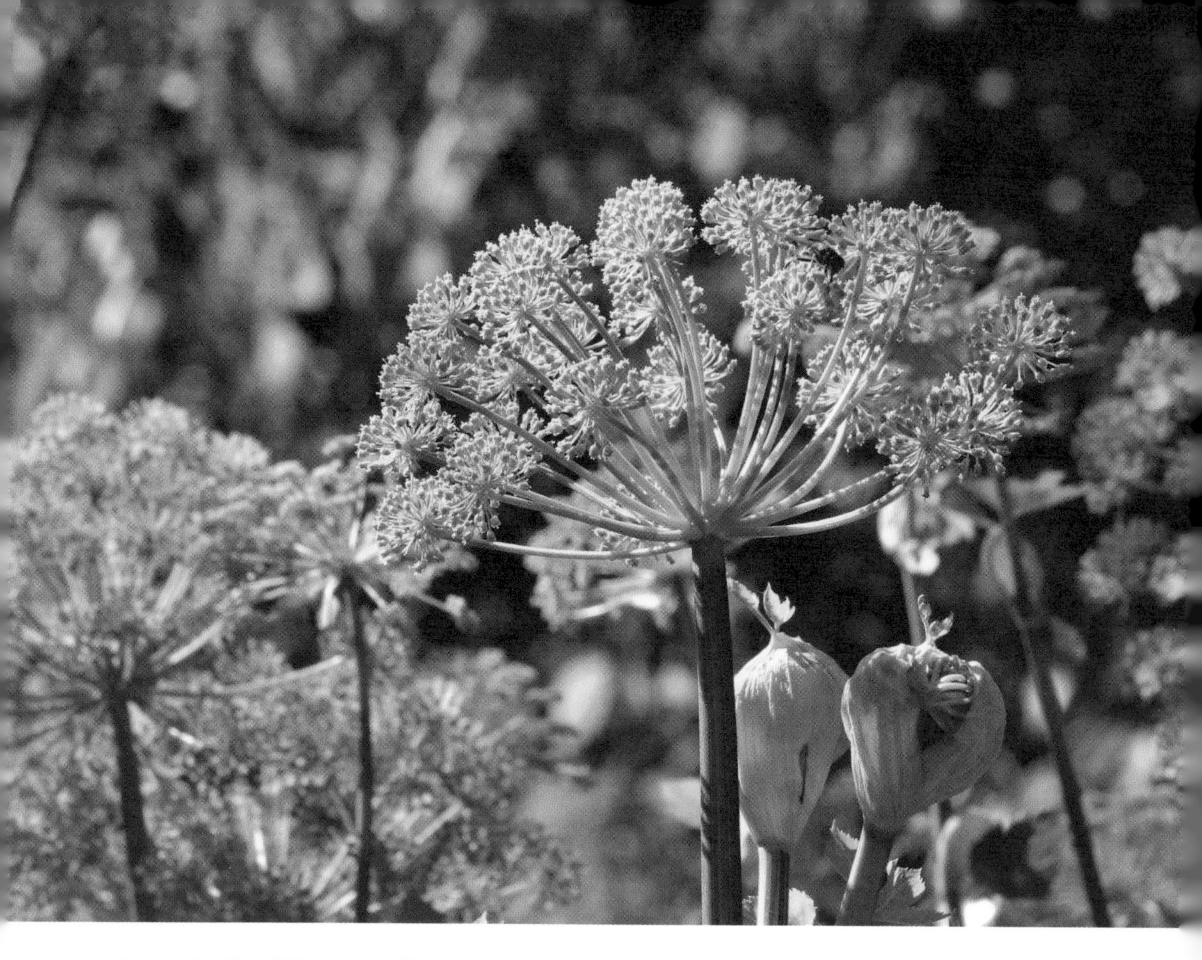

ANGELICA

Alternative names: St Michael's flower, herb of angels, Holy Ghost plant, garden angelica

HOW TO IDENTIFY: Angelica can grow to over 2 metres (6½ feet) tall. It has striking globe-shaped umbels of small yellowy green flowers.

Angelica is easily confused with other similar plants such as hemlock, which is poisonous – only use a plant that you have grown yourself or bought from a reputable garden supplier.

HISTORY: During the Middle Ages every part of angelica was seen as a defensive plant against evil and witchcraft. It was burned during exorcisms, grown in gardens for protection and added to bathwater to remove hexes. This statuesque plant is also known as "St Michael's Flower", as it is often in flower on May 8, the day that, according to Christian legend, St Michael the archangel appeared on Mount Gargano in Apulia, Italy in around AD 490.

FOLKLORE: Legend has it that a medieval monk was visited in a dream by the archangel Raphael who revealed that chewing angelica would not only cure the plague but also protect against witchcraft.

The leaves can be scattered on the floor to purify an area and also burned in cleansing smudge sticks and healing incenses.

In North America an infusion of crushed roots is still used by the Iroquois tribes as a wash to remove ghosts from the home and to aid childbirth.

FOLK MEDICINE: Culpeper, the seventeenth-century herbalist, recommended angelica for curing "virtually everything under the sun", including snakebites, deafness, ulcers and the easing of wind.

Known to be a "warming plant", angelica is still used to stimulate the circulation of people who suffer with cold hands and feet in winter.

Causing distaste for alcohol, angelica root is used in Chinese medicine as a deterrent to those who like to drink a little more than they should.

Tobacco made from angelica is smoked by the Sami in Lapland, with the belief that it will prolong life, and in France the chewing of angelica root was thought to have the same benefit.

OTHER COMMON USES: The seeds and stems are used to flavour the alcoholic drinks Dubonnet, Benedictine and Chartreuse. Young stems can be used in salads and the older stems are candied for cake decorations.

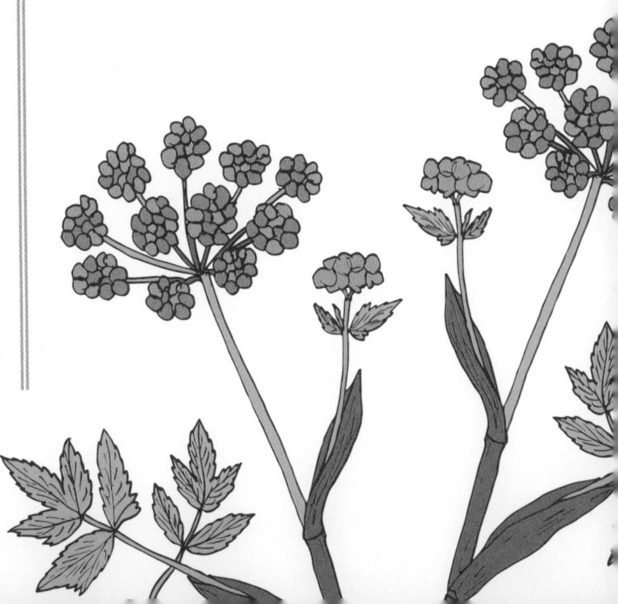

ANGELICA AND GINGER INDIGESTION SYRUP

Both angelica and ginger are known for their tummy-calming properties by relieving intestinal gas and easing nausea. Angelica contains anti-inflammatory, antioxidant and painkilling properties, which can also soothe heartburn caused by acid reflux.

Makes approx 800ml

INGREDIENTS

50g sliced angelica root

200g sliced organic fresh ginger

150g sugar

500ml water

Equipment needed

Clean, sterilized bottle

Fine sieve

METHOD

Gently simmer the angelica and ginger in a saucepan with the sugar and water for 45 minutes.

Remove from heat and allow to steep for an hour.

Strain the syrup through a fine sieve.

Pour into a sterilized bottle.

Keep in the fridge for about a month, take a spoonful as required.

Can also be diluted with still or sparkling water.

Not recommended for use when pregnant or if diabetic.

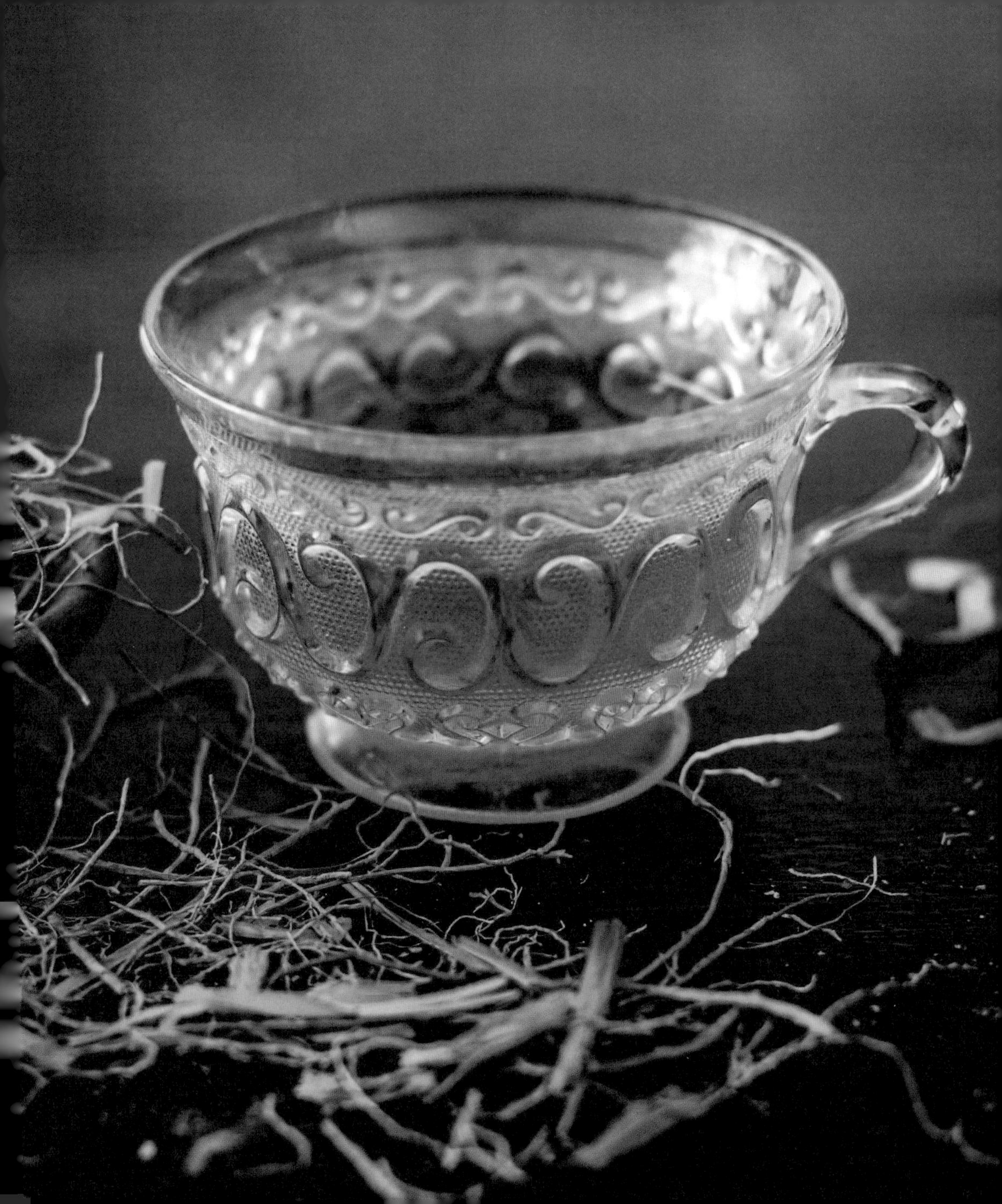

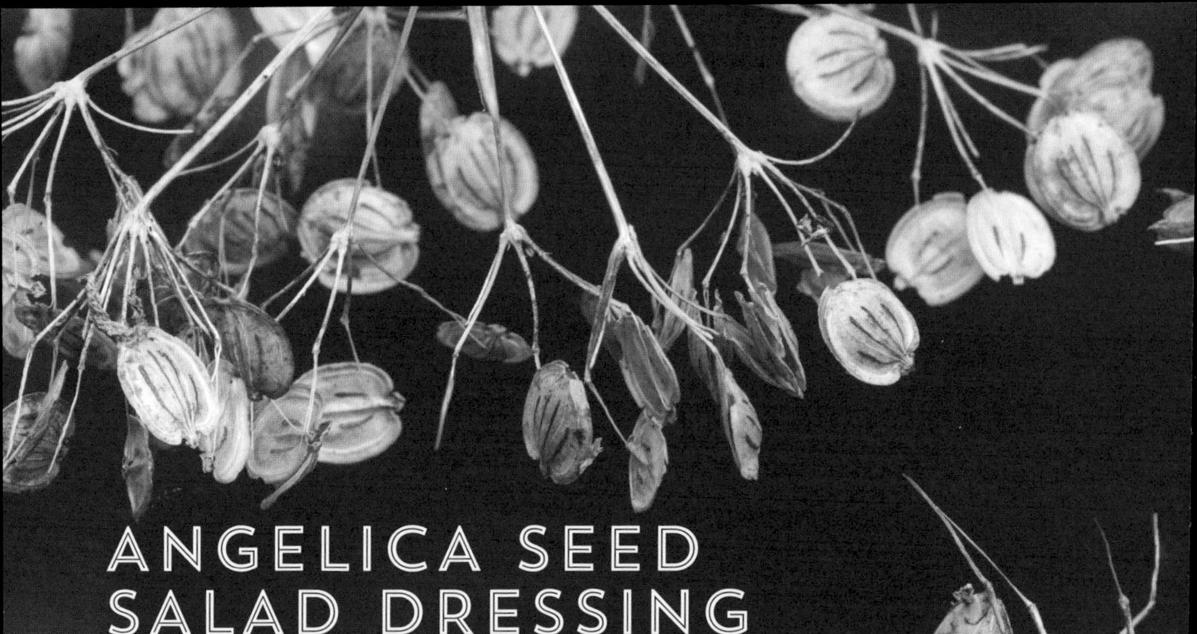

ANGELICA SEED SALAD DRESSING

Angelica seeds make a sweet and woody tasting dressing that goes perfectly with edible leaves and flowers foraged from your garden – try nasturtium leaves, young dandelions or you may be lucky enough to find some chickweed or purslane. If you prefer, just toss the dressing through some salad leaves from your local organic grower.

Makes approximately 50ml

INGREDIENTS

2 tsp angelica seeds

2 tbsp organic olive or rape seed oil

Zest and juice of 1 organic lemon

1 tbsp organic white wine vinegar

METHOD

Place all the ingredients in a clean jam jar and shake until combined.

Pour over your salad and combine.

Best to use the dressing straightaway, but can be kept in the jar for a couple of days if necessary.

Not recommended for use when pregnant or if diabetic.

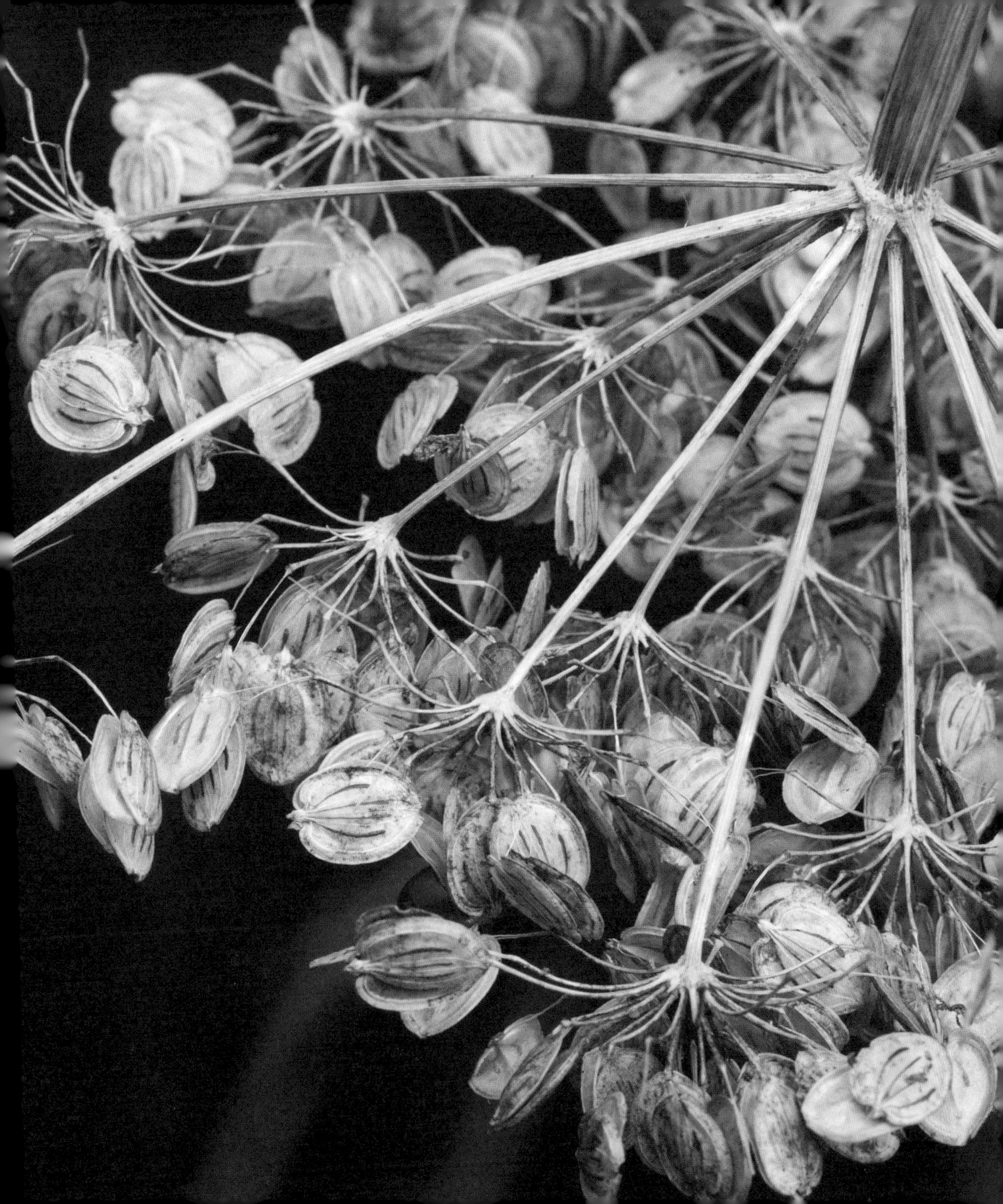

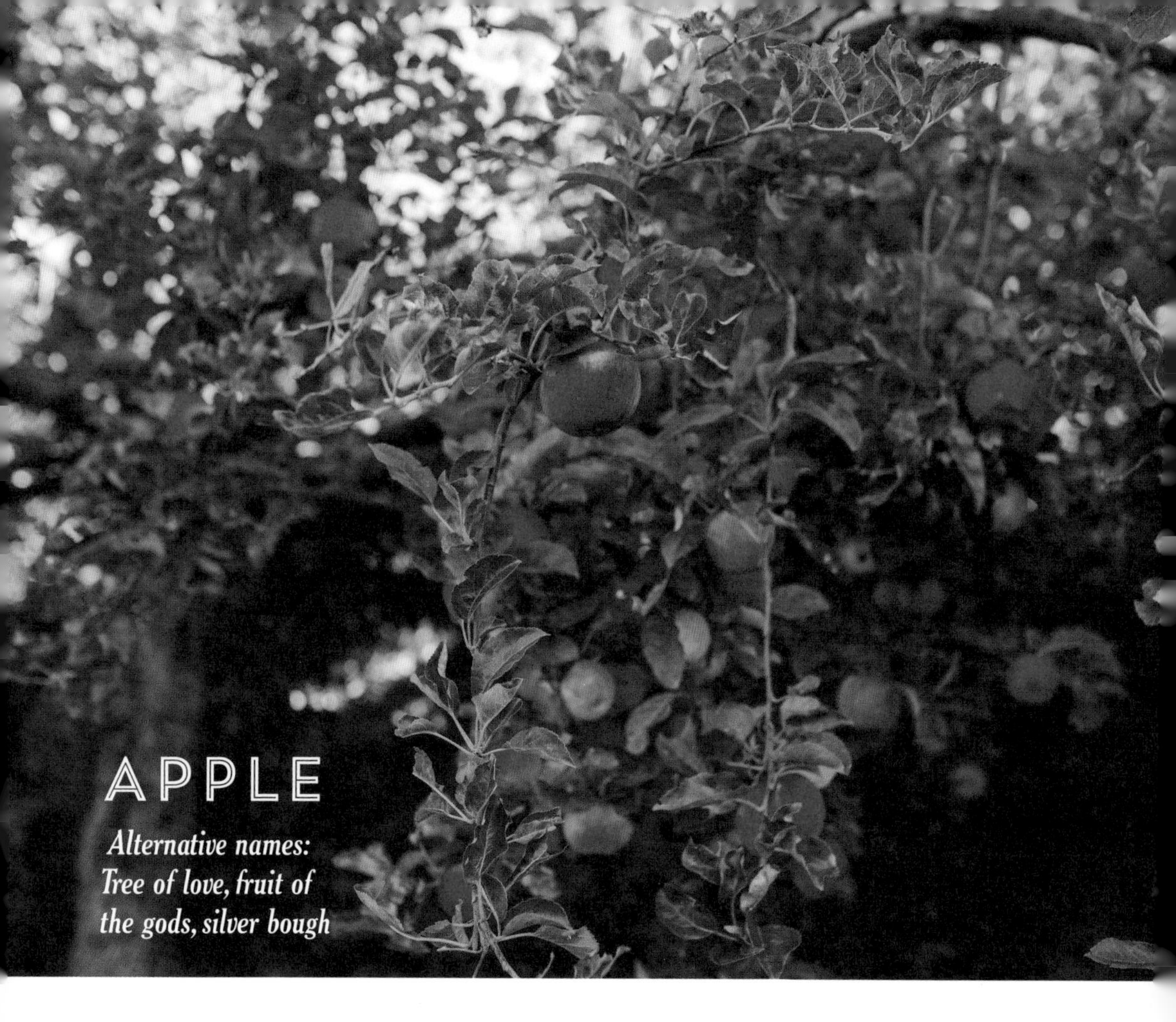

APPLE

Alternative names:* *Tree of love, fruit of the gods, silver bough

HOW TO IDENTIFY: The trunk of an apple tree is usually grey with ridges and bumps. Large sweet or sour fruits are harvested in late summer and, depending on the variety, can be many shades of red and green, varying widely in flavour from very sweet eating apples to deliciously tart cookers.

HISTORY: Crab apples, known as wildings, are the only apple variety native to the UK, the pips having been discovered in Neolithic sites inhabited thousands of years ago. Roman soldiers carried apples across Europe, planting pips as they marched northward. Unfortunately, most of these varieties weren't suited to the British climate and it fell to the Normans in the eleventh century to introduce our most loved varieties from France such as Golden Delicious, Gala and Pink Lady.

FOLKLORE: Most people hope for dry weather on St Swithun's Day (15 July), but not if you are an apple grower. If it rains on this day, also known as "Apple Christening Day", the crop will be blessed and no matter how small or green the apples are they will be ready to eat and will keep well through the winter. As told in the anonymous text *Notes and Queries* in 1896, *"When I was a lad we were told not to eat apples before St. Swithun's day or they would make us ill, as they had not been christened."*

Apple and other fruit trees that blossom out of season are believed to predict death or misfortune as it is thought to be going against nature.

Apples have a strong association with magic, particularly in the art of divination and for love potions. To discover your future partner cut up an apple in front of a mirror in a dark room, lit only by one candle, just before midnight. Throw one piece of the apple over your right shoulder and eat the rest while brushing your hair, and at midnight your lover's reflection will appear in the mirror.

FOLK MEDICINE: Culpeper writes: "a poultice of roasted sweet apples, with powder of frankincense, removes pains of the side... roasted apples are good for the asthmatic, either raw, roasted or boiled."

The nineteenth-century Welsh saying *"Eat an apple before going to bed and you'll keep the doctor from earning his bread"* became shortened to the more familiar *"An apple a day keeps the doctor away."*

Apple sauce was, and still is, eaten with rich foods such as pork or goose as the acids in the apple help with digestion.

Rotten apples were used as a poultice for sore eyes and a ripe juicy apple eaten at bedtime will cure constipation.

OTHER COMMON USES: Green or under-ripe apples contain a high amount of soluble fibre called pectin. This can be used when making jam with fruits that are low in pectin, such as strawberries and cherries, to help them set.

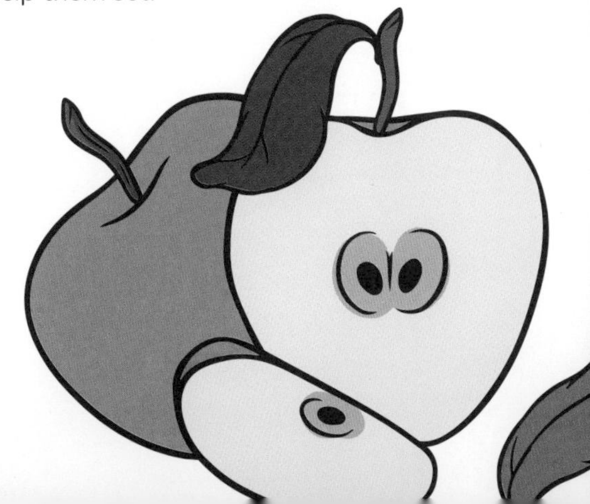

ORGANIC APPLE CIDER VINEGAR

We seem to have only recently discovered the wonderful health benefits of apple cider vinegar; it can be easily purchased in supermarkets although raw vinegar containing the "mother" is quite expensive. It only costs pennies to make at home with the added benefit of using up all those excess apples in late summer. The probiotic qualities of apple cider vinegar help with digestion and boost the immune system. Antibacterial properties are useful in a natural cleaning spray around the house, or for treating smelly feet and even nail fungus. Mix a spoonful of apple cider vinegar with honey and a little hot water to soothe a sore throat. High in phosphorus, calcium, potassium and magnesium and made using basic kitchen equipment and a simple fermentation process, apple cider vinegar is really worth the time and effort it takes to make it.

Makes 1 litre

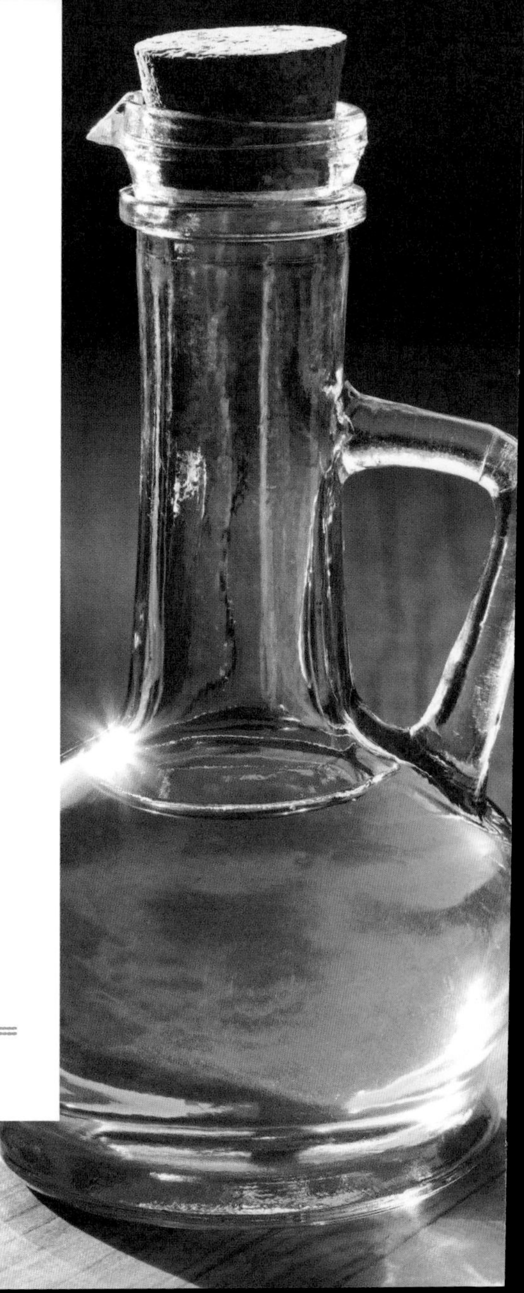

INGREDIENTS

3 small organic apples chopped and washed (including the peel and core)

3 tsp sugar

Approx. 1 litre of filtered or mineral water

Equipment needed

Large glass jar

Muslin or cotton cloth

String

METHOD

Place your chopped apples into a clean wide-mouthed jar.

Mix the sugar with 200ml of the water until dissolved.

Pour this on top of the apples.

Add as much of the remaining water is needed to cover the apples completely.

Put a non-metallic weight on the apples to keep them submerged. I find that a plastic freezer bag filled with water will do the job nicely.

Cover the jar with the cloth and secure with string – this allows the mixture to ferment and keeps bugs out.

Place the jar in a warm dry place out of direct sunlight for three weeks. After this time the liquid should smell fairly sweet with bubbles on the top – congratulations you have achieved fermentation!

Strain out the apples and put in the compost, return the liquid to the jar.

Cover the jar with the cloth again and put it back in the warm dry place for 4 to 6 weeks stirring as often as you can remember with a wooden spoon. You will be able to taste and smell when your apple cider vinegar is ready as it will be distinctly vinegary.

Decant it into sterilized bottles ready to use.

There should be a cloudy "mother" that has floated to the top of your jar, this is gold dust and can be used to kickstart your next batch of apple cider vinegar!

ELIXIR NO. 9

This is my nine-ingredient twist on traditional "Fire cider", an immune-boosting, anti-viral, anti-inflammatory, decongestant, antioxidant and antibacterial powerhouse of a remedy. There are many recipes out there and the one thing they have in common is the use of organic apple cider vinegar, along with ingredients that you may well have growing in your garden. This elixir takes at least four weeks to mature so it's a good idea to start a batch at the end of summer in readiness for those inevitable winter coughs and colds. If you don't "grow your own" try to source pesticide-free ingredients from your local farm shop or social enterprise – not only is it good to support small independent businesses but it's probably local and fresher, too.

Makes approx 900ml

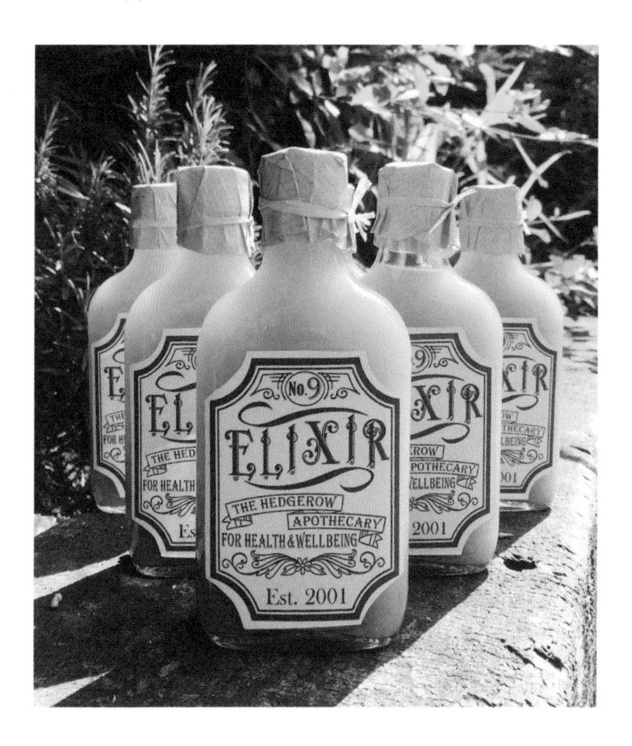

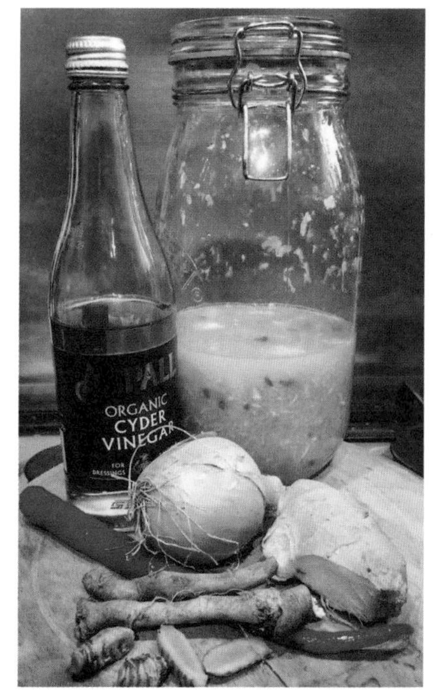

INGREDIENTS

800ml organic apple cider vinegar

50g peeled and grated root ginger

50g peeled and grated fresh horseradish

50g peeled and grated turmeric root – careful, this will stain everything that it touches!

1 medium-sized onion, peeled and chopped

4 large garlic cloves, peeled and grated

2 chillies, seeds included, chopped – go as hot as you dare!

2 lemons, zest and juice

½ tsp black peppercorns

Equipment needed

A 1.5 litre Kilner type jar with glass lid or a wide-mouthed plastic bottle

Fine sieve or muslin

METHOD

Pack all of the ingredients, apart from the vinegar, into a clean jar.

Slowly pour in the apple cider vinegar making sure that it completely covers the fresh ingredients.

Shake well and store in a cool dark place for at least 4 weeks.

Shake weekly ensuring that everything is staying under the vinegar.

Strain the elixir through a fine sieve or muslin squeezing out every drop. Don't discard the solids as they can be frozen into ice cubes and used in stir-fries.

Bottle and label your liquid gold.

Keeps for well over a year in a cool dark place.

We take our elixir neat by the tablespoon as soon as we feel a cough or cold coming on. If that's not for you then dilute it in warm water with a spoon of raw honey and it will be just as effective.

Avoid taking large amounts of apple cider vinegar if you take insulin.

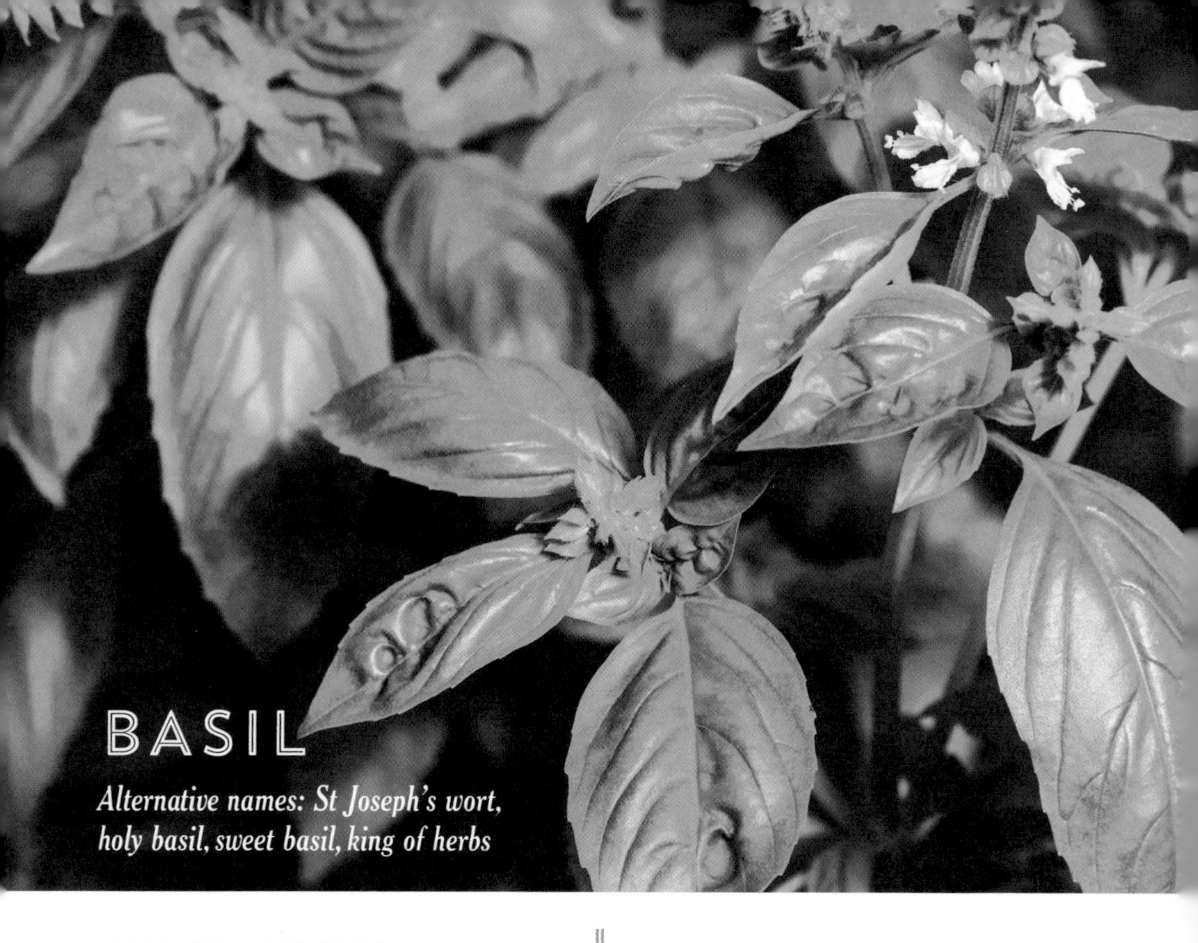

BASIL

Alternative names: St Joseph's wort, holy basil, sweet basil, king of herbs

HOW TO IDENTIFY: A tender plant with glossy green leaves and a peppery liquorice flavour and scent.

HISTORY: Originating in South East Asia we can once again thank the Romans for introducing basil to our kitchens and medicine cabinets. Pliny the Elder, the Roman author, recommends it as an aphrodisiac, not just for people but for horses and donkeys, too! The Ancient Greeks strangely believed that to grow extremely fragrant basil you should shout and swear angrily as you sow the seeds into the ground.

In India it is believed that a basil leaf placed on the tongue will aid the passage of the dead to heaven. It was also regarded as so sacred that criminals once had to swear an oath on basil in a court of law.

FOLKLORE: In Roman mythology the Basilisk was a mythical fire-breathing dragon that could kill you just by looking at you. Luckily, though, basil was just the antidote you needed to counteract the Basilisk's venom.

The Ancient Greeks used basil to detect witches; while burning basil they called out the names of suspected witches, and if the leaves crackled on a particular name then they were undoubtedly a witch.

Basil will shrivel if held in the hands of an unfaithful wife; however carrying it on your person will bring you good luck and wealth.

In John Parkinson's *The Expert Gardener,* published in 1640, he states that "*basil must be sown in March when the moone is olde*" – the phase of the moon in its last quarter before a new moon.

In seventeenth-century England, basil was hung above doorways and strewn on the floor to ward off evil spirits – "*where basil lays no evil can enter.*"

FOLK MEDICINE: In the seventeenth century there appears to have been a strange belief that smelling basil would cause scorpions to grow in your brain and that placing basil under a stone and waiting for two days would turn it into a scorpion!

Even Culpeper believed that basil "*... being laid to rot in horse-dung, it will breed venomous beasts.*" Hilarius, a French physician, affirms upon his own knowledge, that an acquaintance of his, by common smelling to it, had a "*scorpion bred in his brain.*"

Rue was believed to be a reliable remedy for poisons. Basil would not grow near rue causing Culpeper to be suspicious that "*something is the matter with this herb... we know that rue is a great enemy to poison.*"

OTHER COMMON USES: Basil is the perfect companion plant for tomatoes, not just because the two cook beautifully together, but because it also keeps away tomato hornworms, aphids and whitefly. Basil shortbread is delicious – just substitute two tablespoons of chopped fresh basil instead of calendula and thyme in the recipe on page 56.

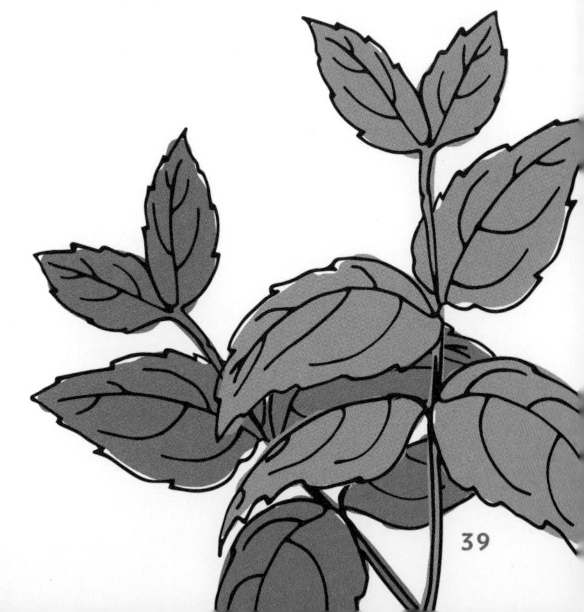

BASIL STEAM FOR HEADACHES

Basil is analgesic and a muscle relaxant so is especially effective on tension headaches and sinus pain. It also has the added bonus that you get to smell like an Italian kitchen for the rest of the day!

INGREDIENTS

2 tbsp fresh basil, or 1 tbsp dried

1 litre boiling water

Equipment needed

Heat resistant bowl

Clean towel

METHOD

Add the basil and the boiling water to the heatproof bowl and stir.

Cover your head with the towel, carefully lean over the pot and breathe in the steam for 5–10 minutes or until your headache starts to ease.

Follow this with a cup of basil, lemon and honey tea to really reap the soothing benefits of basil.

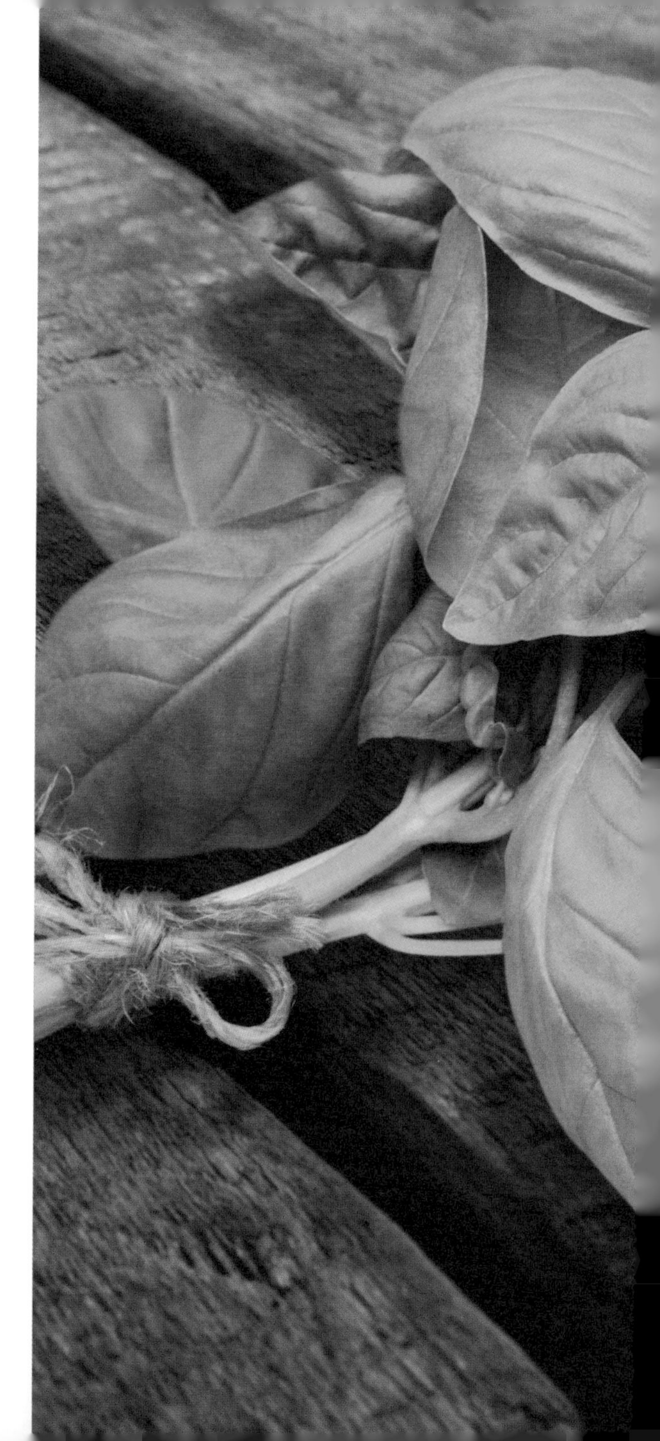

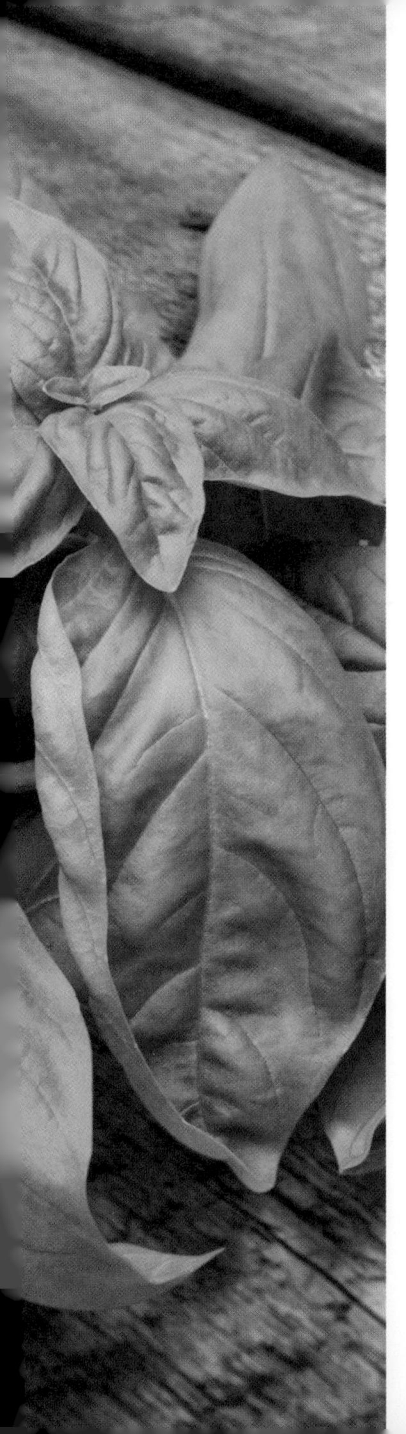

BASIL AND LEMON SURFACE CLEANER

Basil is antibacterial and anti-fungal, while lemon is antibacterial, antiseptic, smells great and is a gentle natural bleach. Vinegar can remove grease and grime, dissolve lime-scale, effectively kill germs and best of all is totally natural and cheap!

Makes 1 litre

INGREDIENTS

1 pesticide-free whole lemon, chopped

Handful of fresh basil leaves, torn into pieces

500ml white vinegar

500ml water

Equipment needed

Large jar

Fine sieve or muslin

Spray bottle

METHOD

Put the chopped lemon in the jar.

Add the basil and pour over the vinegar.

Leave for at least 2 weeks in the fridge, shaking occasionally.

At the end of two weeks:

Strain the infused vinegar into a jug.

Add 500ml water.

Pour into a clean spray bottle and use as needed in the kitchen and bathroom.

I've also found that this is a fabulous streak-free window cleaner – just spray on and polish off with old newspaper.

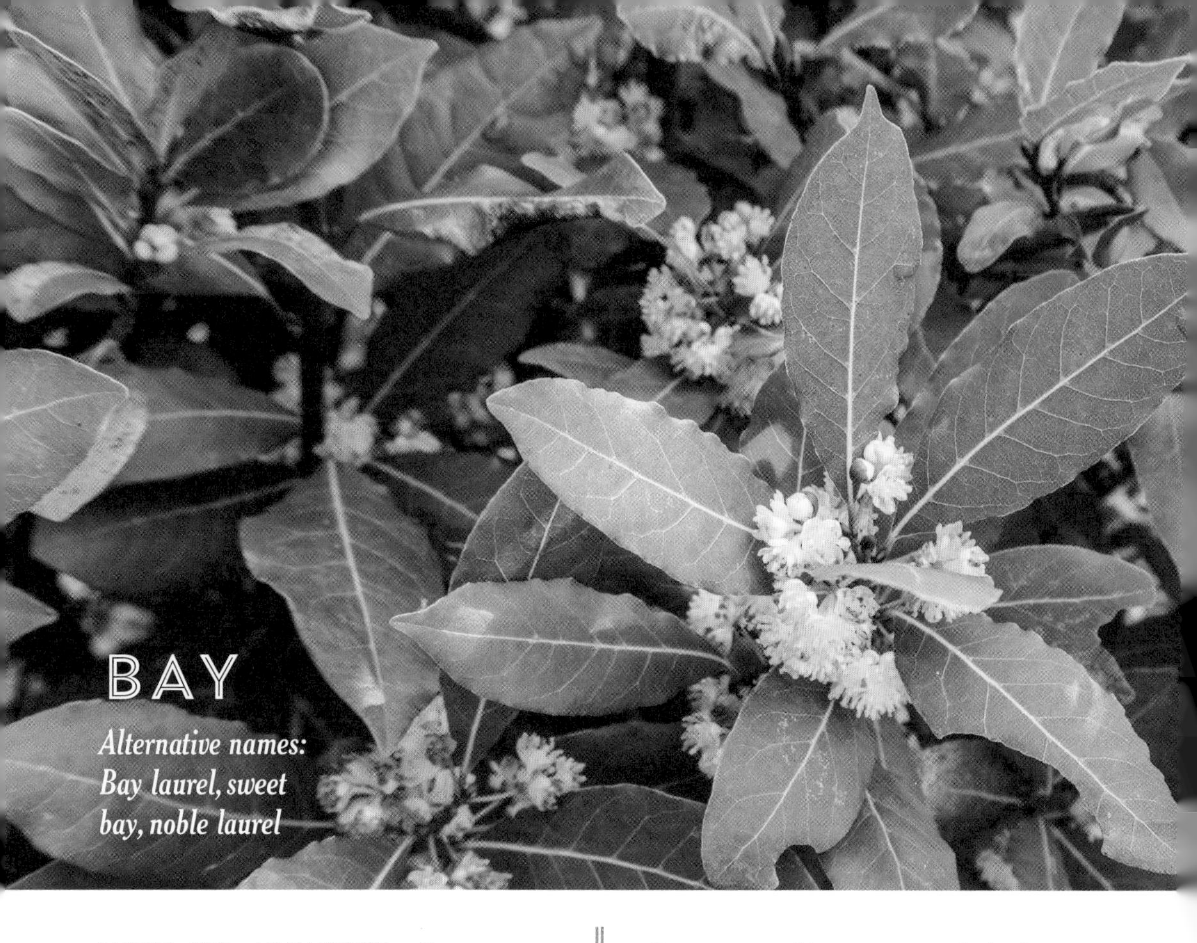

BAY

***Alternative names:* Bay laurel, sweet bay, noble laurel**

HOW TO IDENTIFY: Bay trees can grow up to 18 metres (60 feet) high, with glossy leaves, small yellow flowers and minute edible black berries that are a great favourite of birds, so I like to let them enjoy them.

HISTORY: Laurel fashioned into a wreath was considered to be the highest honour awarded to winners in the Pythian games of ancient Greece.

Romans used bay as a symbol of victory and also believed that it was inhabited by a "fire demon" that would protect anyone who carried it from thunder and lightning.

FOLKLORE: An old charm from the West Country, recorded in Chope's 1938 volume of *Report and transactions of the Devonshire association for the advancement of science*, says that to attract love the following should be performed before bed on Valentine's Eve:

"Take five bay leaves, and pin them to your pillow, one at each corner and one in the middle. Then, lying down, say the following seven times, and count seven, seven times over at each interval:

'Sweet guardian angels let me have
What I most earnestly do crave
A valentine endued with love.
Who will both true and constant prove.'"

Do this carefully and your future husband will appear in your dreams that night.

Bay leaves crackle loudly as they burn. If you write your wishes on the leaves and toss them into the fire and they smoulder rather than crackle, the omens are not good.

If your bay tree suddenly begins to wilt it is an omen that there will be a death in the house or that bad luck is just around the corner, or that a reigning monarch has died:

"Tis thought the king is dead, we'll not stay. The bay tree in our country is withered."
Richard II,
William Shakespeare

Bay leaves are burned during exorcisms, hung in houses to banish ghosts and if made into a broom can be used to "sweep away" ex-spouses, unwelcome visitors or lodgers who have outstayed their welcome.

FOLK MEDICINE: Culpeper tells us that: "*The berries are very effectual against the poison of venomous creatures, and the stings of wasps and bees, as also against the pestilence, or other infectious diseases…*"

The leaves and fruit were strewn on the floor to repel insects, used to treat flatulence and hysteria and to ease the pain of arthritis.

OTHER COMMON USES: Bay leaves repel moths, flies and ants and can be folded into clothing or put into storage containers of dried goods to keep them pest free.

They are commonly used in soups and stews to add a fragrant flavour.

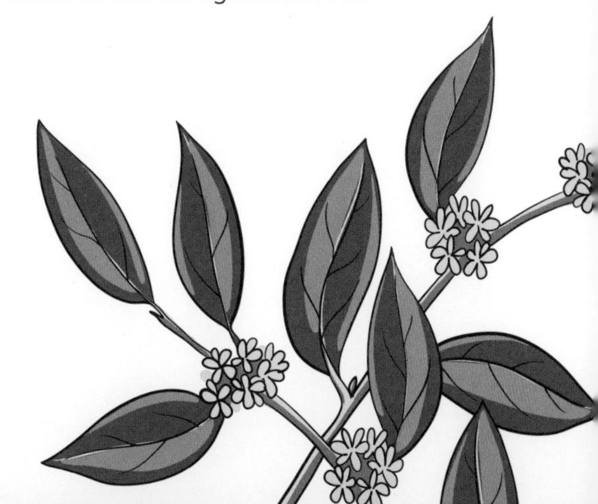

BAY LEAF AND CLOVE RINSE FOR DANDRUFF

Bay leaf is a natural anti-inflammatory and antioxidant, which can ease dryness and itchiness of the scalp. Cloves are antiseptic, growth stimulating and will help to cleanse the hair of any bacteria.

Makes enough for two good rinses

INGREDIENTS

1 litre water

24 clove buds

6 bay leaves

Equipment needed

Sieve or muslin

Bottle or jar

METHOD

Add the cloves and water to a saucepan, bring to the boil for 10 minutes with the lid on.

Tear the bay leaves and stir into the clove water.

Boil for another 10 minutes.

Allow to cool then strain the liquid.

After using shampoo, pour over the hair and massage in thoroughly. Leave for 15 minutes, then rinse out with cool water.

Store in the fridge and use within 1 month.

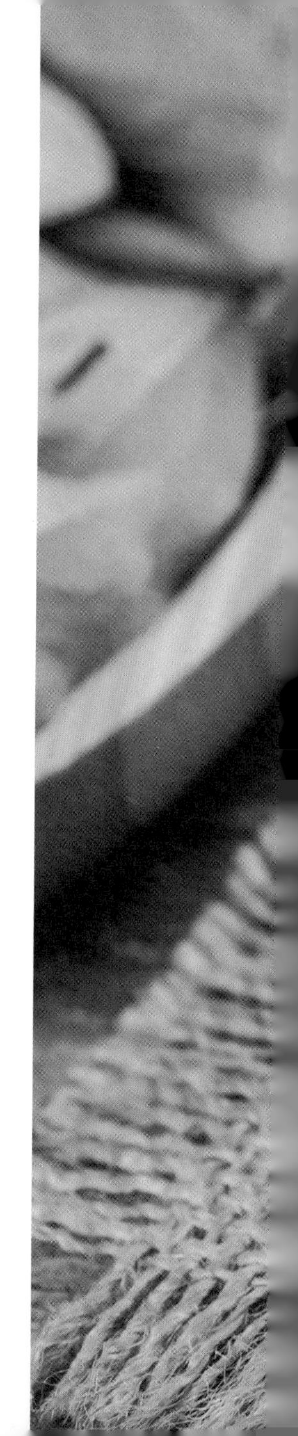

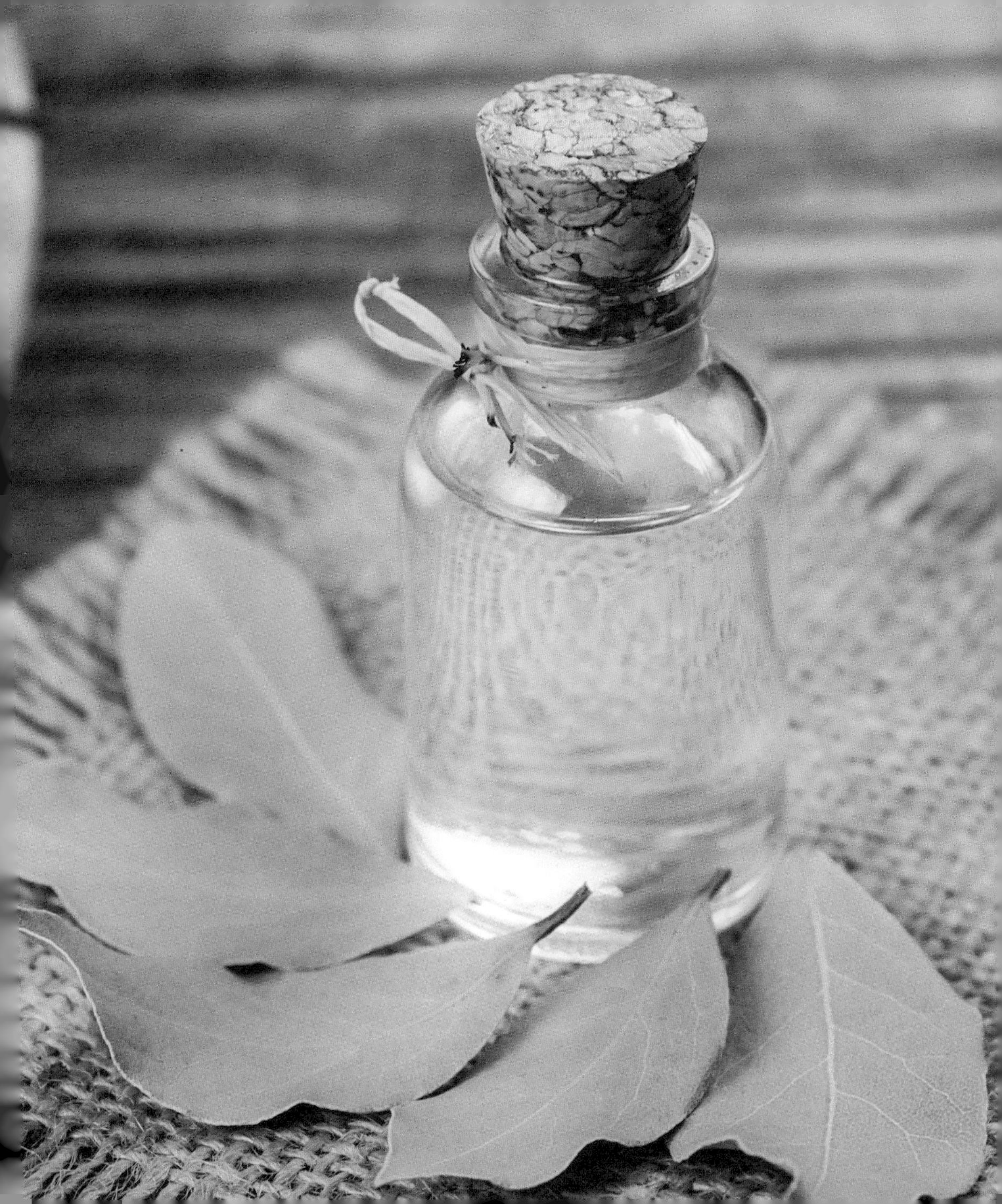

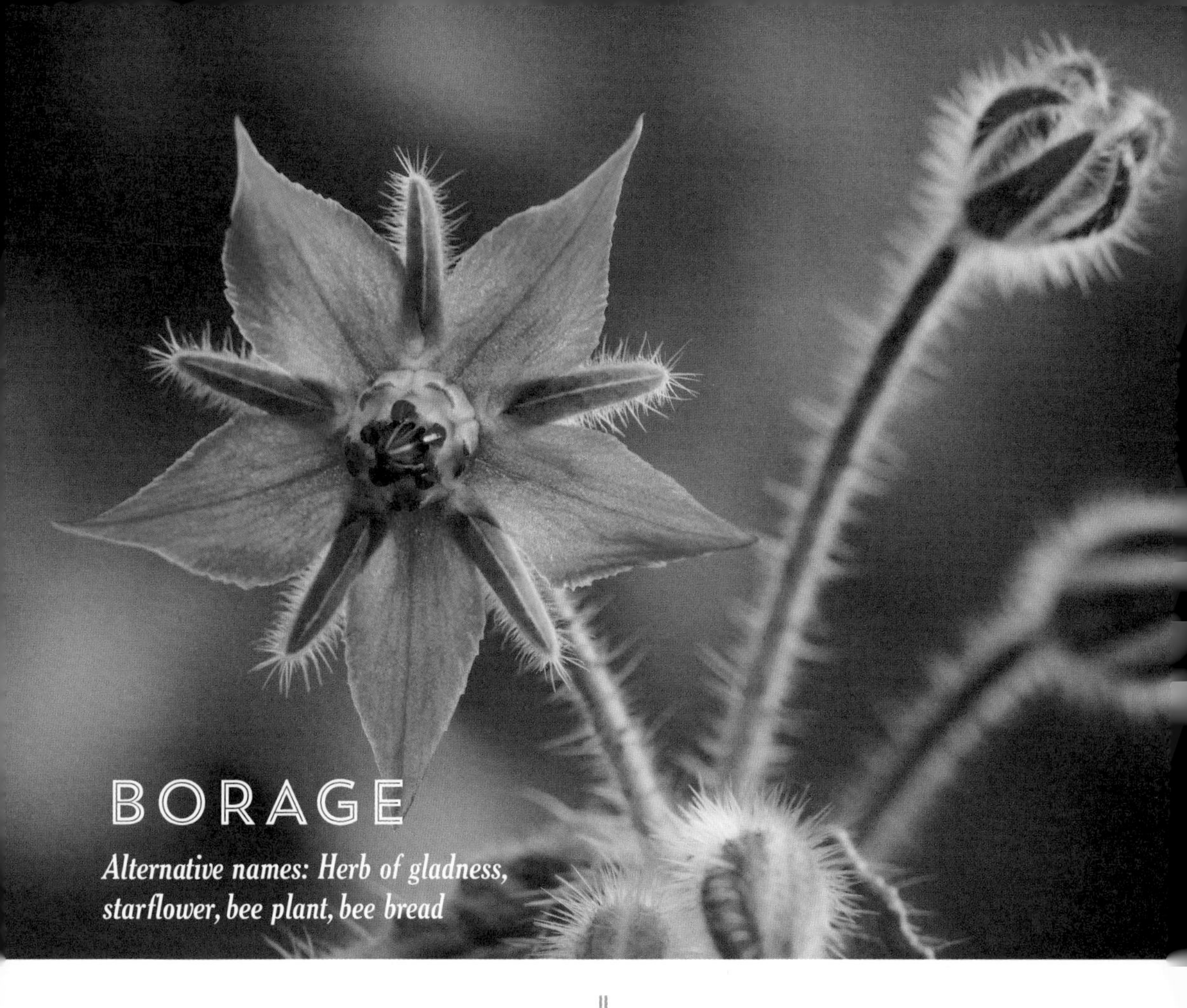

BORAGE

Alternative names: Herb of gladness, starflower, bee plant, bee bread

HOW TO IDENTIFY: Borage is easily identified by its beautiful star-shaped blue flowers, which have cone-like black anthers in the centre. The leaves and stems are covered in white, prickly bristles.

HISTORY: The brilliant blue colour of borage flowers is so beautiful that it is said to have inspired Renaissance painters to reproduce it when painting the robes of the Virgin Mary.

Borage comes from the Gaelic word *borrach* meaning "courage". A drink made with borage flowers was often drunk by Roman soldiers and Celtic warriors before battle to make them fearless. Knights heading off to the Crusades had borage flowers embroidered onto their scarves for the same reason.

Interestingly, modern research has discovered that borage increases the body's production of adrenalin, preparing it for "fight or flight" should you need the courage to escape a dangerous situation.

FOLKLORE: Borage flowers slipped into the drink of a potential suitor will give him the courage to propose.

Dried borage leaves sprinkled around the home will bring peace and harmony, and drinking a tea made from the flowers will increase your psychic powers.

Harvest and dry a few flowers to place in a little medicine bag or pouch to carry with you when you need inner strength and bravery.

FOLK MEDICINE: John Gerard writes in his book *Herball* in 1597:

> *"Those of our time do use the flowers in salads to exhilarate and make the mind glad. There be also many things made of these used everywhere for the comfort of the heart, for the driving away of sorrow and increasing the joy of the mind."*

He also says that the leaves and flowers put into wine will make "*men and women glad and merry and drive away all sadness, dullness and melancholy.*" I'm not sure we can attribute that solely to the effects of borage though!

OTHER COMMON USES: Borage flowers look beautiful frozen into ice cubes when you make a jug of Pimm's in the summer. Use boiled water to keep the ice crystal clear. The flowers can also be added to salads or crystallized to decorate cakes.

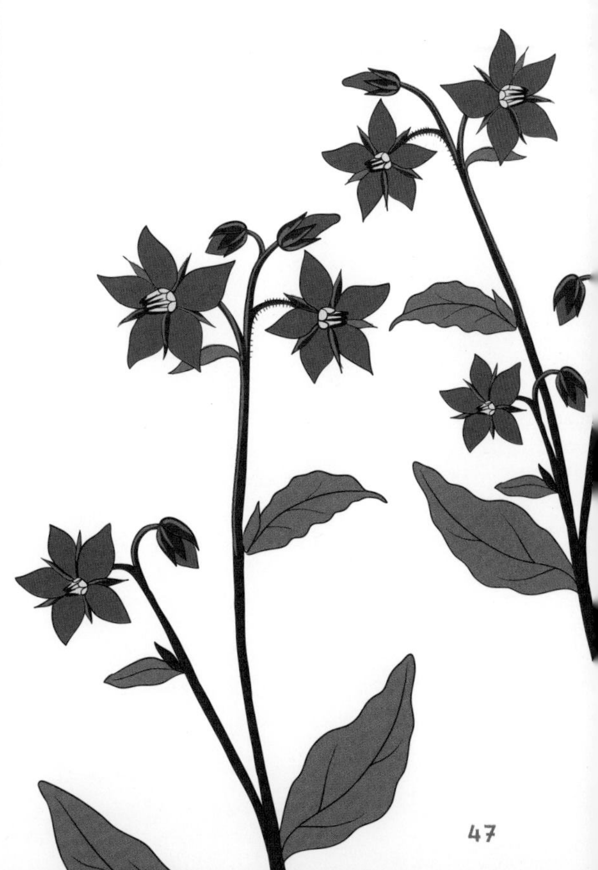

BORAGE INFUSION FOR TIRED EYES

Borage leaves are cooling and soothing and will help to reduce the puffiness of tired eyes.

INGREDIENTS

Handful of young borage leaves, chopped

Just-boiled water

Equipment needed

Cotton make-up removal pads

METHOD

Put the chopped leaves into a cup and pour over the water.

Allow to cool completely in the fridge before straining out the leaves.

Soak some cotton pads in the borage infusion, lay back, place them over your closed eyes and relax.

The anti-inflammatory properties of this cold infusion can also help relieve the itchiness of insect bites and eczema.

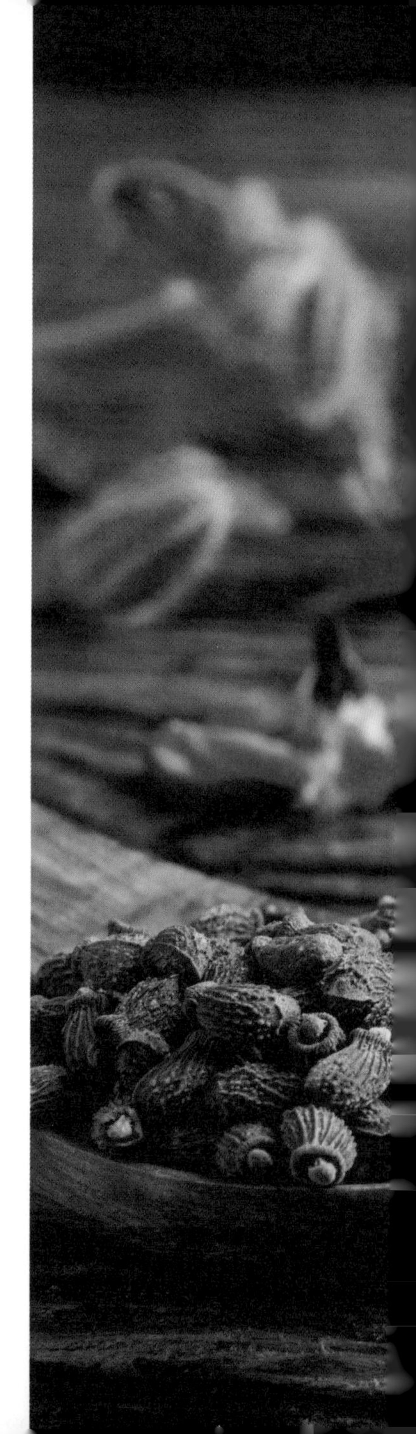

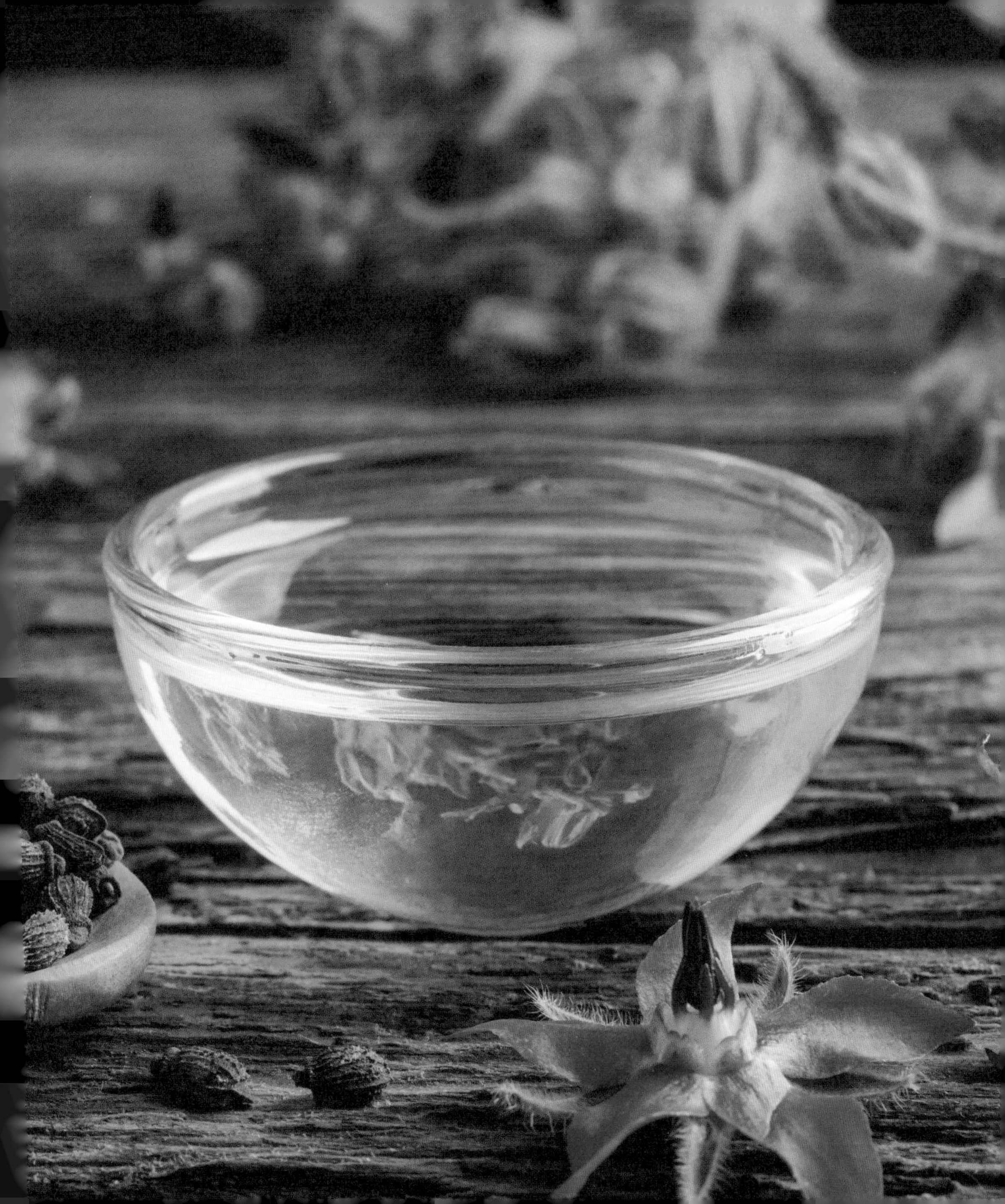

UPLIFTING BORAGE COCKTAIL

This delicious summer drink uses flowers straight from the garden. The mild mood-lifting properties are sure to make it a party favourite. The flowers have a delicate cucumber-like taste enhanced by making them into syrup. If you haven't made your own elderflower cordial for this recipe, a shop-bought version works just as well.

Serves 6

INGREDIENTS

For the borage syrup:

200ml water

250g white sugar

100g fresh young borage flowers

Equipment needed

Fine sieve

Glass bottle

METHOD

Put the water and sugar in a small saucepan over a medium heat.

Stir continually until all the sugar is dissolved then bring to a gentle boil.

Stir in the borage flowers, reduce the heat, cover the pan and simmer for 15 minutes. Don't let it burn.

Remove from heat and put it aside for at least an hour to allow the flavour to infuse.

Strain the borage from the syrup squeezing the flowers to get the maximum flavour, bottle the syrup and refrigerate until needed.

For the cocktail:

150ml gin or vodka

50ml borage syrup

50ml homemade elderflower cordial

Juice of half a lime

250ml sparkling water, tonic or Prosecco

Borage and other edible flower ice cubes

METHOD

Pour all the cocktail ingredients into a glass jug and stir well.

Garnish with borage ice cubes and fresh borage flowers.

For a non-alcoholic version for children just leave out the gin.

Guaranteed to lift the spirits!

Overconsumption of borage oil can be harmful to the liver if used over long periods of time, always consult a qualified herbalist before using.

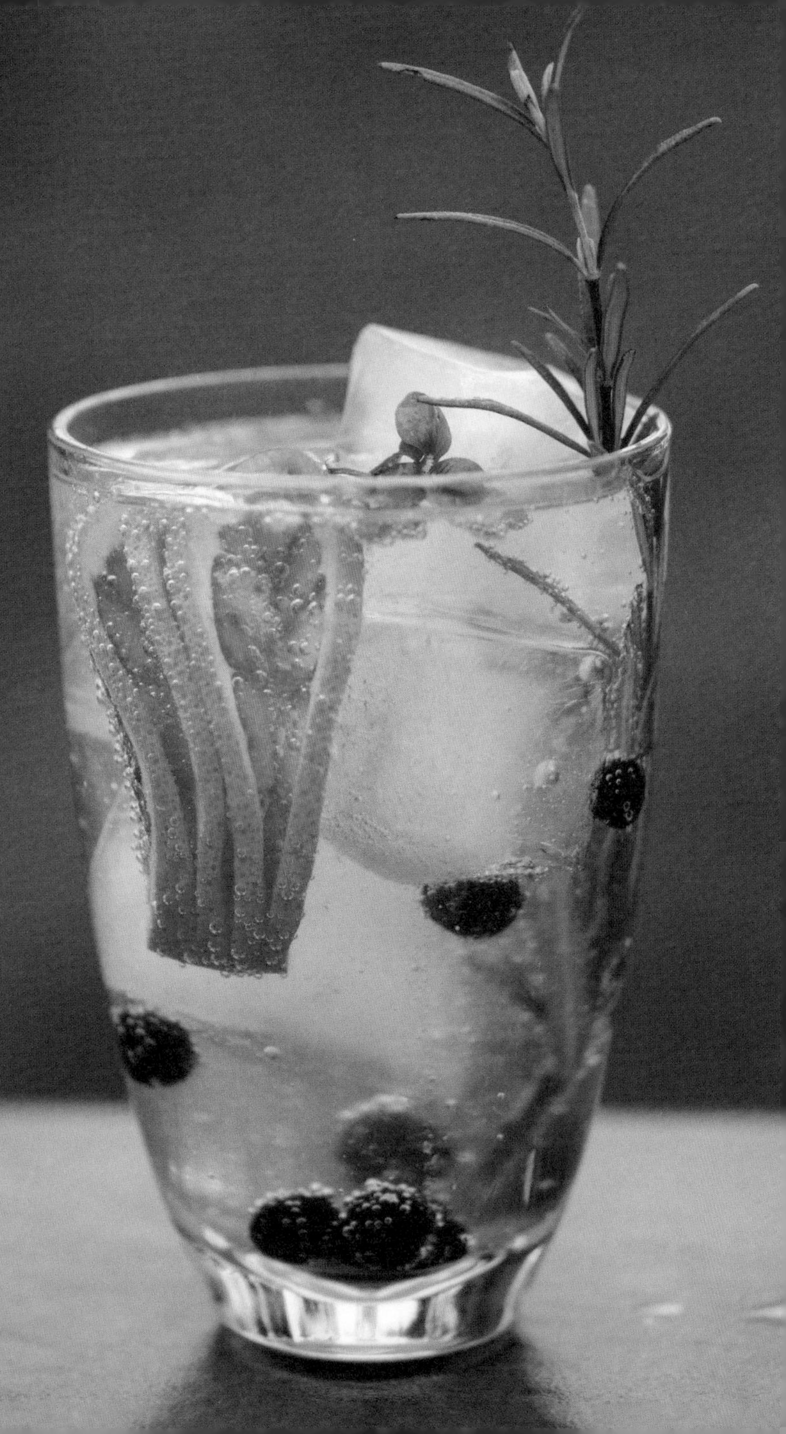

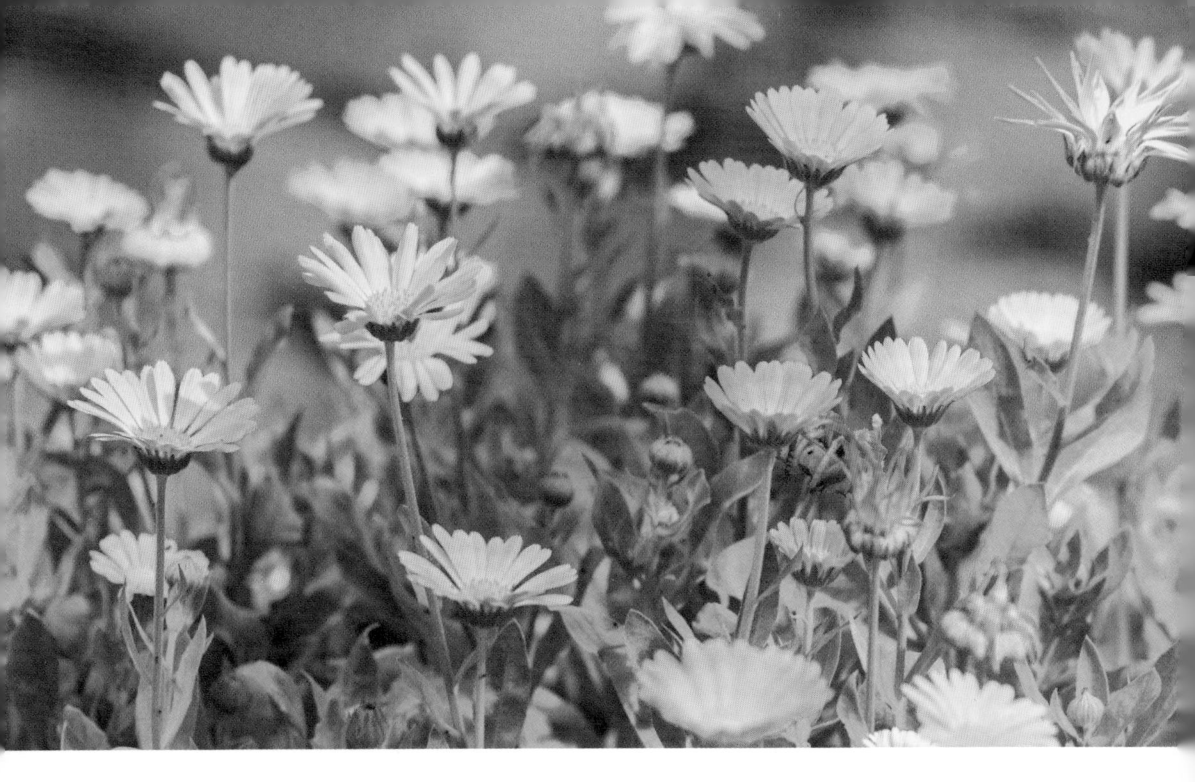

CALENDULA

Alternative names: Pot marigold, summer's bride, Mary gold, holigold, Jack on horseback, measle flower, drunkards

HOW TO IDENTIFY: An absolute must for the English cottage garden, this cheerful daisy-like flower comes in many shades from pale creamy yellow to deep burnt orange. Calendula blooms from early spring until autumn, producing many flower heads that can be dried for use in the medicine chest all year round.

HISTORY: Calendula was prized by the Greeks, Romans and Egyptians for its wonderful healing properties and used as a food colouring, in cosmetics and to dye cloth shades of lemon yellow through to light brown.

Gertrude Jekyll, the renowned British horticulturist, grew an abundance of calendula during World War One to be sent to field hospitals in France. The cleansing and antiseptic properties of calendula were harnessed to speed up the healing of wounds. Used by country folk to tell the time, calendula blossoms open up at about 9 o'clock each morning to welcome the sun and close again at 3 o'clock in the afternoon signalling the end of the working day in the fields.

FOLKLORE: Hang a garland of calendula over the entrance to your home to remove all powers from witches and prevent evil from entering your house.

Eating calendula petals will allow you to see the faery folk or if you place them under your pillow your dreams will surely come true.

Scatter calendula petals in your bathwater to give yourself a healthy, sunny glow guaranteed to draw many admiring glances.

FOLK MEDICINE: A dozen calendula heads steeped in boiling water made a soothing "measle flower" tea that was traditionally given to children to ease the misery of measles.

Add a handful of calendula blossoms to your daily bath to soothe sunburned skin and ease the itch of insect bites or rashes.

OTHER COMMON USES: The petals have a slightly peppery flavour and can add a little sunshine and tang to salads and bakes.

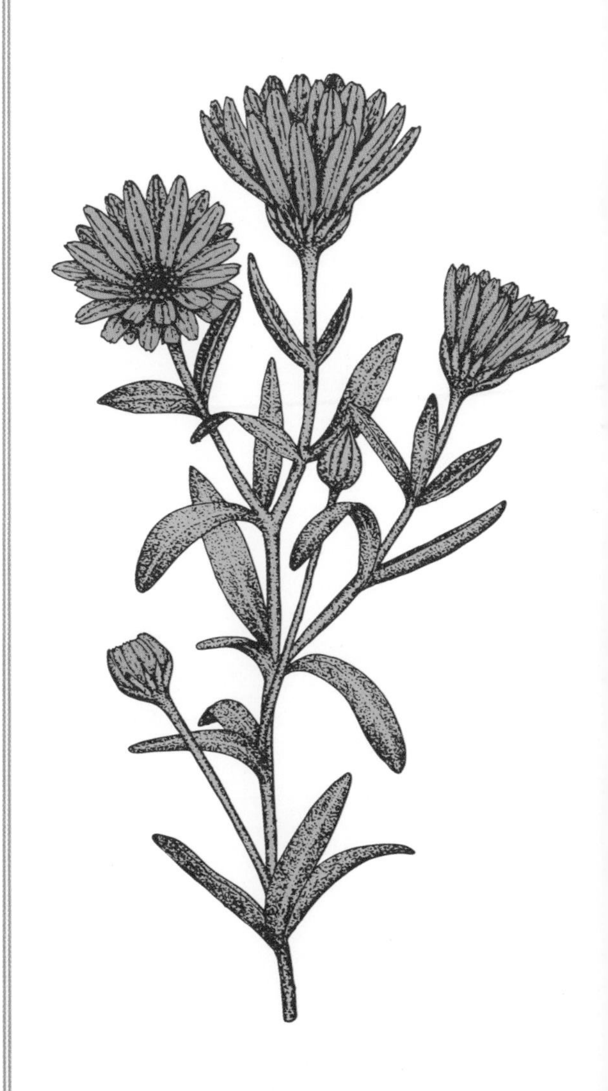

CALENDULA HEALING HAND BALM

Fresh or dried calendula can be used in both of these recipes making it an incredibly versatile plant to grow in the garden and use all year round.

With two nurses in the family who have to constantly wash their hands, I wanted to gift them something natural that was free from parabens and petroleum jelly.

Calendula is anti-inflammatory, antiseptic and antibacterial. It nourishes and hydrates the driest of skin and is gentle enough for use on the most sensitive of skin conditions such as eczema.

Lavender oil has natural anti-inflammatory and healing properties, while tea tree contains a natural antiseptic, helping to calm redness and inflammation.

My apothecary research led me to discover a traditional American homesteading recipe used on farm animals to help soothe sore udders. My mum and mother-in-law experimented using it on their faces and tell me that it keeps their skin super hydrated and soft. They've got me doing it now, too!

I took the essence of that recipe as a basis for this truly soothing balm; it really does the job and my nurses and the rest of the family can't get enough of it.

Makes approximately 150ml

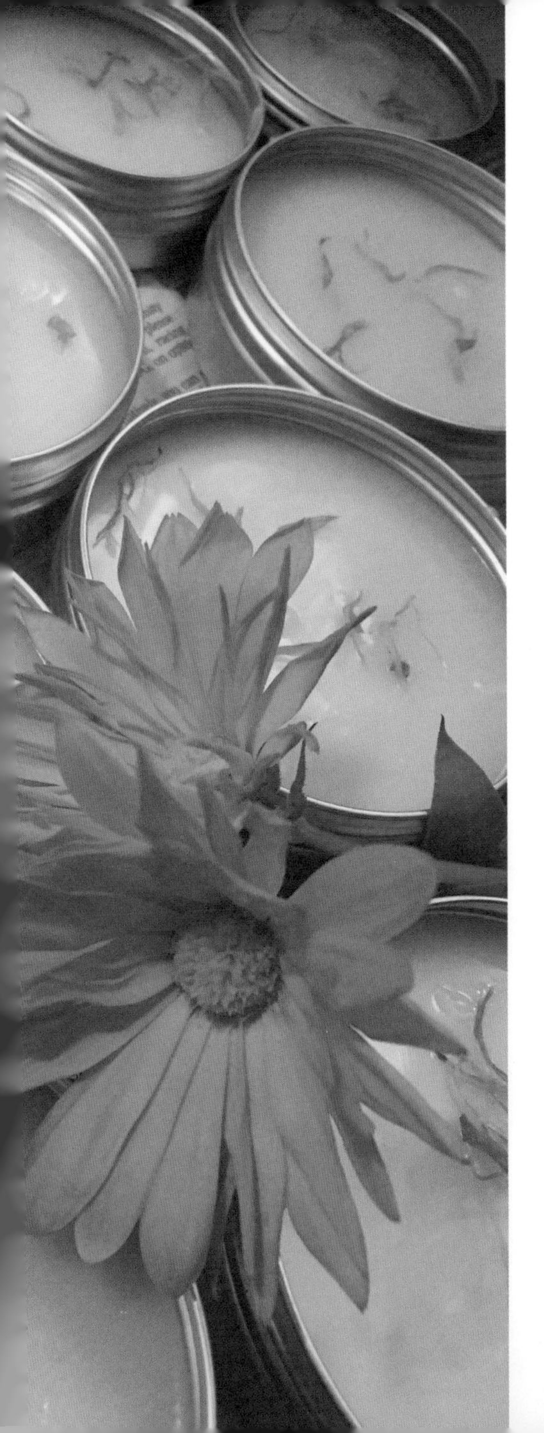

INGREDIENTS

14g unrefined beeswax, or soy wax for a vegan alternative

28g organic shea butter

28g organic coconut oil

90ml calendula infused carrier oil

5 drops lavender essential oil

5 drops tea tree essential oil

Equipment needed

Heatproof bowl

Shallow tins or jars

METHOD

Melt the beeswax, shea butter, coconut oil and calendula oil in a heatproof bowl placed over a pan of boiling water.

Once melted, take the mixture off the heat, combine and stir in the essential oils.

Pour into sterilized jars or tins, sprinkle a few dried calendula petals over the balm for decoration. (See pages 10–11 for how to dry flowers and herbs.)

Allow to cool completely before putting on the lid.

Always do a skin test before using.

Keeps for about 6 months or longer if refrigerated.

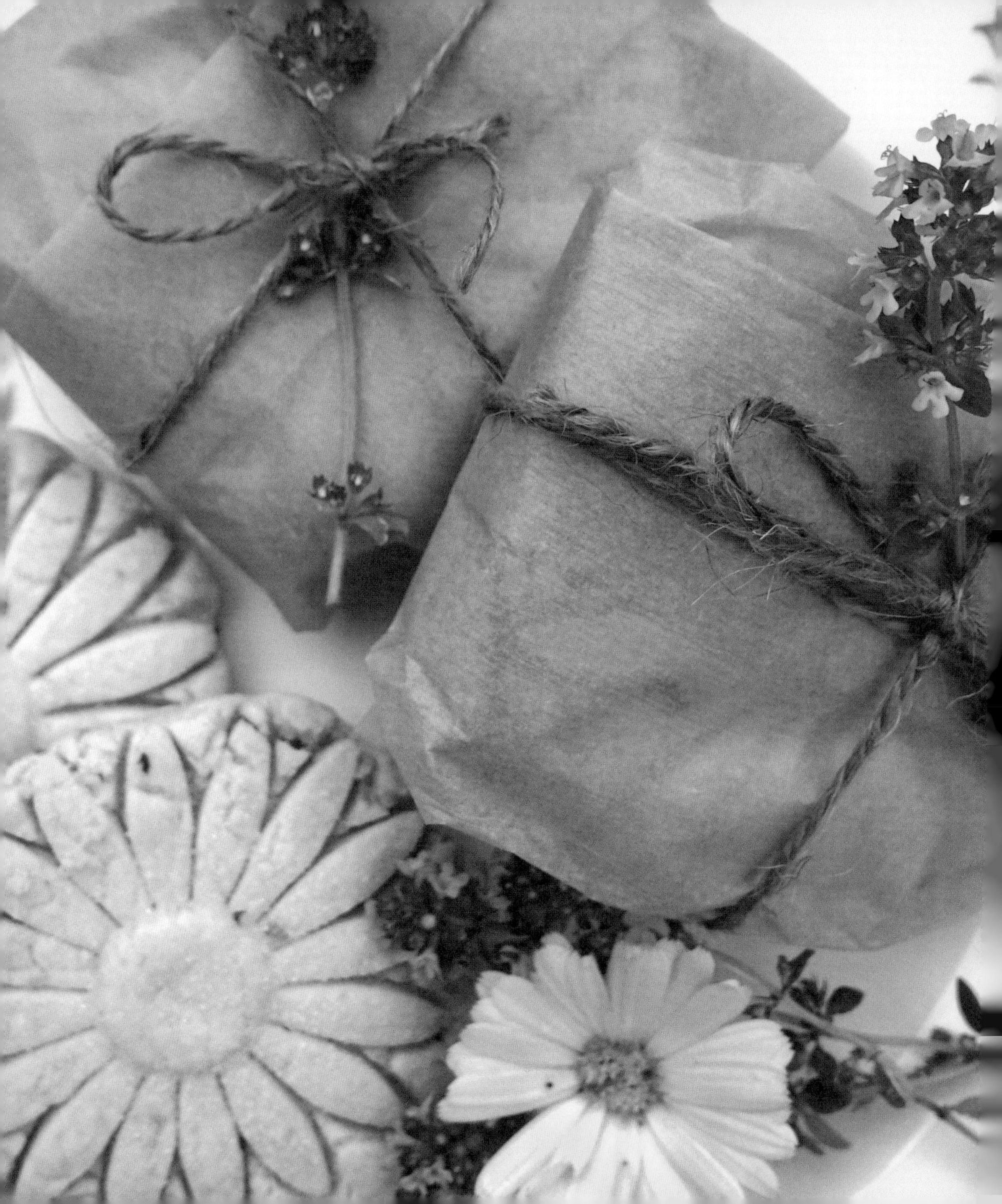

CALENDULA AND THYME SHORTBREAD BISCUITS

Everyone loves a good home-baked shortbread biscuit, and the addition of calendula and thyme means these buttery and slightly minty peppery treats are just a little bit different. Family and friends will love them.

Makes 10–20 biscuits depending on size

INGREDIENTS

225g softened unsalted butter (you can use a plant-based alternative)

110g caster sugar

225g plain flour

110g cornflour

Pinch of fine salts

3–4 tbsp chopped fresh calendula petals

2 tbsp chopped fresh thyme

Equipment needed

Biscuit cutters

Baking trays

METHOD

Line two baking trays with baking paper.

Cream the butter and sugar together until light and fluffy using a mixer or a wooden spoon.

Sift in the flour and cornflour and add the salt. Mix until combined into a stiff dough.

Tip the dough onto a lightly floured worktop.

Add the calendula and thyme and gently knead until combined.

Roll the dough out to about 1cm (½ inch) thickness; this can be made easier by rolling the dough between two sheets of baking paper.

Cut dough out into generous-sized rounds or shapes. Place the rounds onto the prepared baking trays and chill for at least 30 minutes (this stops them spreading).

Preheat oven to 170°C. Bake for about 20 minutes or until the edges of your biscuits turn golden brown.

Allow to cool on the baking trays for 5 minutes to crisp up, then transfer onto a wire rack and dust with a little extra caster sugar.

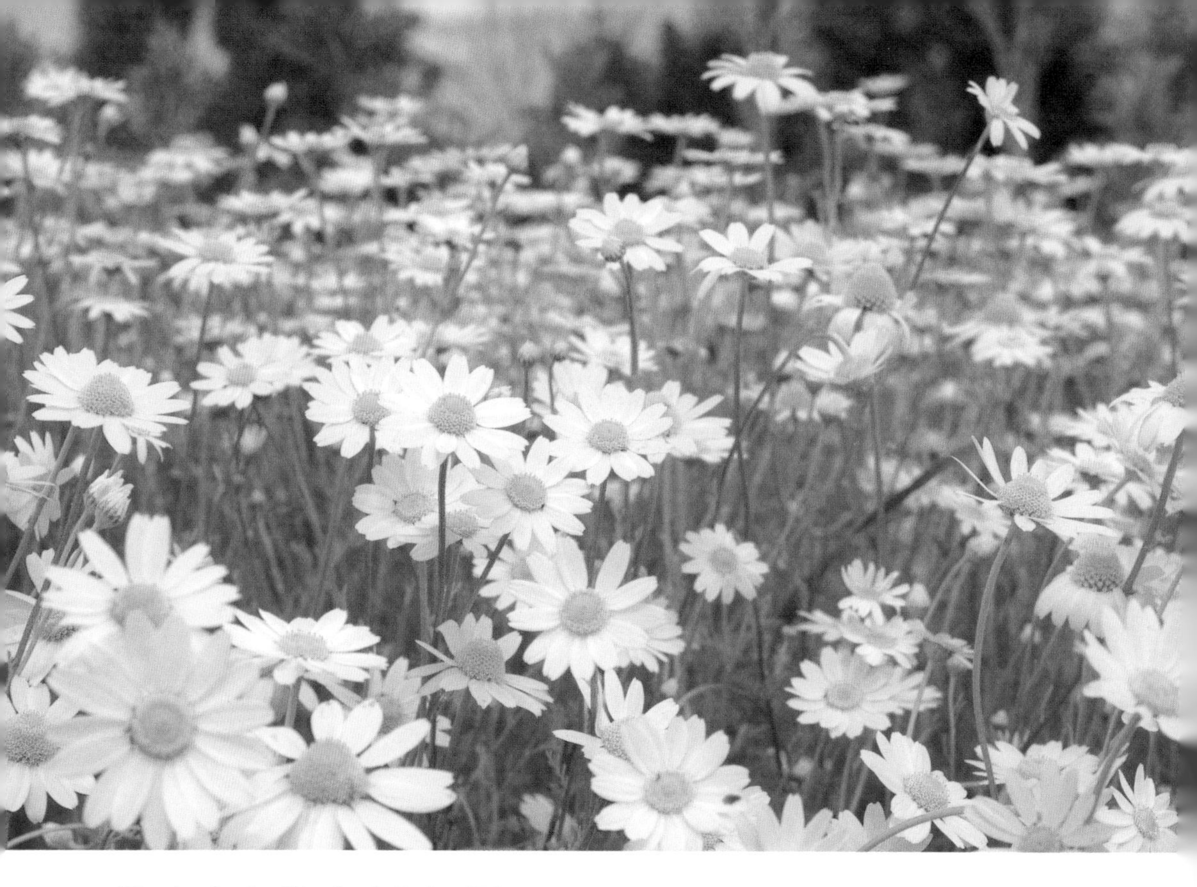

CAMOMILE

Alternative names: Earth apple, whig plant, Roman chamomile

HOW TO IDENTIFY: Camomile is a low-growing herb, commonly found in lawns. It has small daisy-like flowers, feathery leaves and an apple-like scent when crushed.

HISTORY: Camomile was the most prized of herbs to the Ancient Egyptians, believed to be capable of curing all known ailments. It has been depicted in hieroglyphics dating back over 2,000 years and was used as an offering to the sun god Ra. Ancient Egyptian women made camomile poultices for their eyes to reduce puffiness, while camomile oil was widely used in the embalming process.

Camomile was one of the sacred herbs of the Anglo Saxons along with plantain, watercress, fennel, chervil, nettle, mugwort, crab apple and betony. These beneficial herbs made up the sacred nine herbs charm, which was traditionally recited over a sick person to call upon the healing power of the Anglo Saxon god Woden. Camomile lawns became fashionable in Elizabethan England where genteel ladies enjoyed the sweet fragrance that was released as they crushed the herb under their feet as they walked.

FOLKLORE: Washing your hands with water infused with camomile will ensure good luck at the gambling tables.

Wearing a garland of camomile will attract love. If this doesn't work bathe in an infusion of the flowers and you will become irresistible.

Blending dried camomile with lavender to burn as incense will guarantee a good night's sleep and peaceful dreams.

Carry camomile with you if you feel that you are in physical or magical danger and place the plant on your doorstep and windowsills to ward off evil.

FOLK MEDICINE: In *The Tale of Peter Rabbit*, after being chased out of Mr McGregor's vegetable garden Beatrix Potter recounts that: "*Peter was not very well during the evening. His mother put him to bed and made some camomile tea*" and she gave a dose of it to Peter to calm his tummy.

Peter's mother must have taken her advice from Culpeper: "*...it helps to dissolve the pains in the belly... It easeth all pains of the cholic and stone, and all pains and torments of the belly, and gently provoketh urine.*"

To make a healing charm, place dried camomile, eucalyptus, cinnamon, sage and garlic into a blue bag and sprinkle with sandalwood oil.

OTHER COMMON USES: An infusion of camomile flowers has long been used as a rinse to brighten blonde hair.

Camomile is known as the "plant's physician" as it can have a healing effect if planted next to any sickly plants in your garden.

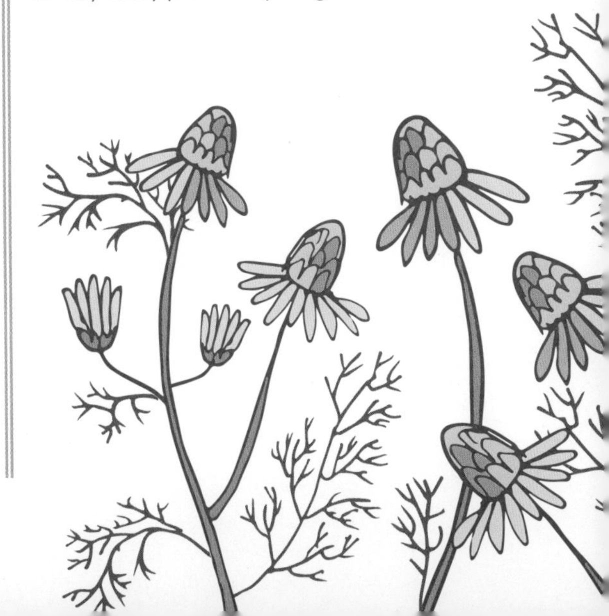

CAMOMILE AND NETTLE TEA FOR HAY FEVER

Camomile contains natural antihistamine as well as being anti-inflammatory and antioxidant. Nettles can also help your fight against seasonal itchy eyes and sniffles as well as containing vitamin C, iron and calcium. A little local raw honey can be added for sweetness – although the jury is out as to whether or not local honey can ease hay fever symptoms I still like to use it. I grow a patch of pesticide-free nettles in the garden specifically as a habitat for wildlife but also to use for remedies and in baking.

Makes 3–4 cups

INGREDIENTS

4 tsp fresh pesticide-free camomile (or 2 tsp of dried)

3 tbsp nettle tops (or 2 tbsp dried)

Raw honey to taste

Boiled water

Equipment needed

Teapot or heatproof jug

METHOD

Wash the nettles and chop roughly (wear gloves to avoid being stung!).

Put the camomile and nettles into a teapot or jug and pour over the boiling water.

Allow to steep for 5 minutes.

Strain into a teacup and add raw honey to taste.

Drink three times a day for as long as you need to.

Any leftover tea can be cooled and used to soak cotton pads for tired and itchy eyes, or used as a final rinse for blonde hair.

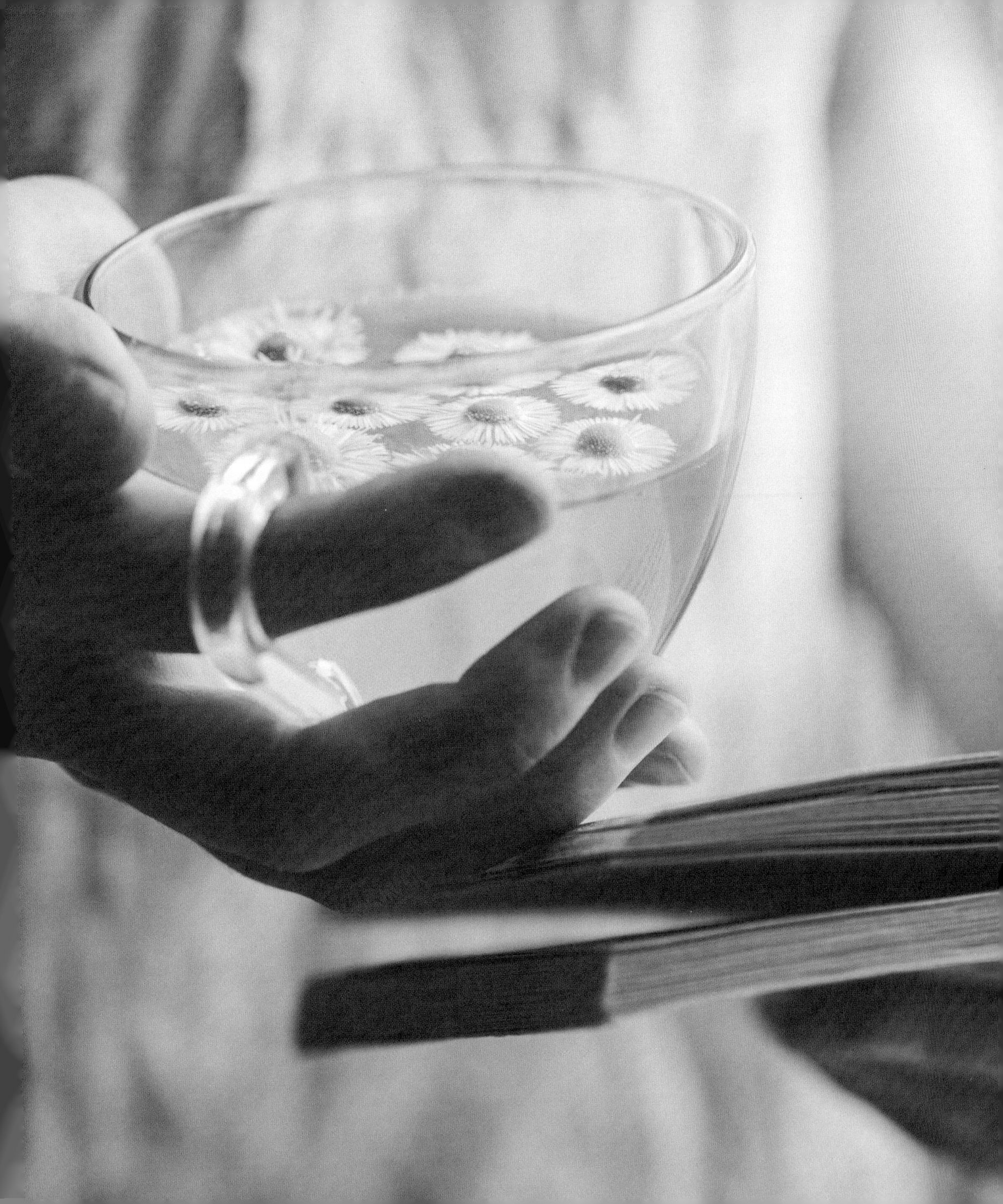

CAMOMILE-INFUSED HAIR OIL

Not just for blondes, camomile is soothing on scalps, can help treat dandruff and promote healthy hair growth. I would use dried camomile for this or allow fresh to wilt for a couple of days before using.

Choose a carrier oil that suits your hair type and use once a month to keep those locks in tip-top condition. Try to buy organic if possible, as this oil will penetrate your skin and enter your bloodstream taking any pesticides and chemicals with it.

Makes 200ml

INGREDIENTS

200ml of your chosen carrier oil: Apricot kernel to strengthen hair, Argan oil for taming frizz, coconut oil for deep shine or olive oil for curly hair

20g dried camomile flowers

Equipment needed

Heatproof bowl

Fine sieve or muslin

Jar

METHOD

Place the camomile and oil in a heatproof bowl over a pan of boiling water and heat for 30 minutes to give the herbs time to infuse.

Allow to cool before straining through a fine sieve or muslin, squeezing to extract the maximum amount of oil.

Pour into a clean jar.

I like to apply this when in the bath as it gives me a reason to stay a little longer.

Pop your sealed jar of oil in the bathwater with you to warm up before pouring a little into your hands and applying it to the hair.

Wrap your hair in a towel or shower cap, lay back and relax for 30 minutes or longer while the oil works its magic.

Perhaps make some cornflower and camomile compresses for tired eyes (see page 72) for an extra treat as you bathe.

Rinse the oil from your hair and shampoo as usual; if your hair tends to be greasy you may not need to use conditioner.

Will keep for about a year in a cool dry place.

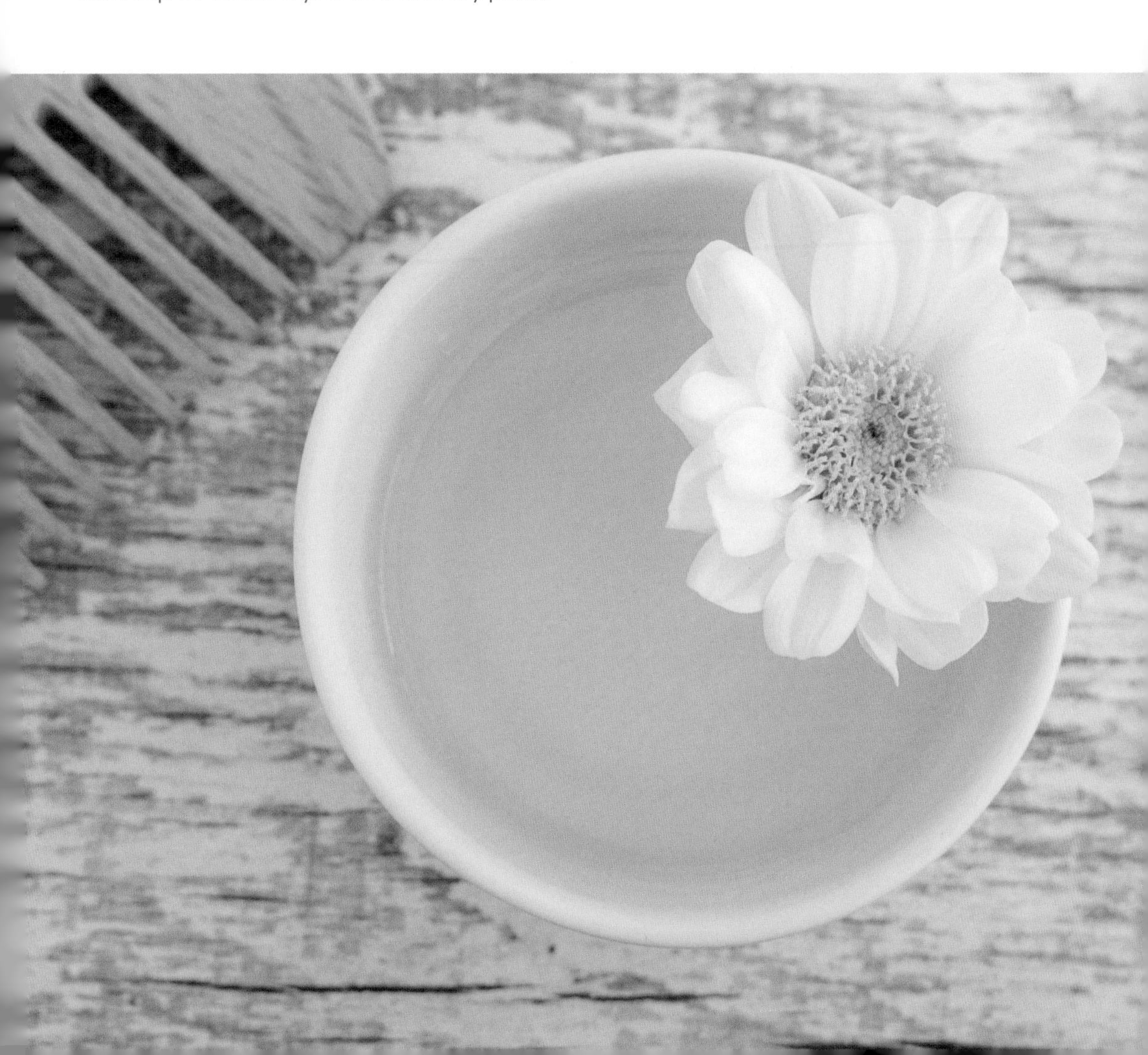

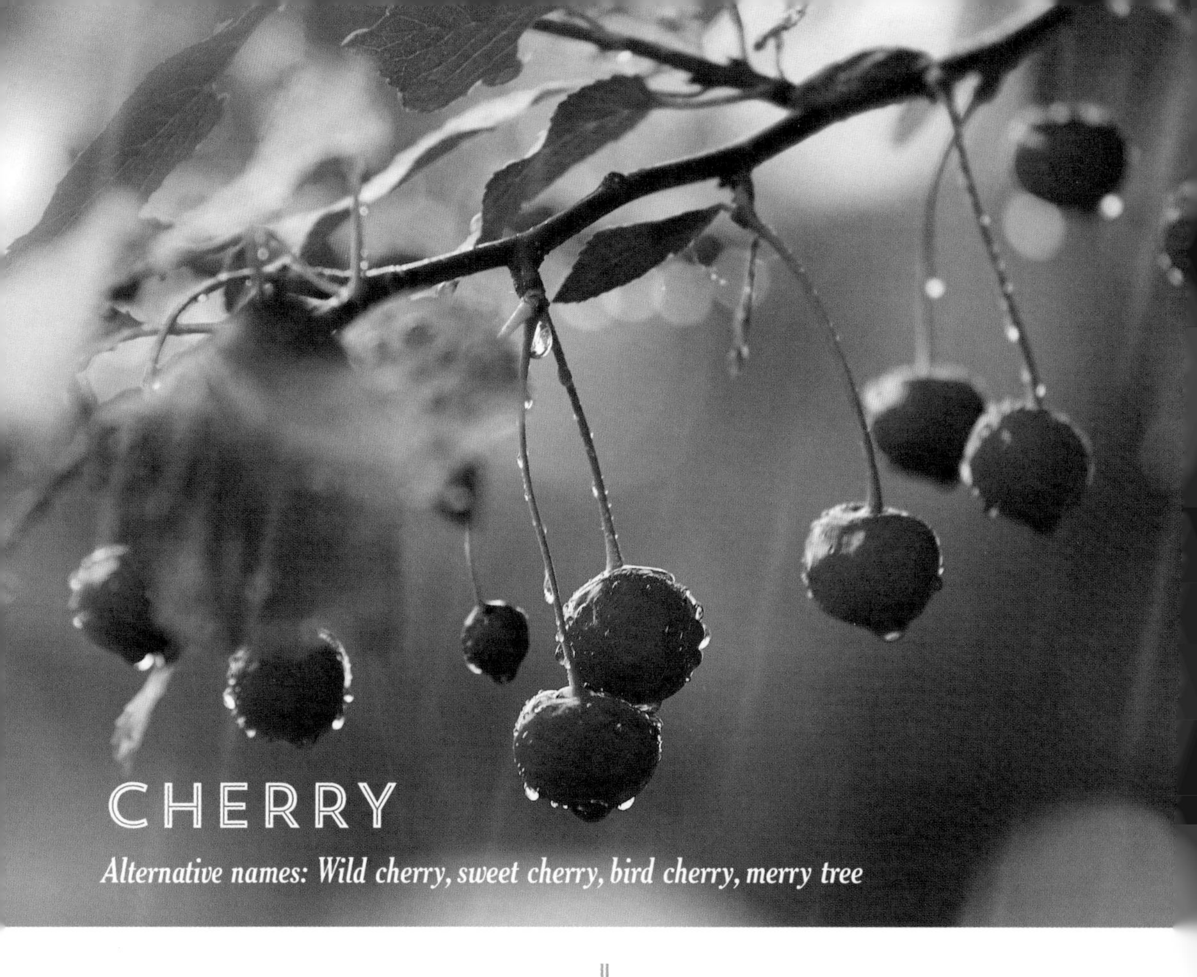

CHERRY

Alternative names: Wild cherry, sweet cherry, bird cherry, merry tree

HOW TO IDENTIFY: A tall tree that can reach up to 5 metres (16 feet) with masses of snowy white or pink blossom in the spring, turning into delicious red fleshy fruits in early summer.

HISTORY: Native wild cherries, sometimes known as hags, were foraged by our ancestors for thousands of years, cherry stones having been found in early Bronze Age settlements dating back to 2000 BC.

Henry VIII introduced cultivated cherries, which taste much better than wild ones, to his farm near Sittingbourne in Kent in the sixteenth century. Having tasted cherries on a trip to Flanders he enjoyed them so much that he decreed they should be grown for him in the UK.

FOLKLORE: Cherries were often used in fortune telling. Children sang around a cherry tree in a twentieth-century nursery rhyme from Yorkshire: "*Cuckoo, cuckoo cherry tree, good bird tell me, how many years before I die?*" Each child then shook the cherry tree, and the number of cherries that fell symbolized the number of years left before the child died!

In medieval England the bark of the cherry tree was placed by the front door to ward off the plague.

To attract love, tie a strand of your hair to a cherry tree as it begins to blossom.

Count cherry stones after your meal to reveal the occupation of your future spouse:

"Tinker, tailor, soldier, sailor, rich man, poor man, beggar man, thief."

FOLK MEDICINE: Culpeper lists the attributes of the cherry tree as:

"The gum of the cherry tree dissolved in wine, is good for a cold, cough and hoarseness of the throat; mendeth the colour in the face, sharpeneth the eyesight, provoketh appetite..."

Cherry root was used to treat intestinal worms, skin ailments, cold sores and burns. Cherry bark was an ingredient in herbal cough syrups.

OTHER COMMON USES: The bark of the cherry tree has been used to produce a cream fabric dye, and the roots will create a red dye.

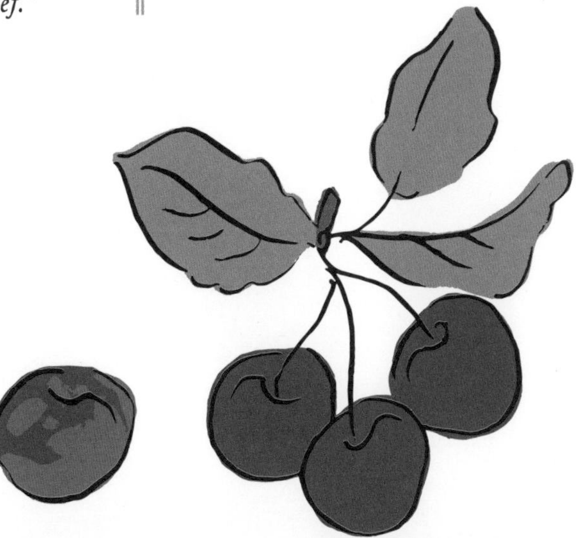

CHERRY MOON MILK FOR RESTFUL SLEEP

Moon milk is rooted in the Hindu tradition of Ayurvedic medicine, which is used to restore balance to the mind, body and spirit. Warm milk is well known to promote restful sleep, and cherries have natural tryptophan that can increase the production of serotonin. The spices are all recognized for their calming properties and also give the moon milk a lovely flavour. Finally, honey, when combined with milk, is guaranteed to give you the best chance of a peaceful night.

For a plant-based alternative, almond milk contains melatonin, tryptophan and magnesium, oat milk is a source of tryptophan and magnesium, and cashew or coconut milk also work beautifully as they are rich in magnesium, which supports relaxation and a good night's sleep.

Makes enough for two people

INGREDIENTS

150ml milk – plant-based if preferred

150ml tart cherry juice

Pinch of ground nutmeg

¼ tsp ground cinnamon

Pinch of ground cardamom

Honey or maple syrup to taste

Equipment needed

Fine sieve

METHOD

Combine all ingredients except for the honey in a saucepan and whisk together until well incorporated.

Warm over a medium heat for 5 minutes stirring occasionally.

Pour through a fine sieve and whisk again using a stick blender to create froth.

Add honey or maple syrup as needed.

Drink before bedtime.

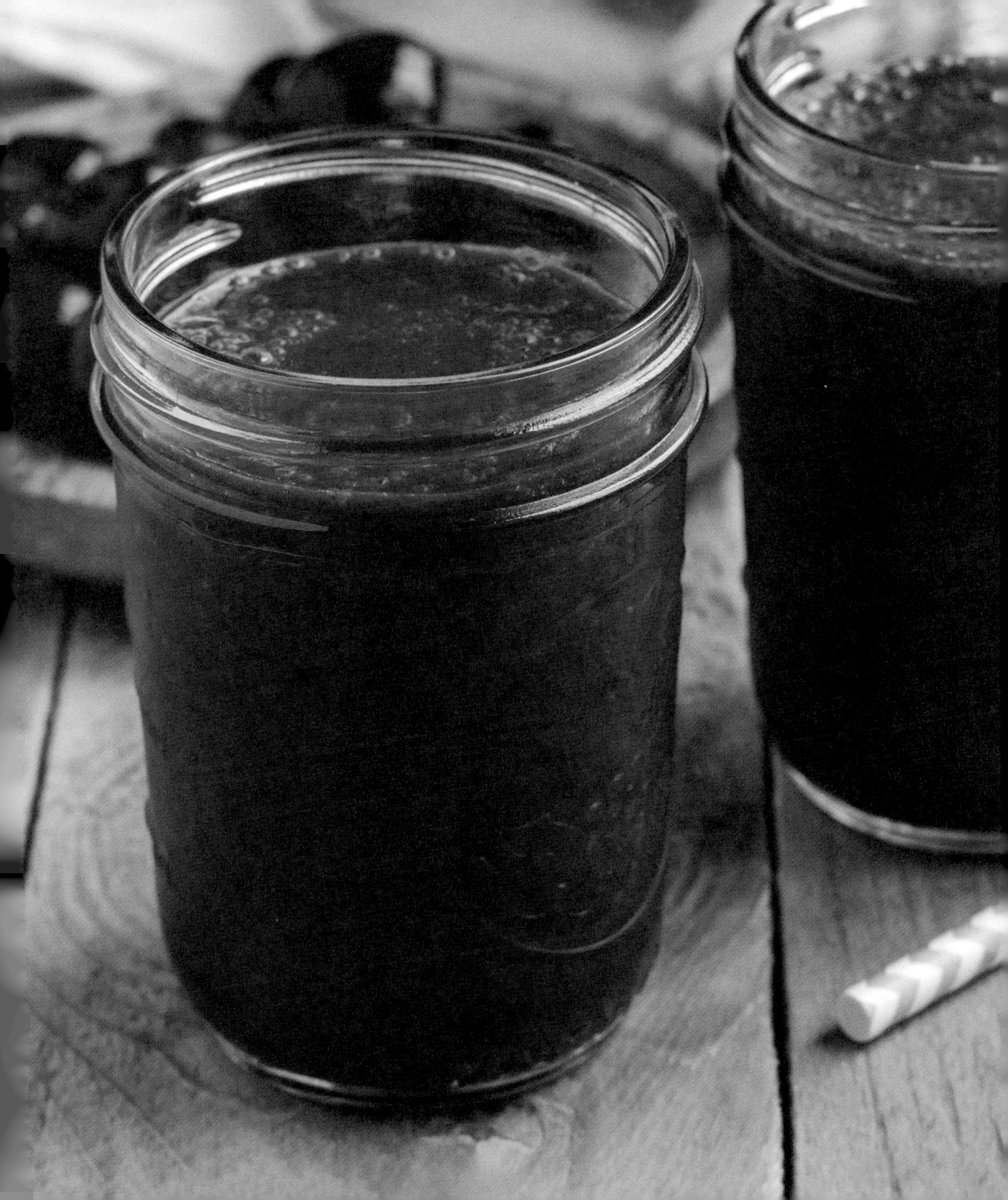

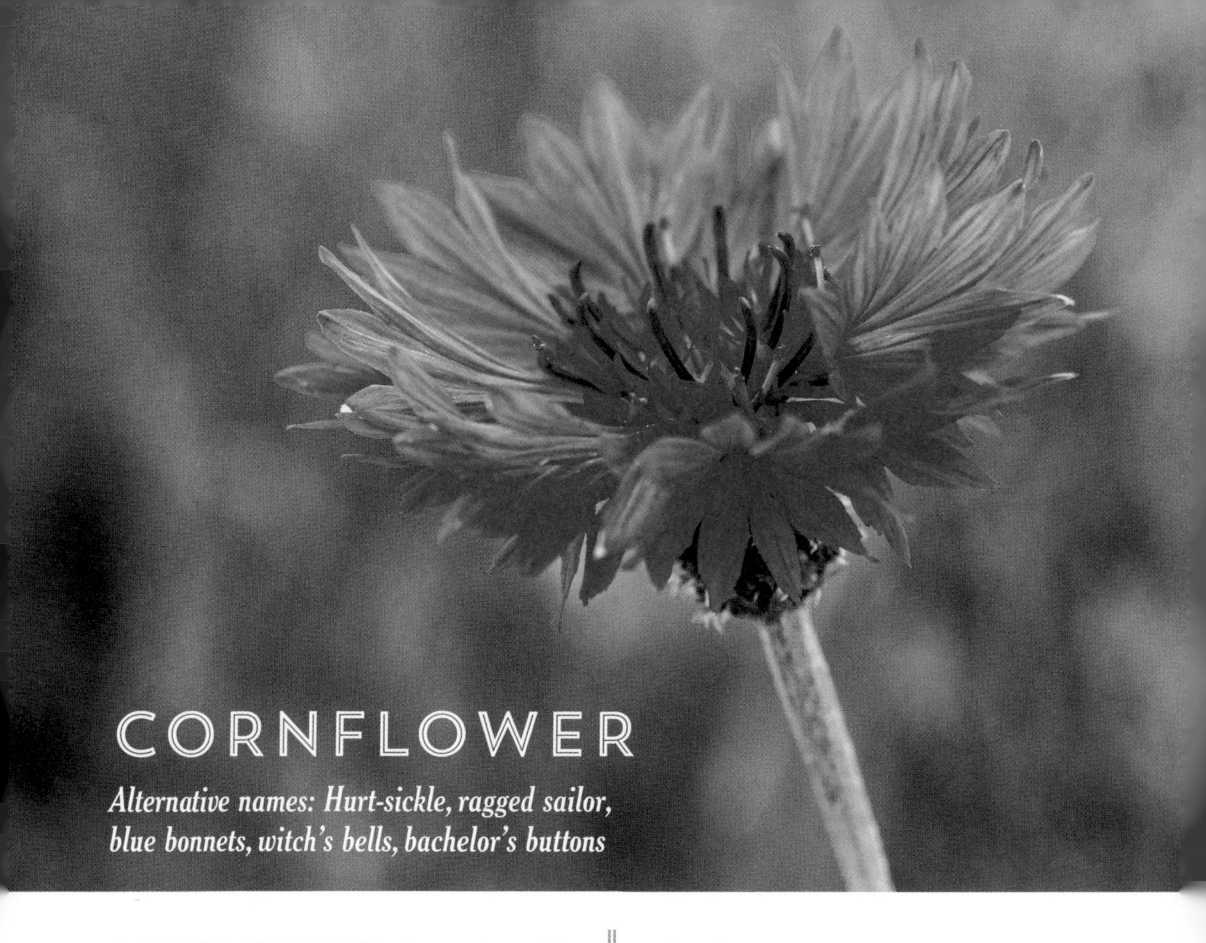

CORNFLOWER

Alternative names: Hurt-sickle, ragged sailor, blue bonnets, witch's bells, bachelor's buttons

HOW TO IDENTIFY: A member of the daisy family, the cornflower is recognized by its striking blue colour and star-like petals.

HISTORY: Floral collars consisting of cornflowers represented new life and fertility to the Ancient Egyptians. Cornflowers, olive leaves and poppies were found in terracotta storage jars in the tomb of Tutankhamen and were still identifiable after 3,000 years.

Cornflowers were once considered by farmers to be a nuisance growing amongst the corn in arable fields, and they were almost wiped out in the 1970s by the overuse of pesticides. Thankfully they have been saved by becoming a garden favourite.

In France, cornflowers are worn for remembrance on Armistice Day in much the same way as poppies are worn in the UK.

FOLKLORE: Cornflowers are used in folk magic for fertility and abundance, placed by doors and in cupboards to prevent negative energy from entering and worn as a charm to attract love. Rolling in a field full of cornflowers was believed to attract youth, happiness, beauty and suitors.

Young men wore cornflowers when they were in love. Unfortunately, if their love was not reciprocated the colour would gradually fade.

Victorian spinsters wore cornflowers on their clothing to indicate that they were single and looking for love, which gave the flowers the nickname "bachelor's buttons".

People covered their eyes with cornflowers in the belief that their sight would be strengthened, with the added benefit that they could also enable them to see faeries.

The flower would be burned while saying a prayer for protection if a storm was known to be coming.

FOLK MEDICINE: Cornflowers can stop a nosebleed but only if picked on Corpus Christi Sunday (the first Sunday 60 days after Easter).

A distillation of the petals can soothe tired eyes and it was used as a remedy for fever, plagues and poison. Culpeper advises:

"The powder or dried leaves of the cornflower is given with good success to those that are bruised by a fall, or have a broken vein inwardly... The seed or leaves taken in wine is very good against the plague, and all infectious diseases... The juice dropped in the eyes takes away the heat and inflammation in them."

Eau de Casse Lunettes was a popular French eyewash made from cornflower petals to combat infection and cataracts. Evidently it was particularly effective on blue eyes.

OTHER COMMON USES: The plant and flowers are edible but are fairly bitter.

Cornflowers are also used to make a natural blue ink or dye.

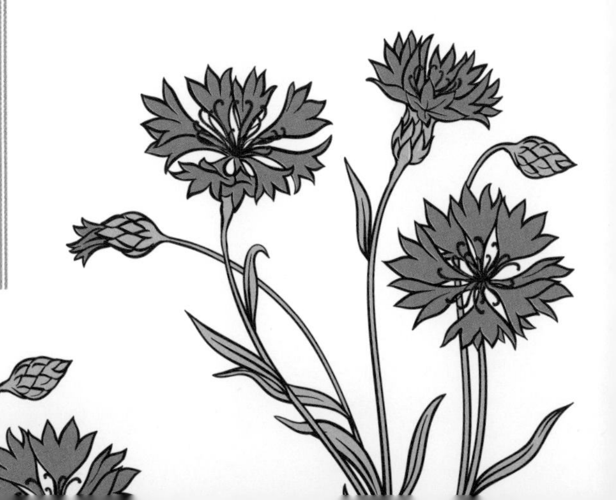

CORNFLOWER INK

This is something fun to make with children or for yourself if you are creative. Gather cornflowers to make turquoise blue ink, poppies for red ink, buttercups for yellow ink and use different leaves to make green ink – the method remains the same.

INGREDIENTS

Enough petals to loosely fill a jam jar

2 jam jars of water

1 tsp white vinegar

Pinch of salt

Equipment needed

Paintbrush or dip pen

METHOD

Bring the water to the boil and stir in your petals – use a non-metallic container if possible.

Simmer until the liquid has changed colour and reduced by half.

Add the vinegar and salt to "fix" the colour.

Strain out your petals and your ink is ready to use either with a paintbrush or a dip pen.

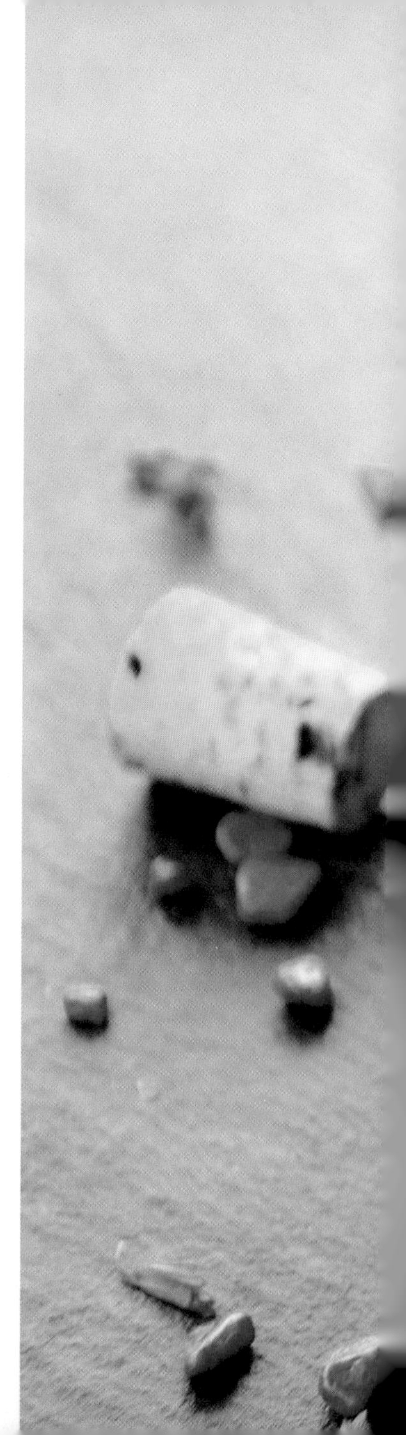

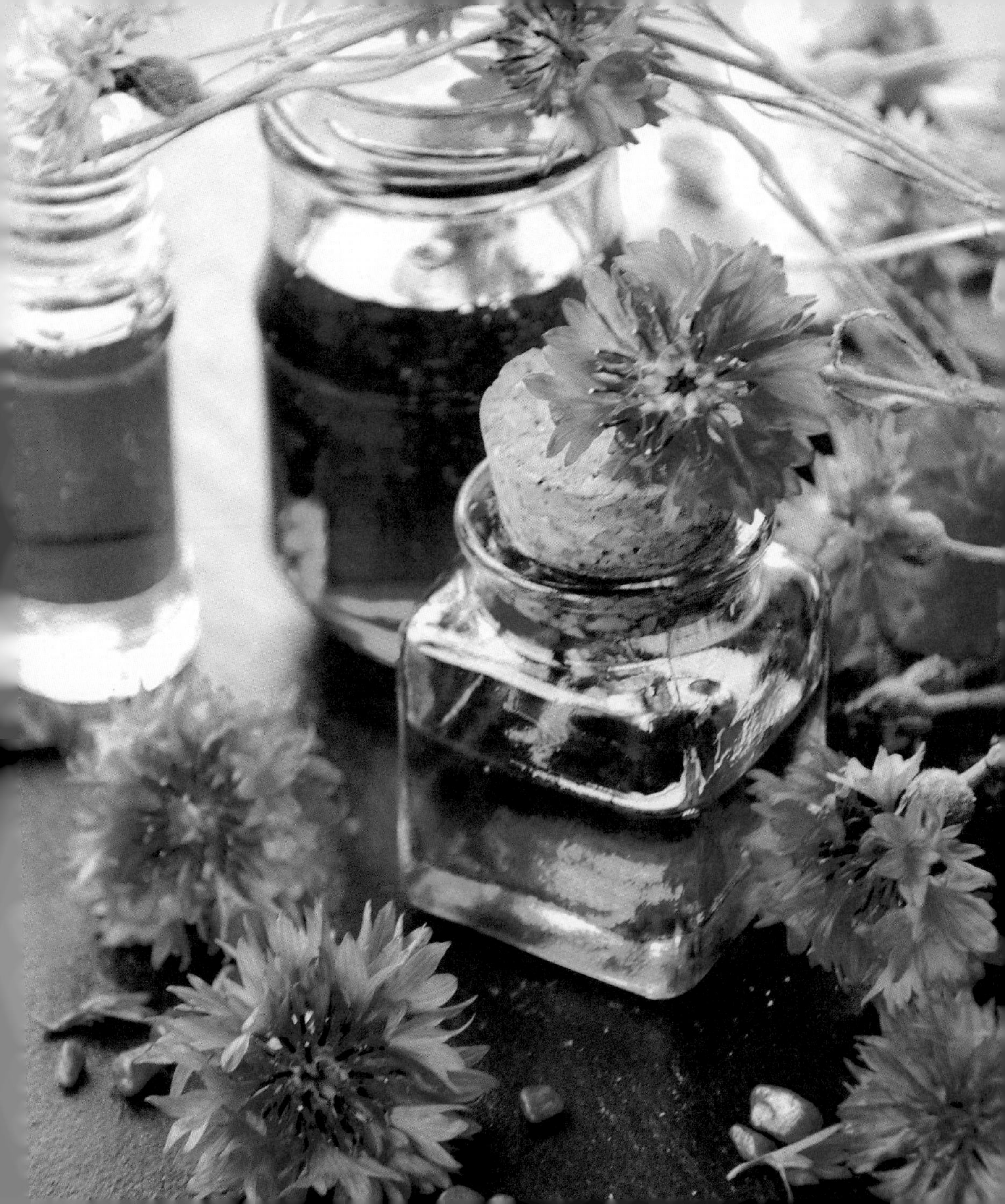

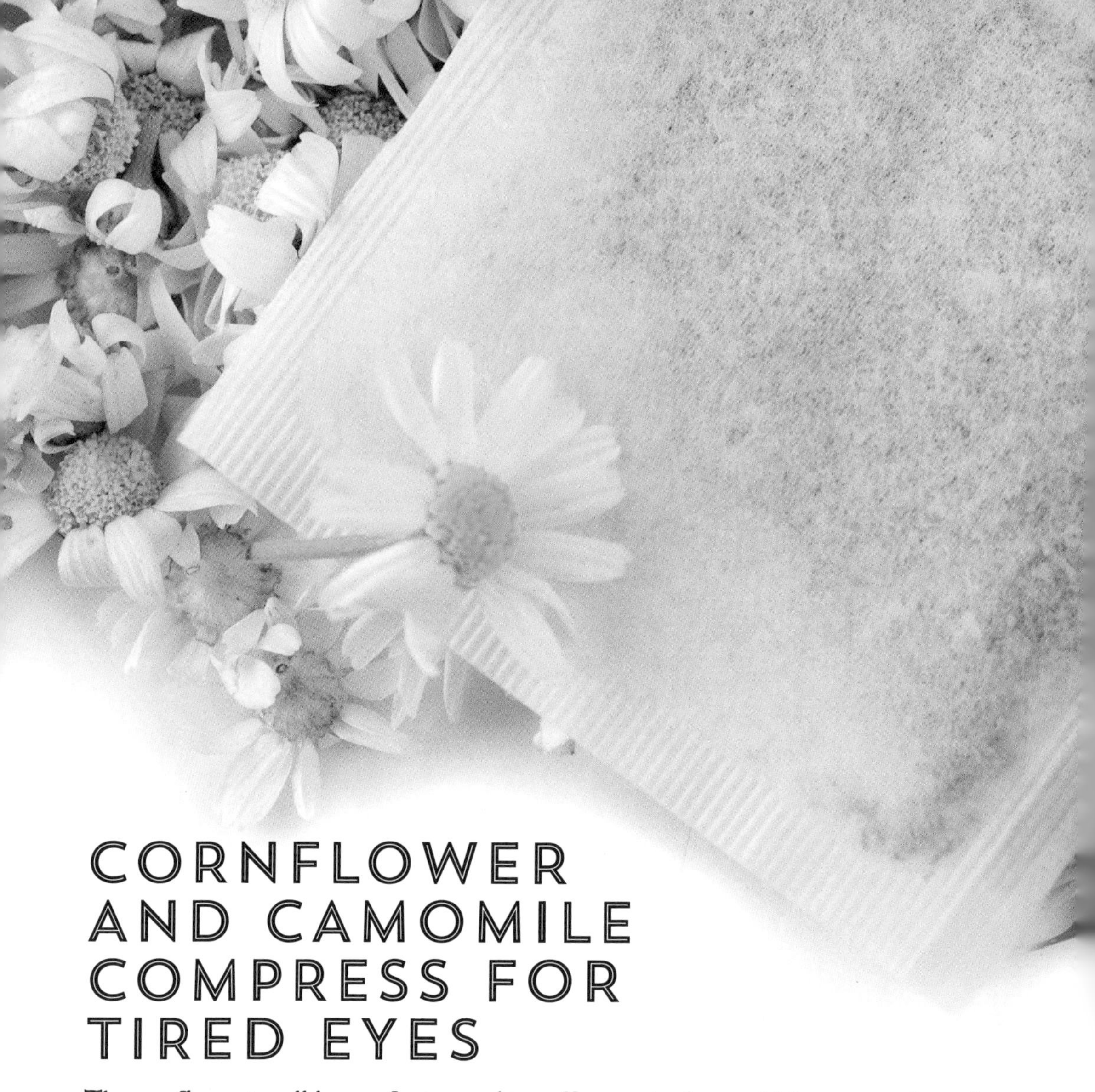

CORNFLOWER AND CAMOMILE COMPRESS FOR TIRED EYES

The cornflower is well known for its soothing effect on tired eyes. Adding camomile to the mix will reduce dark circles and puffy skin under eyes – you might just see some faeries too.

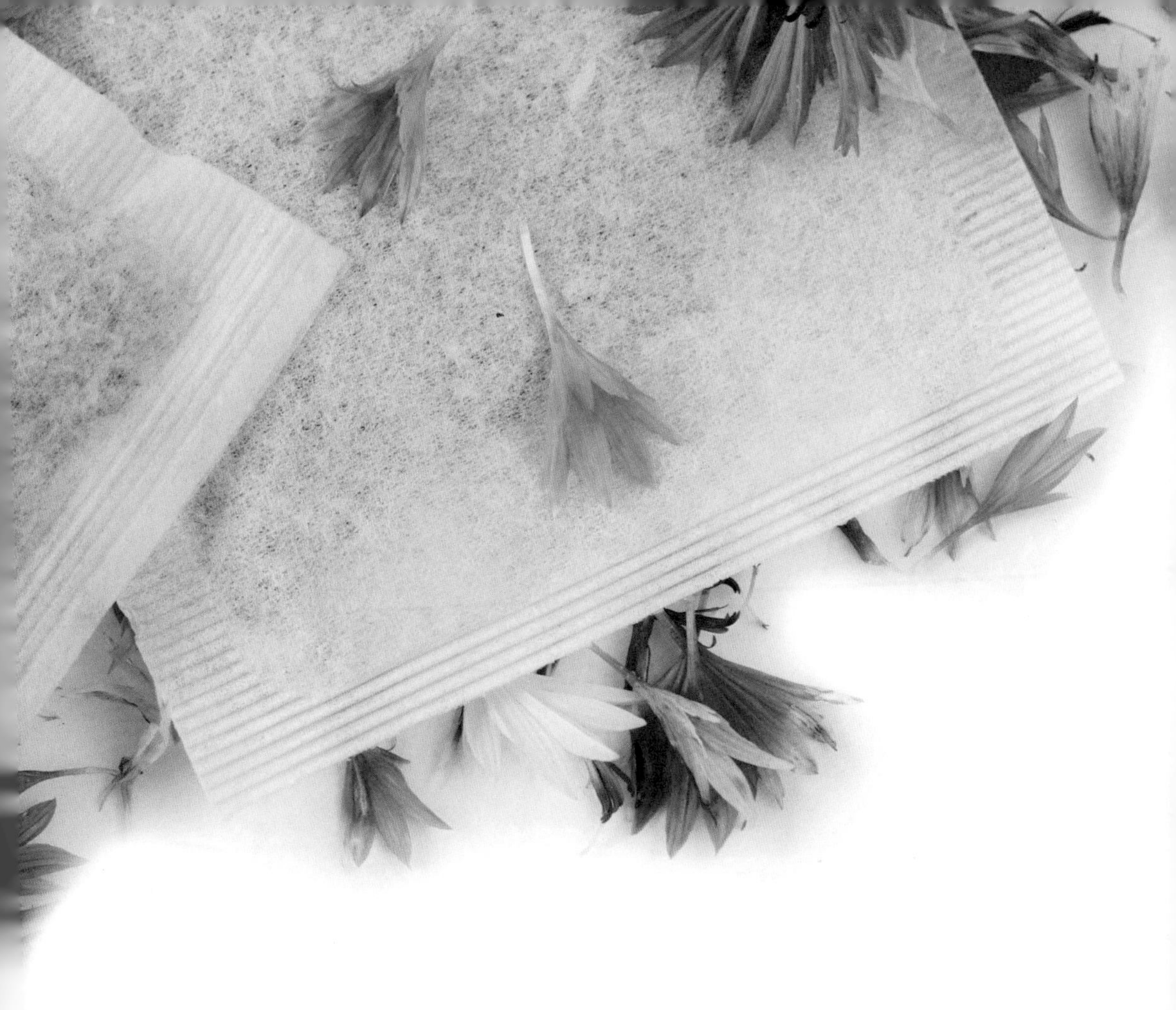

INGREDIENTS

2 organic camomile tea bags

2 or 3 cornflower heads, fresh or dried

250ml boiling water

METHOD

Put the cornflowers and camomile tea bags in a heat resistant jug or mug. Pour over the boiling water.

Allow to cool completely, or even better pop into the fridge.

Squeeze out the tea bags, lie back and place them over your closed eyes. Relax for 30 minutes.

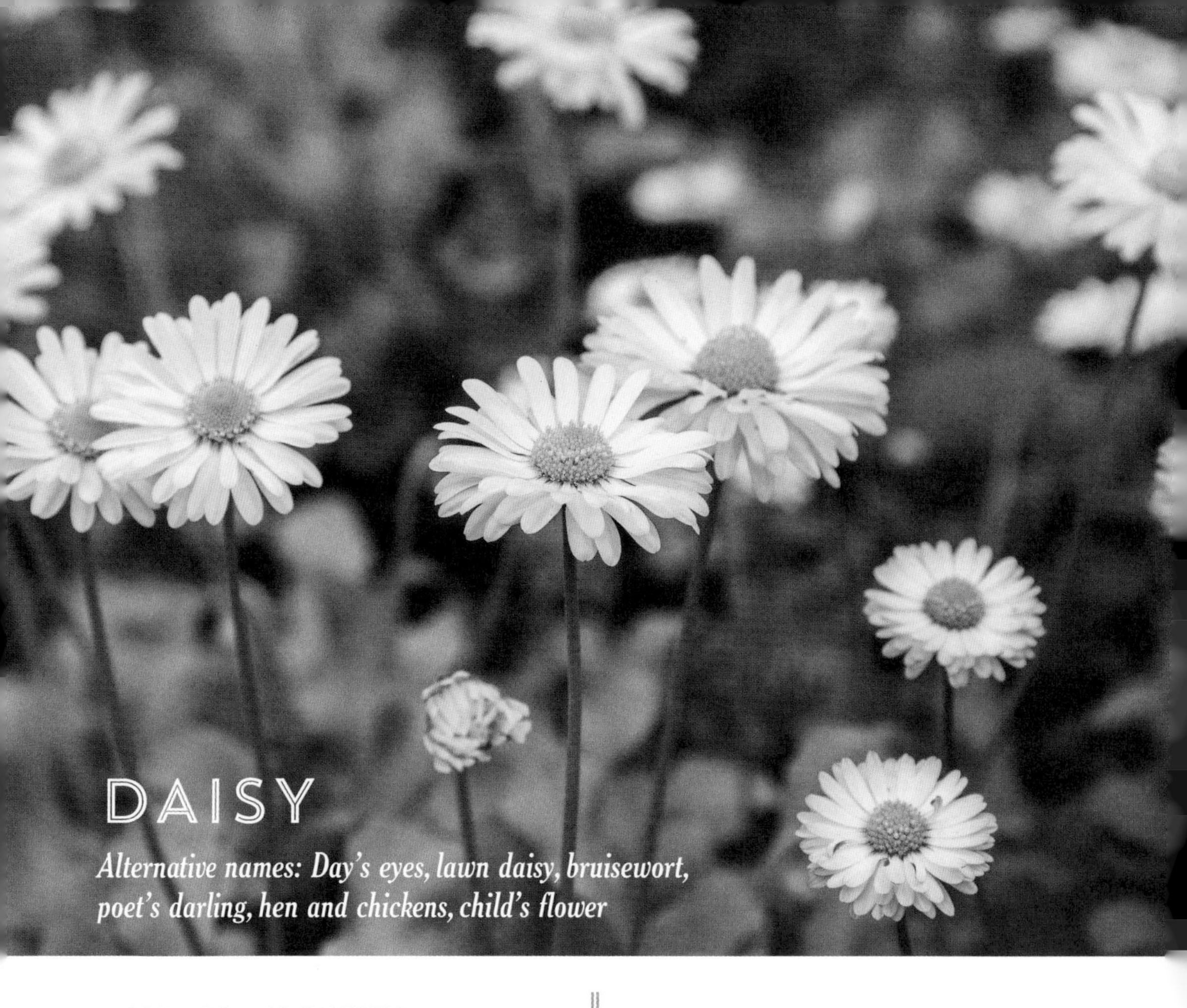

DAISY

Alternative names: Day's eyes, lawn daisy, bruisewort, poet's darling, hen and chickens, child's flower

HOW TO IDENTIFY: Daisies are commonly found in lawns and grassy areas. These tiny yellow-centred flowers have pretty white petals which are often tipped with pink.

HISTORY: Roman legions instructed their slaves to fill sacks with daisies, which were then squeezed to extract juice. This juice was then used to soak bandages for strapping up wounds caused in battle, helping to prevent infection and speed up healing.

A nineteenth-century English proverb tells us that *"mild spring weather is only assured when daisies are flowering thickly on the grass."*

FOLKLORE: In the Middle Ages it was believed that if puppies were fed milk infused with daisies it would *"keepeth them from growing great"* – John Gerard, sixteenth-century herbalist.

Placing daisy chains around the necks and on the heads of children was thought to protect them from being carried away by faeries, a tradition carried on in school playgrounds even now.

"He loves me, he loves me not" has been chanted by many, if not all, lovesick teenagers as they resolutely pluck the petals from a daisy hoping for a favourable answer. If the result is hopeful, another daisy can be stripped saying "*this year, next year, sometime, never*" to discover when they will marry.

A maiden should walk into a meadow where daisies grow and, with her eyes closed, pluck a handful of flowers. The number of daisies that she has pulled is the number of years that she will have to wait before she marries.

An amulet filled with dried daisies hung above a child's bed will keep them protected from evil influences. Daisies scattered around the home will create a feeling of security and happiness.

FOLK MEDICINE: The medieval practice of the "doctrine of signatures" suggests that you should treat an ailment with a plant that most resembles the afflicted body part. For example, walnuts were recommended for brain health and the large lung-shaped roots of lungwort were used for pulmonary diseases. Daisies (or day's eyes) were believed to relieve bloodshot eyes and other eye related problems. This belief was further reinforced by Culpeper: "*The juice of them dropped into the running eyes of any, doth much help them.*"

OTHER COMMON USES: Daisy flowers and leaves are edible and can be added to salads, although they have a somewhat bitter taste. Needless to say, it's best to forage for daisies that are free from pesticides and away from dog-walking areas.

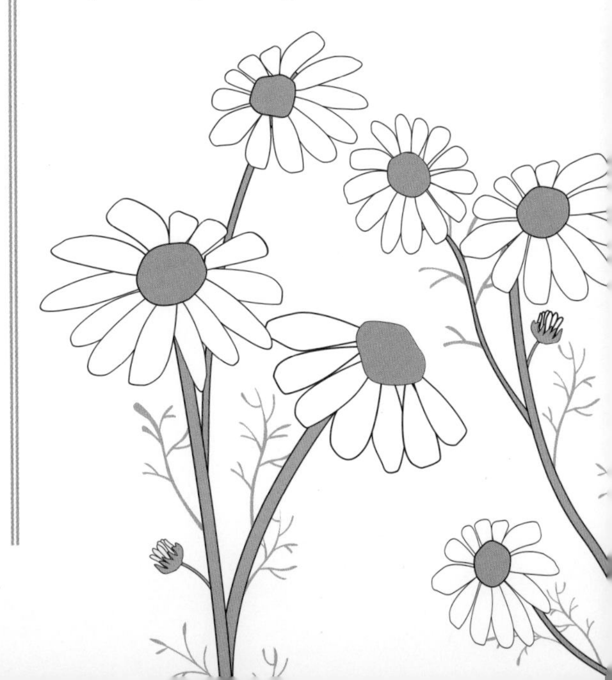

DAISY BUMPS AND BRUISES BALM

Daisies are so easy to find in Europe and contain anti-inflammatory, wound-healing and pain-relieving properties, which are similar to arnica. This balm is an absolute must for your natural first-aid kit and is a great project to make with children. It can also be massaged into the skin to relieve aching joints caused by too much gardening. Camomile is also anti-inflammatory and has pain-relieving properties.

Makes about 110ml

INGREDIENTS

100ml daisy infused oil

10g unrefined beeswax, or soy wax for a vegan alternative

5 drops camomile essential oil

Equipment needed

Heatproof bowl

Sterilized jars or tins

METHOD

Place the daisy infused oil and beeswax in a heatproof bowl over a pan of boiling water.

Once the beeswax has melted, remove from heat and stir in the camomile essential oil.

Pour into sterilized jars or tins and allow to cool completely before popping on the lid.

Do not use if you are allergic to daisies and only put on unbroken skin.

Use within 1 year.

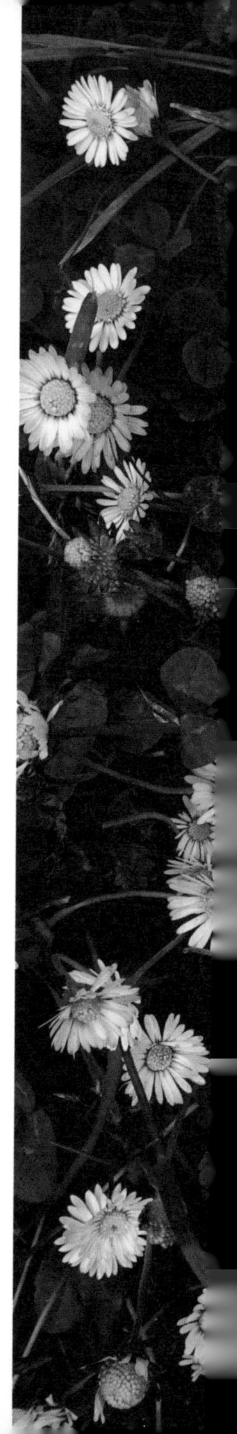

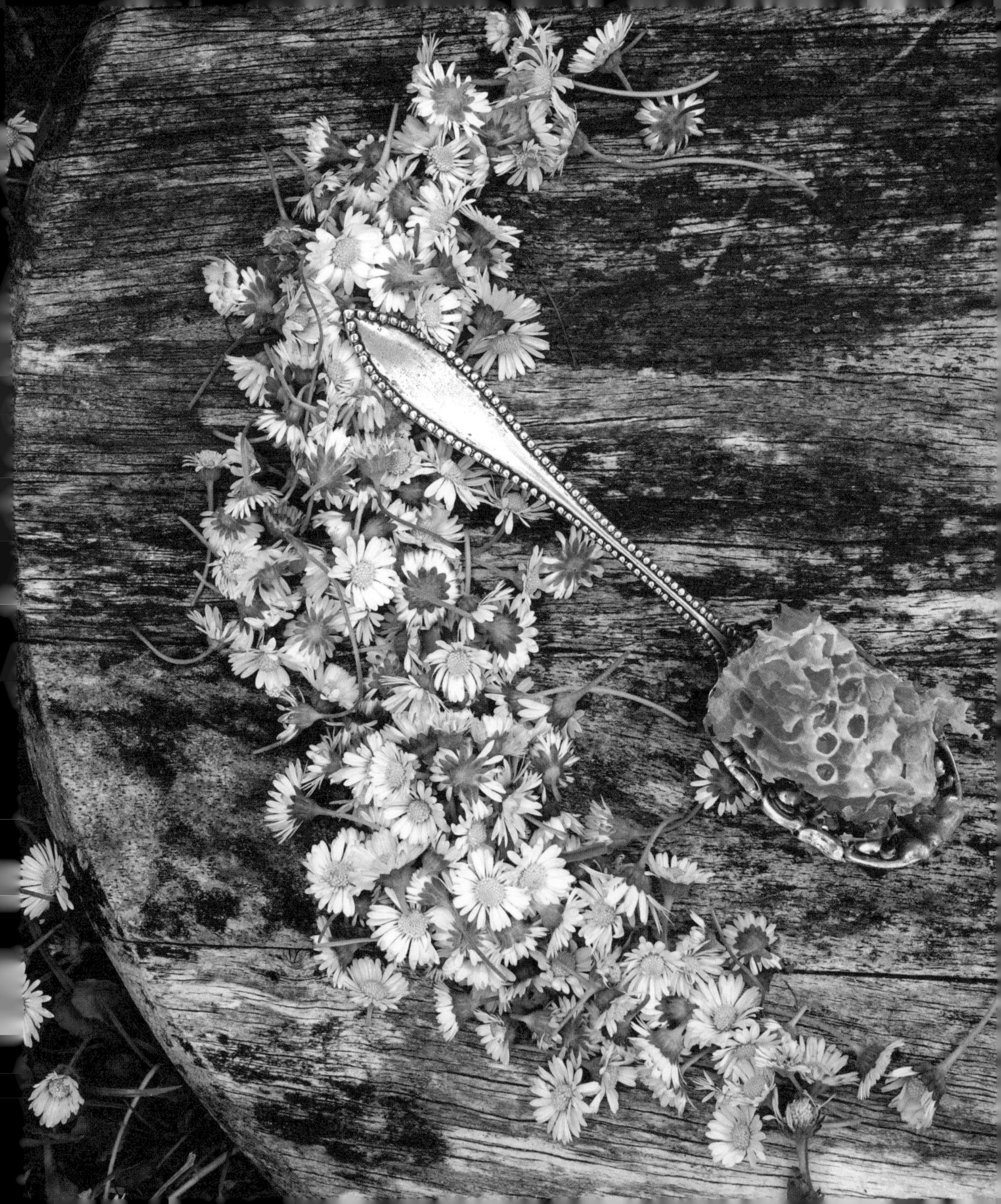

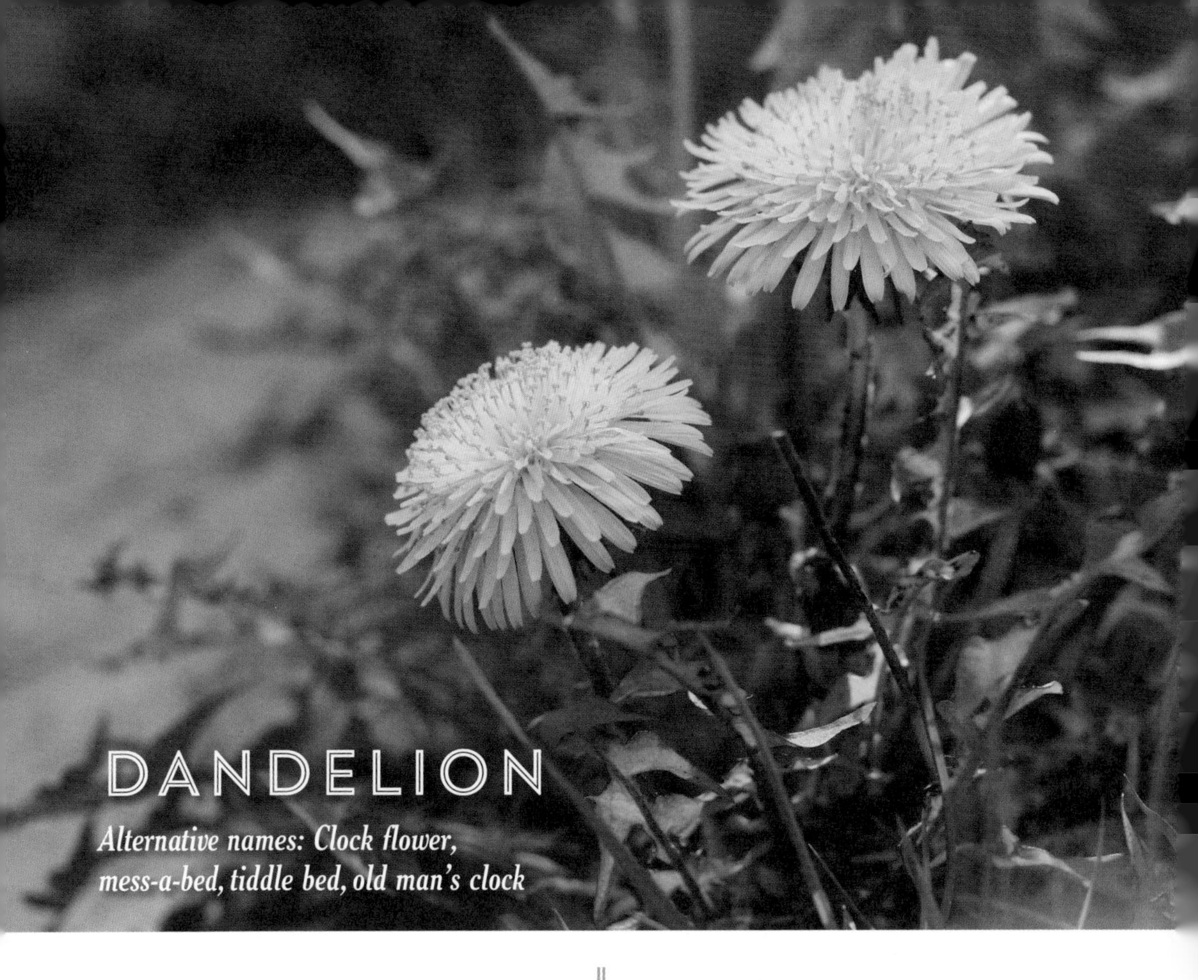

DANDELION

Alternative names: Clock flower, mess-a-bed, tiddle bed, old man's clock

HOW TO IDENTIFY: This plant is probably the most familiar of our wild flowers as it grows rampantly everywhere, especially in lawns and on verges. The beautiful golden yellow flowers shine like little suns in the spring before turning to fluffy dandelion clocks later on in the summer.

The leaves are very distinctive with "lion's teeth" (the French name for dandelion being *dent-du-lion*) edges. The stem is smooth and hollow and will ooze a milky sap once broken open.

HISTORY: Dandelion is regarded as a nuisance nowadays by many keen gardeners, but not so long ago it was possible to make a decent living from digging up the roots for use in medicine.

As recently as the 1930s, teams of "root diggers" would benefit local farmers by ridding their fields of dandelions. These roots were so sought-after for their medicinal properties that a special "green herb" rate was charged for sending them by train to London. A root digger could earn as much as 3d (3 pence) per pound (454g) in weight for washed roots and 1d (1 penny) per pound (454g) in weight for unwashed roots. Dandelion roots were dried and ground coarsely to be used as a coffee substitute during the rationing of World War Two.

FOLKLORE: The childhood joy of gently blowing the seeds off a dandelion globe can not only help you to tell the time, but also tell you how much you are loved. Blow off all the seeds in one go and you are loved with a passion; however, if some seeds remain your partner has some doubts, if lots of seeds remain it might be best to look elsewhere for love.

Blow the seeds in the direction of an absent love to send a message to them.

To give yourself the best chance with all of these superstitions I recommend that you choose a sunny day and a really dry ripe seed head.

If all that wasn't enough, the dandelion globe can also predict the weather. In fine sunny weather the globe is round and fluffy, if rain is on its way the globe shuts like an umbrella until the risk of rain has passed.

FOLK MEDICINE: An important spring tonic, dandelion was regarded as a very powerful cure for many ailments including jaundice and kidney complaints. So effective were dandelion's diuretic properties that children were warned not to touch it or pick it as they would certainly wet the bed that night.

The milky sap from the dandelion stem was rubbed onto warts and allowed to dry; this was repeated until the wart shrivelled away.

OTHER COMMON USES: Dandelion is high in potassium and vitamins A, B, C and D, which can cleanse the blood and stimulate the liver. Young, tender leaves can be mixed into a green salad or made into pesto with pine nuts, olive oil and parmesan cheese. The flowers are traditionally made into wine, beer, cordials and vodka and, of course, the root combined with burdock root makes a delicious tonic.

DANDELION HONEY

Dandelions are one of the first sources of pollen for the bees in the spring, and this recipe for dandelion "honey" makes use of the abundance of dandelions in our back gardens and meadows, as well as being a plant-based treat. Pick your dandelions on a dry day from places that you know to be pesticide free and away from dog-walking areas. Children are particularly good at picking dandelions and will love making this flowery "honey" to eat on toast or scones. I've used teacup measurements for this recipe to make it more child-friendly.

Makes two small jars

INGREDIENTS

2 teacups full of dandelion petals only (discard all greenery as this will make your honey bitter)

2 teacups of water

Juice of 1 organic lemon

250g jam sugar with added pectin

Equipment needed

Muslin cloth or clean tea towel

Sterilized jars

METHOD

Place the petals in a saucepan with the lemon juice and water. Simmer for 30 minutes.

After simmering pour into a covered bowl or jar and leave to steep overnight.

The next day squeeze the entire dandelion infused liquid out through a muslin cloth or clean tea towel into a jug and compost the petals, you should have about 250ml liquid.

Pour into a saucepan and add the jam sugar.

Slowly bring to the boil stirring to dissolve the sugar. Boil for 5 minutes or until it thickens slightly like runny honey.

Pour into sterilized jam jars, pop on the lid and label.

Allow to cool. Once open use within 1 month and keep refrigerated.

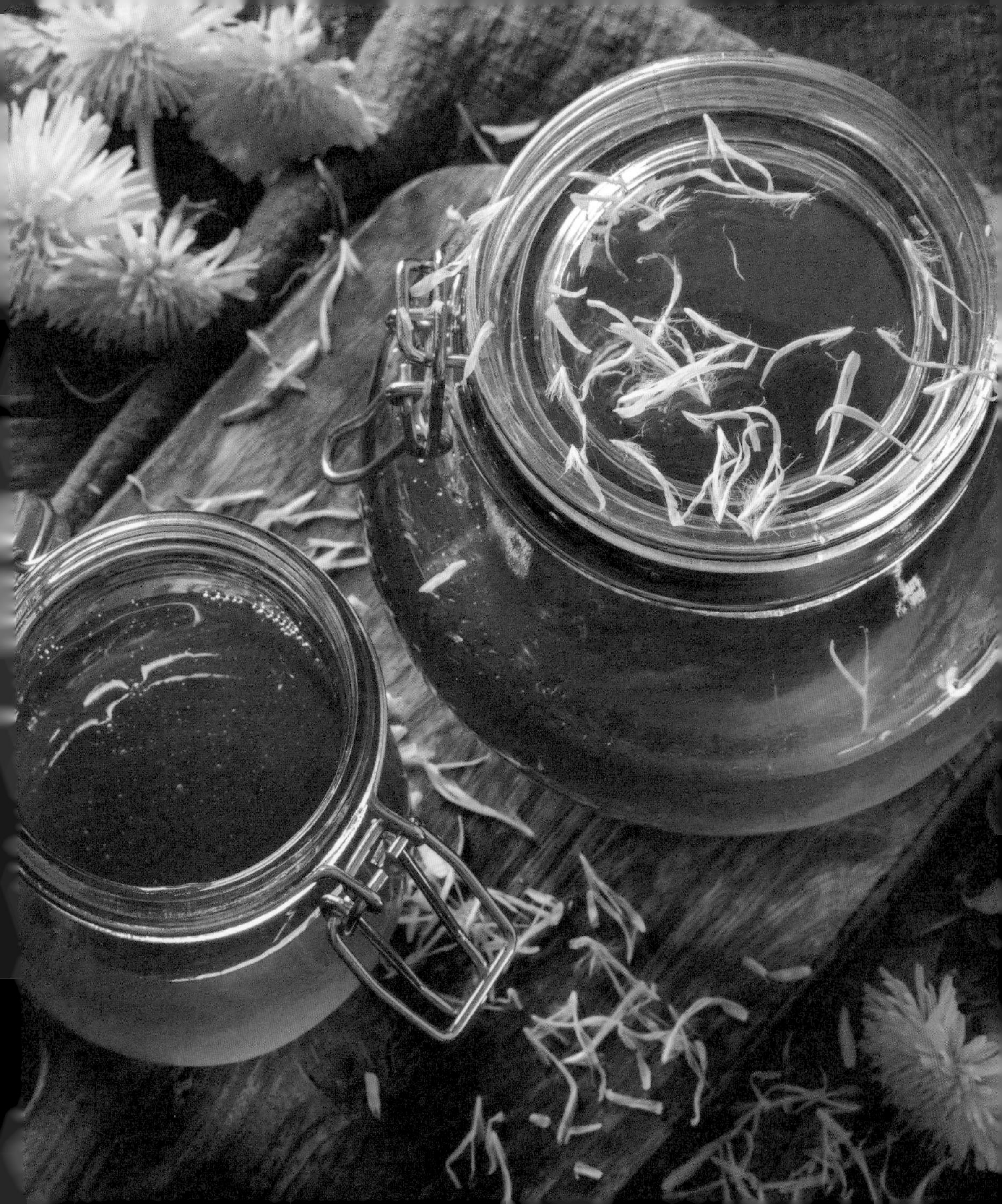

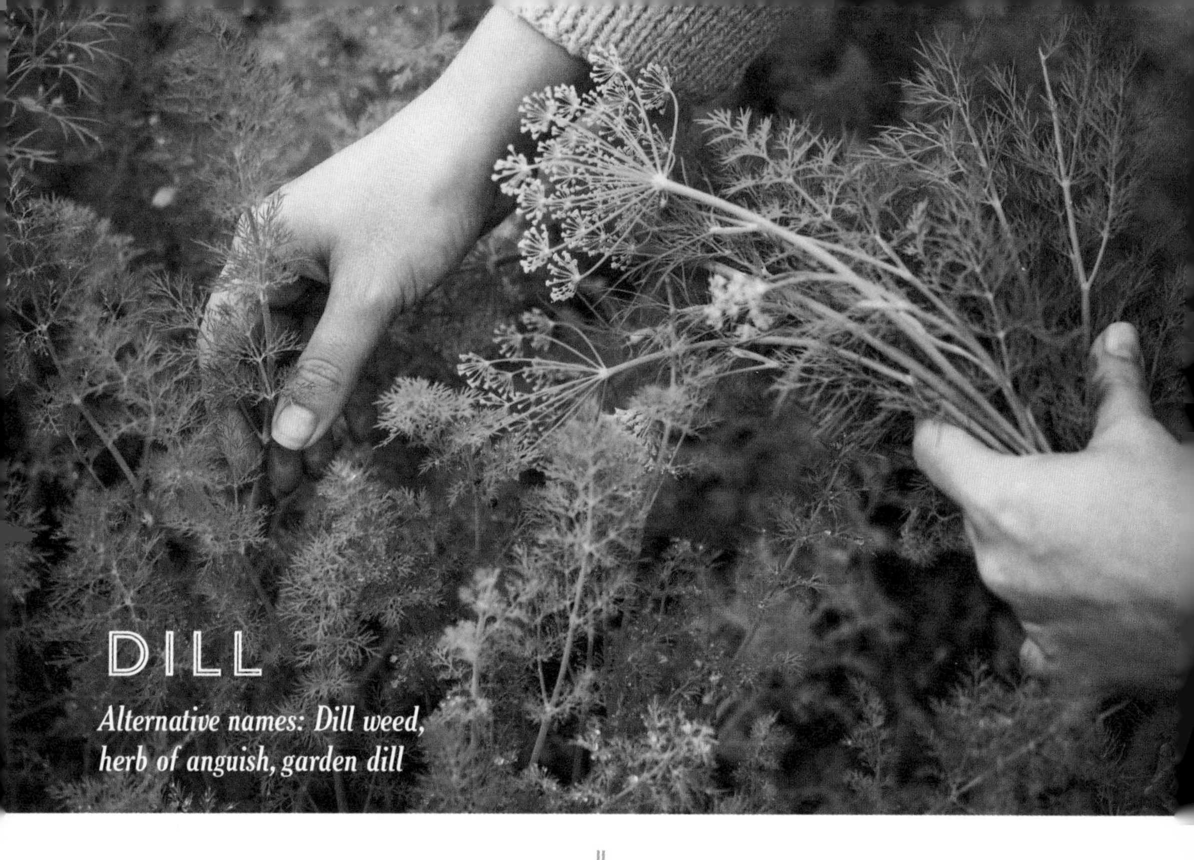

DILL

Alternative names: Dill weed, herb of anguish, garden dill

HOW TO IDENTIFY: Dill is very similar to fennel with feathery blue/green foliage, growing 70–80cm (28–31 inches) tall, with a caraway-like scent.

HISTORY: Ancient Egyptians employed dill to ward off witches as well as using it as an aphrodisiac. Described as "soothing medicine", dill was prescribed to ease tummy troubles. Evidence of its usage has been discovered in Egyptian tombs dating back over 5,000 years.

Roman gladiators rubbed their muscles with dill to ease inflammation and were fed meals containing dill in order to give them the courage to fight.

In the thirteenth century King Edward I imposed import duty on spices and herbs such as dill being shipped into London, in an effort to raise much-needed funds to repair a dilapidated London Bridge.

By the seventeenth century dill was widely grown in monastery and kitchen gardens.

FOLKLORE: Medieval Britons were very superstitious and believed in the power of plants and herbs to protect themselves and their families from supernatural forces. A bundle of dill hung in a doorway would stop witches from entering the house. If you were unfortunate enough to become bewitched a cup of dill tea would speedily remove the curse with the added bonus that it would cure flatulence too!

The seventeenth-century poet John Milton wrote:

"Here holy vervain and here dill,
Gainst witchcraft much availing."

Reinforced by his contemporary Michael Drayton:

"Therewith he vervain and her dill,
That hindreth witches of her will."

European monks believed that dill could reduce fertility and also that it had the power to chase off incubi (demons who preyed on sleeping women).

Brides who wanted to wear the trousers in the relationship would secretly bring dill and mustard seeds to the wedding and repeat:

"I have you mustard, and you dill,
Husband, when I speak, you stay still."

To ensure a favourable outcome should you ever find yourself in front of a judge, tuck a sprig of dill in your shoe. Placing it under the pillow will help to stop snoring and prevent nightmares.

FOLK MEDICINE: Culpeper wrote of dill: "*...and is used in medicines that serve to expel wind, and the pains proceeding therefrom. The seed being roasted or fried, and used in oils or plaisters, dissolve the imposthumes [absesses] in the fundament [bowel] and drieth up all moist ulcers, especially in the fundament.*"

Dill was used to ease colicky pains caused by wind in babies (gripe water still contains dill) and helped stimulate milk production in breastfeeding mothers.

OTHER COMMON USES: Fresh dill is used in many recipes to complement fish, salads, soups, potatoes and vegetable dishes.

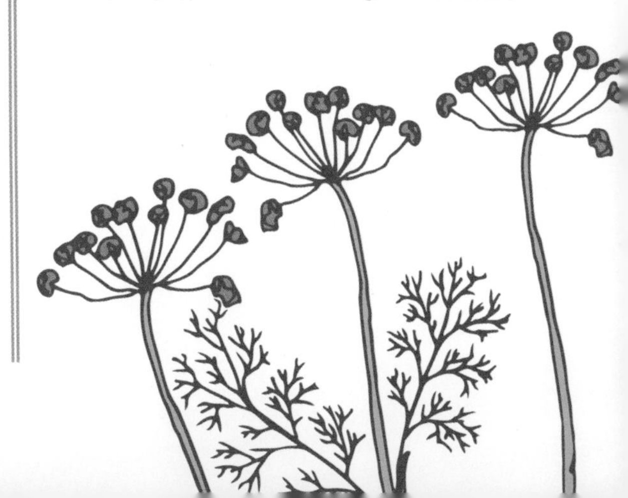

SALT, VINEGAR AND DILL CUCUMBERS

These quick pickled cucumbers are perfect to use up the glut of cucumbers that we all end up with from the veg patch. Pair it with fresh dill from the herb garden for a twist on the American favourite of dill pickles.

The secret to this recipe is giving the flavours time to muddle together, so prepare it at least 30 minutes in advance but ideally overnight.

Makes 6–8 servings

INGREDIENTS

1 large pesticide-free cucumber

50ml white wine vinegar

1 tbsp olive oil

1 tsp granulated sugar

1 tsp sea salt

Freshly ground black pepper

1½ tbsp fresh dill, chopped

METHOD

Thinly slice the cucumber.

Place the vinegar, olive oil, sugar, salt and a few grinds of pepper in a bowl and whisk together.

Add the dill and the sliced cucumber and toss to combine.

Cover and refrigerate for at least 30 minutes.

Keeps in the fridge for 2 to 3 days.

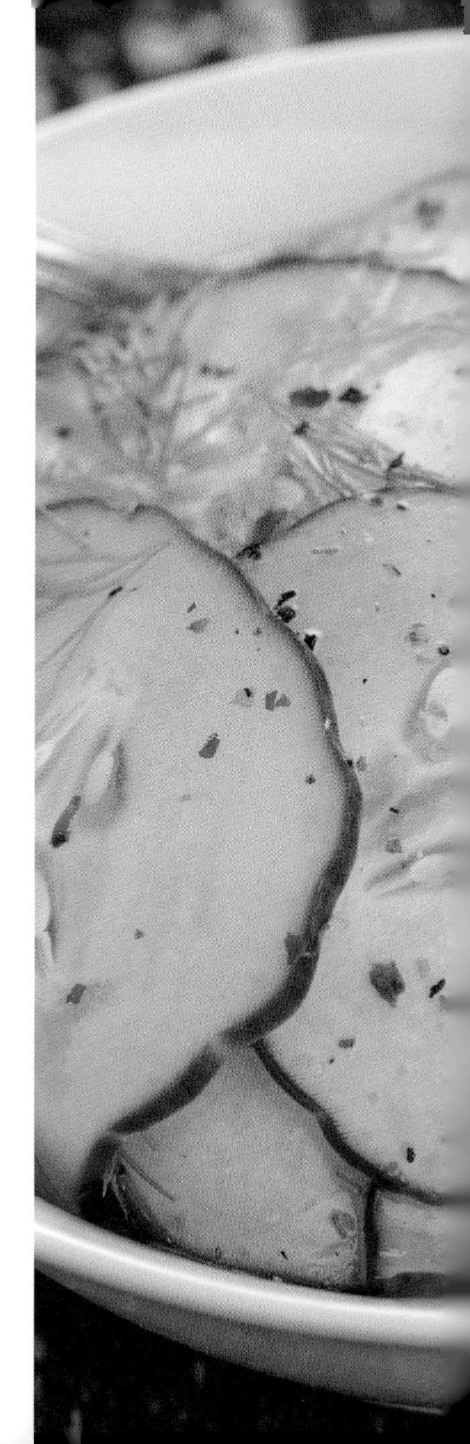

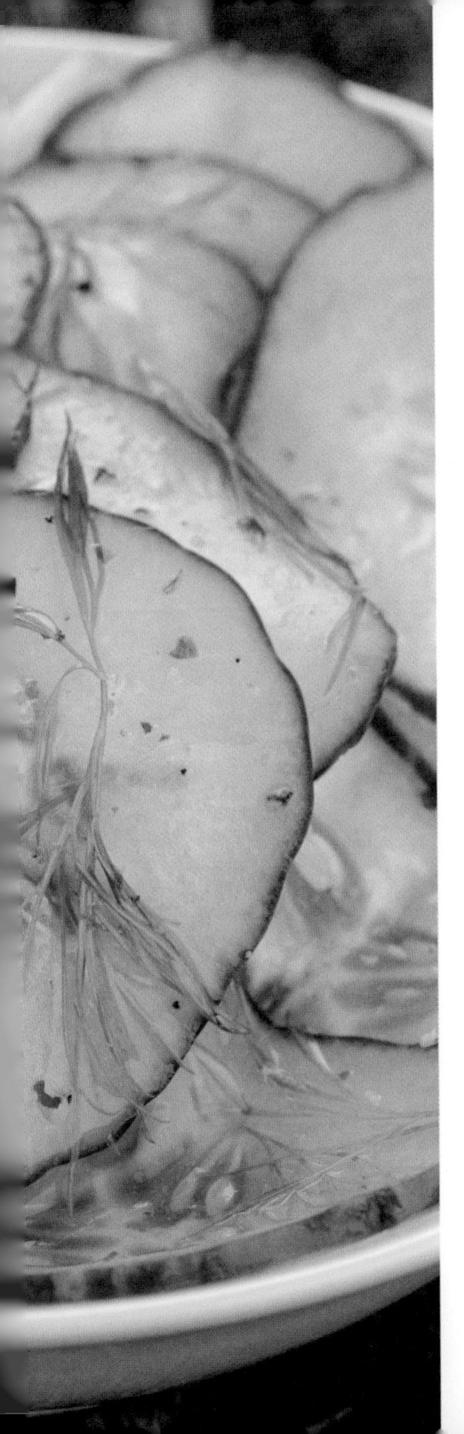

DILL SEED AND HORSETAIL NAIL BATH

Dill seeds are high in mineral salts, such as calcium, which is essential for healthy nails. Horsetail is jam-packed with silica for strong, healthy growth of hair and nails.

Makes 250ml

INGREDIENTS

2 tbsp crushed dill seeds

2 tbsp dried or fresh horsetail chopped

250ml water

METHOD

Boil the herbs in the water until the volume is reduced by half.

Allow to cool to blood heat.

Soak nails in this warm solution for 10–15 minutes three times a week.

Strain any remaining liquid and keep it in the fridge warming it as needed.

Make a fresh solution every week until nails feel stronger.

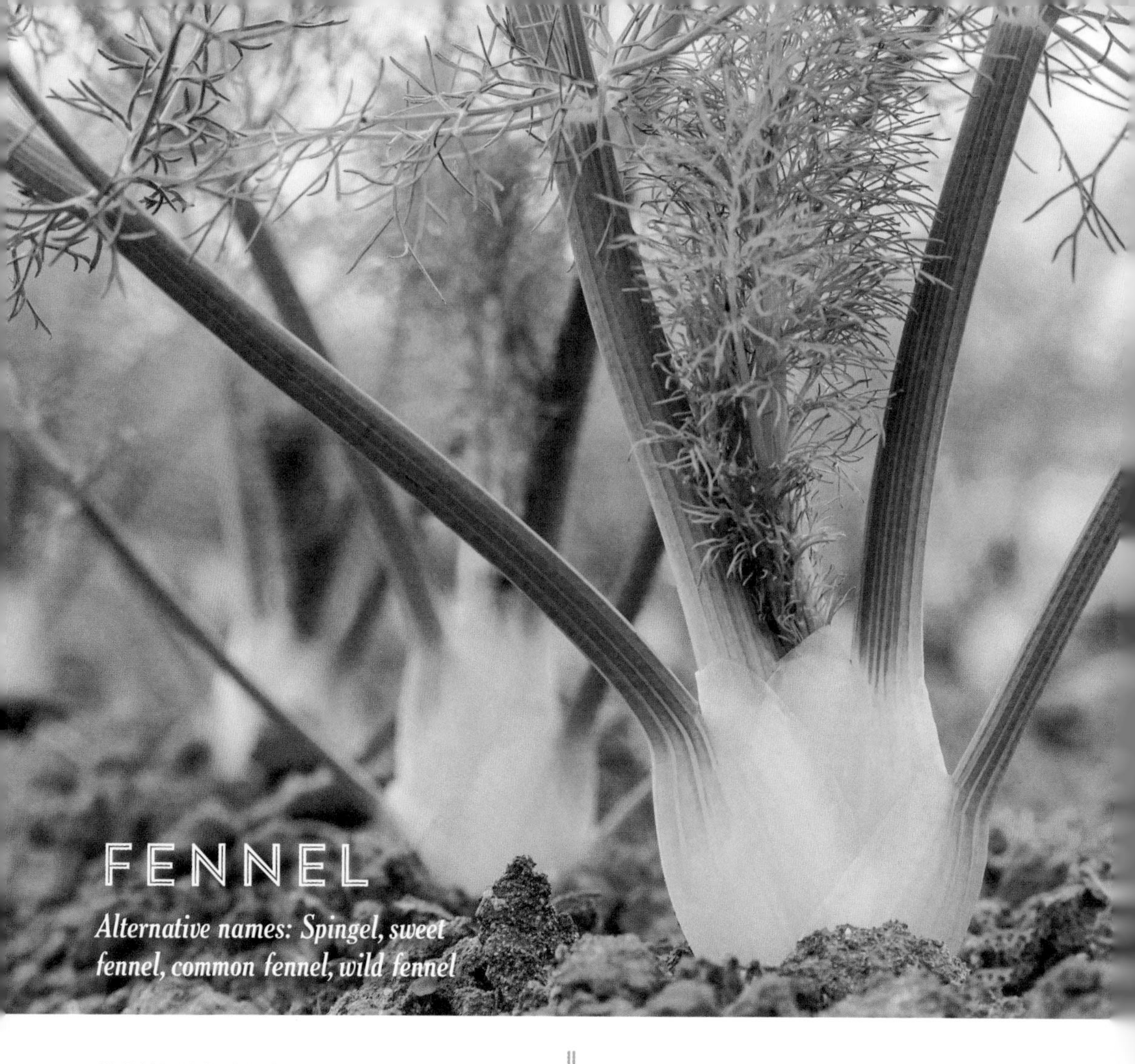

FENNEL

Alternative names: Spingel, sweet fennel, common fennel, wild fennel

HOW TO IDENTIFY: Fennel is a tall, ornamental culinary herb of the carrot family with aromatic seeds, yellow flowers and long feathery leaves.

HISTORY: Infant colic was treated with fennel tea as early as the third century BC. Twenty-first-century babies are still given gripe water containing fennel to ease trapped wind.

Sixteenth-century puritans referred to fennel seeds as "Meeting House seeds" as they were chewed to help stave off hunger and keep children quiet during very long sermons – probably the most fun that the puritans allowed themselves to have!

Fennel has insect-repelling properties and was tucked into horses' bridles to keep flies away and used in dog kennels to deter fleas.

FOLKLORE: Fennel and St John's wort were hung around windows and doors at Midsummer as protection against witches. As an extra precaution, some fennel seeds were put into the keyholes to prevent ghosts from entering, too.

Fennel paste was rubbed into cows' udders in an attempt to protect their milk from being bewitched.

FOLK MEDICINE: The Greeks and Romans drank fennel tea in the belief that it would help them lose weight. Fennel tea was also later prescribed by William Cole, the herbalist, who recommended it "*for those that are grown fat, to abate their unwieldiness and cause them to grow more gaunt and lank.*"

Culpeper says that: "*the leaves or seed, boiled in barley water and drank, are good for nurses, to increase their milk, and make it more wholesome for the child.*" If you were unfortunate enough to have been bitten by a snake or eaten something you shouldn't: "*the seed boiled in wine and drank, is good for those that are bit with serpents, or have eat poisonous herbs or mushrooms.*"

OTHER COMMON USES: As well as still being used in modern remedies for their anti-inflammatory, anti-fungal and antibacterial properties, fennel seeds are found in chorizo, toothpaste and used as flavouring in absinthe.

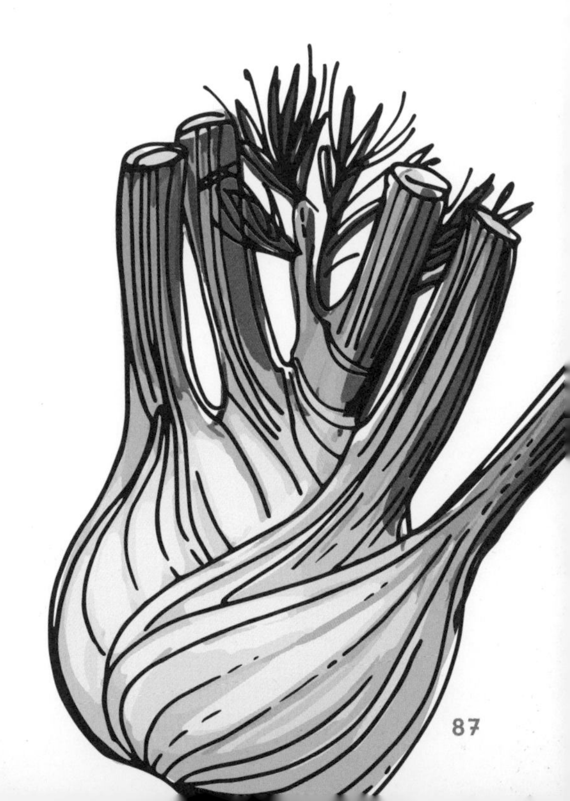

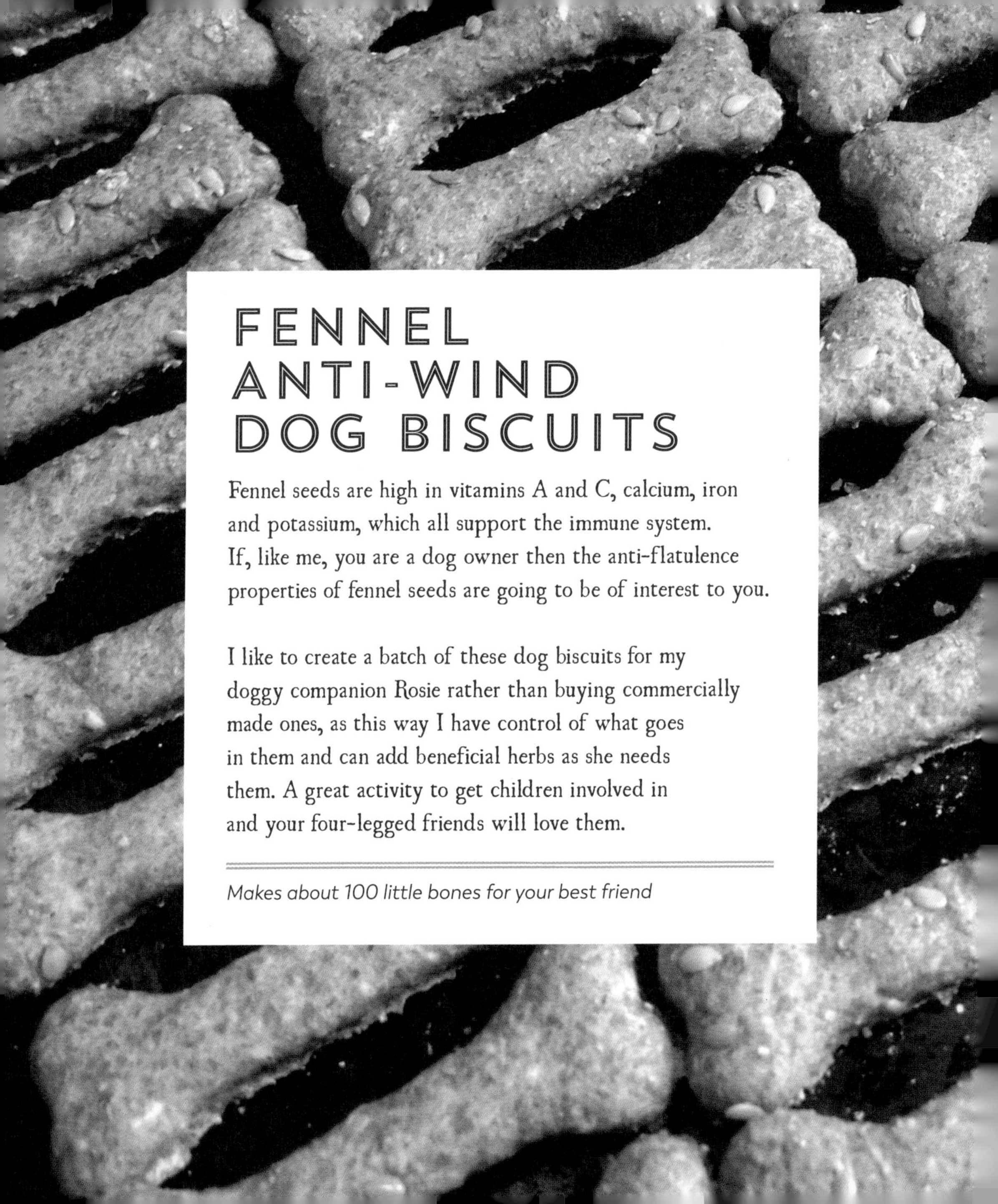

FENNEL ANTI-WIND DOG BISCUITS

Fennel seeds are high in vitamins A and C, calcium, iron and potassium, which all support the immune system. If, like me, you are a dog owner then the anti-flatulence properties of fennel seeds are going to be of interest to you.

I like to create a batch of these dog biscuits for my doggy companion Rosie rather than buying commercially made ones, as this way I have control of what goes in them and can add beneficial herbs as she needs them. A great activity to get children involved in and your four-legged friends will love them.

Makes about 100 little bones for your best friend

INGREDIENTS

400g wholemeal flour (I get this from my local flour mill)

1 large free-range egg, beaten

2 handfuls of porridge oats

6 tbsp vegetable oil

200ml stock made with ½ a low salt stock cube, cooled

1 tbsp crushed fennel seeds*

Equipment needed

Bone-shaped cookie cutter

METHOD

Heat oven to 200°C (400°F).

Mix all ingredients until they come together to form a stiff dough, add more water if necessary.

Dust a clean worktop with flour and roll out the dough to about ½cm thick.

Cut out small shapes – bone-shaped cutters are fun and available online. Place the shapes on a baking tray dusted with flour.

Bake for 20–25 minutes or until the biscuits are golden brown and feel quite dry. Allow to cool on the tray.

Store in an airtight tin, where they will keep crunchy for a couple of months.

*You can add different herbs to the basic dough mixture. Here are some ideas:

- 1 tbsp dried mint and 1 tbsp dried parsley for fresh breath
- 1 tsp ginger powder for motion sickness
- 1 tbsp powdered linseeds for skin problems
- 1 tbsp oregano for upset tummies

FENNEL TEA WITH GINGER, CAMOMILE AND PEPPERMINT

We've all had those days when we feel sluggish and bloated; fennel is packed with fibre and anti-inflammatory properties that will soothe a sore tummy. Ginger aids digestion, calms nausea, is antioxidant and anti-inflammatory. Camomile relaxes the muscle spasms that cause pain and peppermint helps to ease the gas in the bowel.

Makes enough for two cups

INGREDIENTS

1 tbsp crushed fennel seeds

2 tbsp fresh peppermint leaves chopped, or 1 tbsp dried

4 camomile flowers

Thumb-sized piece of fresh ginger, peeled and sliced

500ml boiling water

Honey or maple syrup to sweeten, if needed

METHOD

Put all the ingredients except the honey in a teapot or jug.

Cover and allow to infuse for 10 minutes.

Strain, sweeten with honey if using.

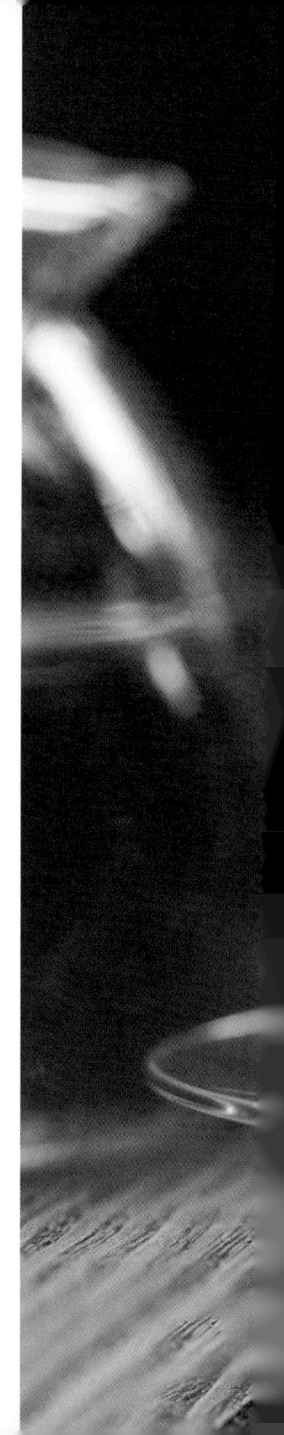

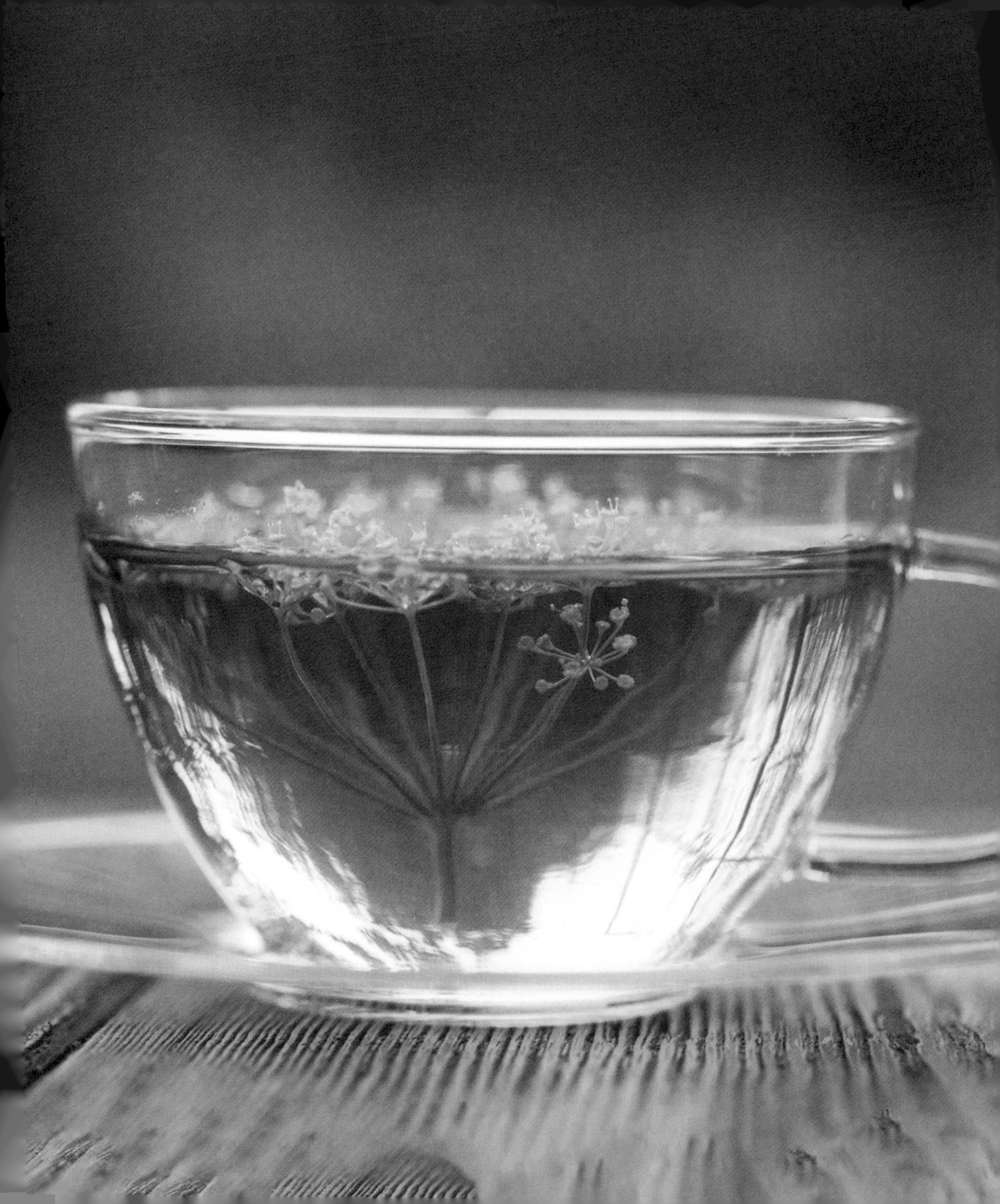

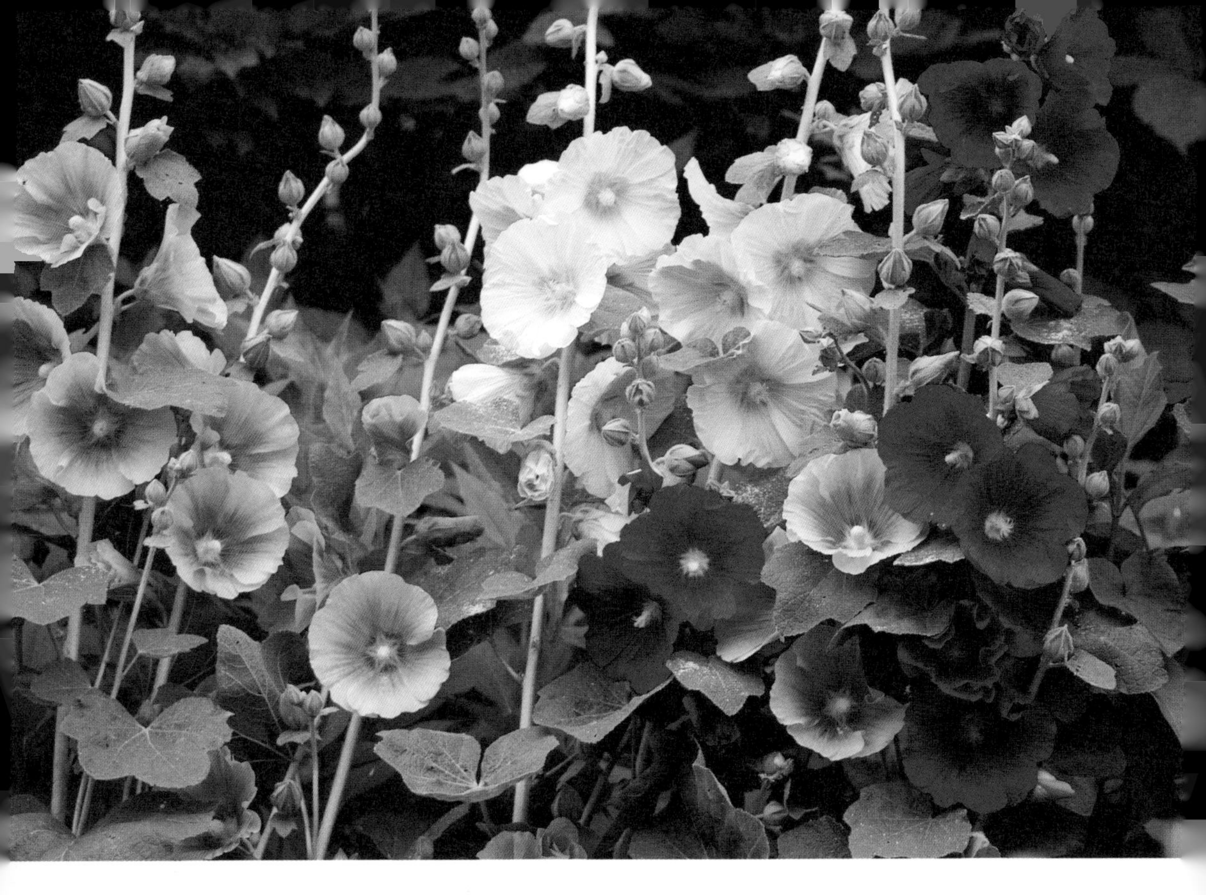

HOLLYHOCK

Alternative names: Rose de mer, malva benedicta, rose papale

HOW TO IDENTIFY: Growing to over 2 metres (6½ feet) in height with colourful blousy flowers along its stem, hollyhocks have long been a cottage garden favourite.

HISTORY: Originally thought to have come from Asia, hollyhocks spread to the Middle East where English crusaders used their medicinal properties to treat injured horses.

The name is derived from "Holy", as in Holy Land, and "hock" from being used to treat horses' hocks.

In Wales in the nineteenth century, fibre from the stalks was used in the manufacture of cloth and the petals made into a blue or green dye.

In Victorian England, tall hollyhocks were grown to obscure the privy, thus saving the blushes of genteel ladies who didn't need to ask where it was – they just looked for the hollyhocks.

FOLKLORE: Faeries use the beautiful blooms as skirts but to be able to see them wearing these, mortals should drink a tea of hollyhock, wild thyme, calendula and hazel buds.

A seventeenth-century recipe for faery salve using hollyhock buds rubbed "*under the eyelids and on the eyelids evening and morning*" will make a faery called Eleby Gathon appear in a glass "*meekly and mildly to resolve him of all manner of questions and to be obedient to all his commands under pain of damnation.*"

FOLK MEDICINE: Culpeper recommended that hollyhock leaves were boiled to make a poultice to cure inflammation and as a gargle for "*swelling of the tonsils*" and that "*it is also of efficacy in the spongy state of the gums, attended with looseness of the teeth and soreness of the mouth.*"

The sixteenth-century herbalist John Gerard tells us that "*the decoction of the floures, especially those of the red, does stop the overmuch flowing of the monthely courses, if they be boiled in red wine.*"

OTHER COMMON USES: Hollyhocks are worth planting just for the fact that they look stunning and their multitudes of flowers are much needed by our native pollinators.

HOLLYHOCK AND THYME COUGH LINCTUS

Hollyhock is a member of the mallow family, which is known for its ability to soothe mucous membranes and ease dry coughs. Thyme is antiseptic, anti-viral, antibacterial, an expectorant and eases congestion. Hollyhocks bloom throughout the summer so it's worth remembering to gather some flowers from the garden to make this in readiness for the onset of autumn coughs.

Makes approximately 300ml

INGREDIENTS

About 20 fresh double bloom hollyhock flowers or 40 single ones

2 tbsp fresh thyme, chopped (try to use young soft stems)

Sugar to cover, around 400g

Equipment needed

Clean and sterilized wide-mouthed jar

Fine sieve or muslin

Measuring jug

Clean and sterilized glass bottle or jar

Brandy, 15ml to each 100ml of resulting syrup

METHOD

Lightly bruise the hollyhock flowers and thyme with a pestle or rolling pin to release their juices.

Put a layer of flowers and thyme in the bottom of the jar and cover with a layer of sugar.

Carry on layering in this way until you have used up all your flowers and thyme, top with a final layer of sugar.

Leave the jar in a warm place until most of the sugar has turned to syrup. This could take up to 4 weeks.

Strain the syrup through a fine sieve or muslin into a measuring jug.

For every 100ml of syrup add 15ml of brandy – this will help to preserve it.

Stir well and pour into a sterilized glass bottle and keep in the fridge.

Take two tablespoons as needed, though not suitable for children due to the alcohol content.

Keeps unopened for about six months. Once opened use within a month.

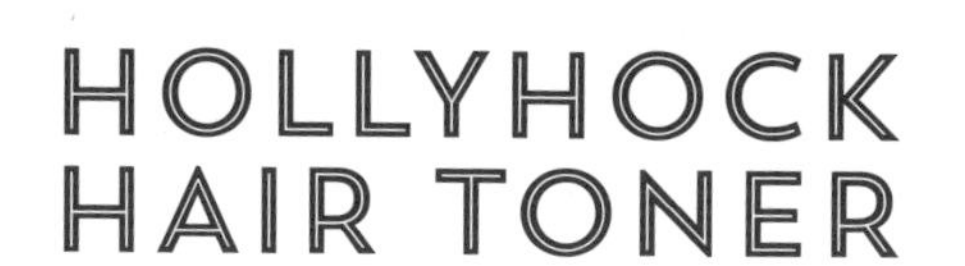

HOLLYHOCK HAIR TONER

If you colour your hair either at home or at the hairdressers, you might find some unwanted brassy tones coming through after a while. Purple hollyhock flowers contain a natural dye that can cancel out these tones, plus the apple cider vinegar is antimicrobial to ease scalp conditions and also adds shine as well as helping to fade yellow tones.

Makes enough for one application, depending on length of hair

INGREDIENTS

2 tbsp fresh purple hollyhock flowers, chopped

2 tbsp apple cider vinegar (see page 34)

250ml water

Equipment needed

Fine sieve

METHOD

In a saucepan boil up the flowers, vinegar and water for about 15–20 minutes until it turns into a thick liquid. Allow to cool completely.

Strain the liquid then apply all over the hair from root to tip.

Leave for 15 minutes, shampoo, rinse and condition as normal.

Always do a strand test before applying this toner.

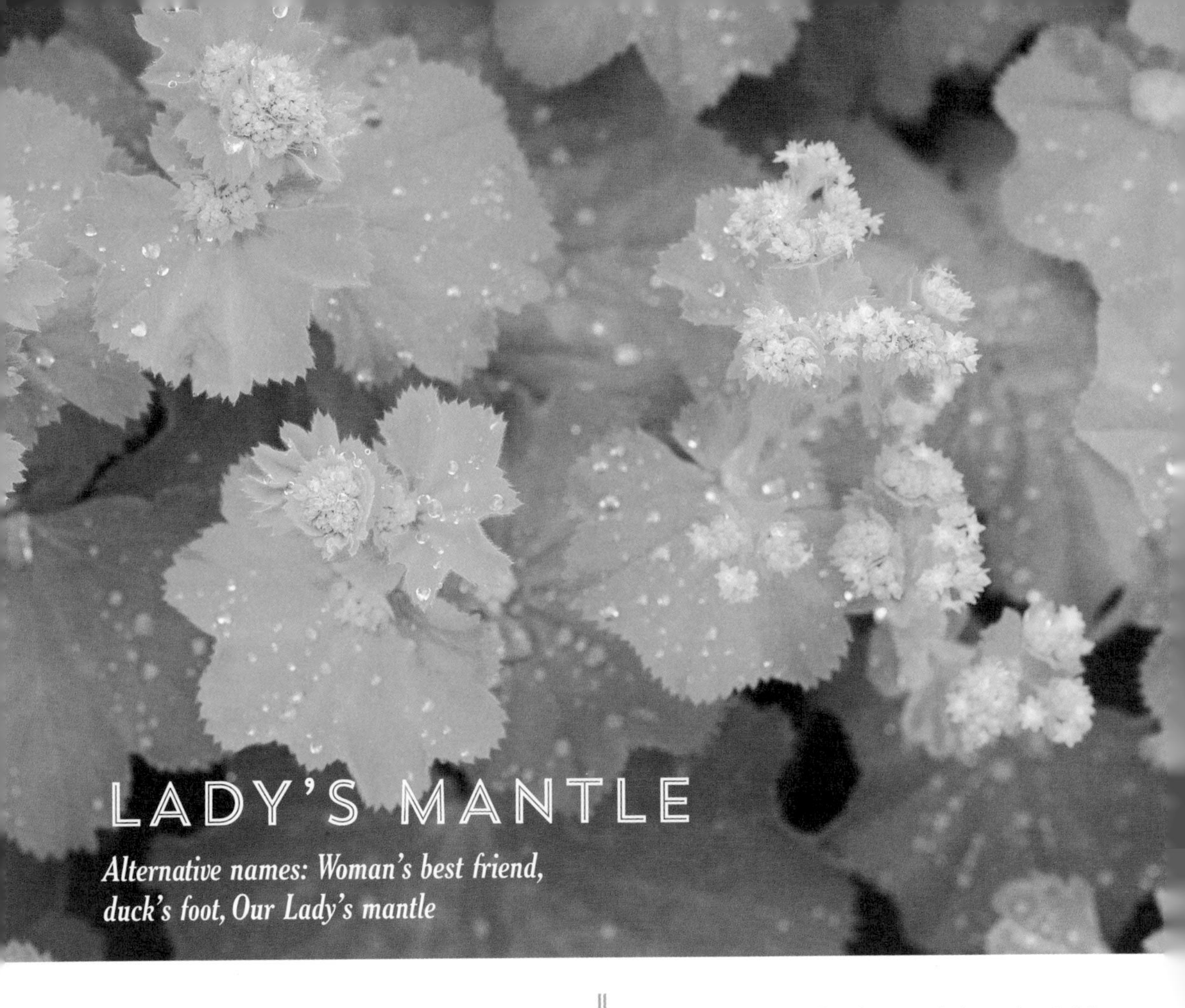

LADY'S MANTLE

Alternative names: Woman's best friend, duck's foot, Our Lady's mantle

HOW TO IDENTIFY: Lady's mantle grows 30–40cm (12–16 inches) tall with neatly pleated jagged leaves and frothy lime green summer flowers.

HISTORY: Native to southern Europe and also known as *Alchemilla vulgaris*, it wasn't until the sixteenth century when botanist Jerome Bock noted that the folds in the leaves resembled the cloak of the Virgin Mary that he named the plant "Our Lady's mantle".

FOLKLORE: Venture out into the garden early to collect the magical silver droplets that emerge from the leaves of lady's mantle. Not only will it restore your youthful beauty "no matter how faded" it will increase your fertility and libido too!

Alchemists thought this powerful "moon water" could help them create the mythical "philosopher's stone", which they believed held the secret of eternal life and was able to transform base metals into gold.

FOLK MEDICINE: Definitely a herb for the ladies according to Culpeper: "*...and such women as have large breasts, causing them to grow less and hard, being both drank and outwardly applied.*"

If you need more evidence the eighteenth-century botanist Sir John Hill tells us that: "*The good women in the north of England apply the leaves to their breasts, to make them recover their form, after they have been swelled with milk.*"

Lady's mantle was also a popular remedy for heavy menstrual bleeding and feminine itching and so effective was it at healing wounds that it could even restore a maiden's virginity!

Culpeper also told women wishing to become pregnant: "*the distilled water drank for 20 days together helps conception and to retain the birth; if the women do sometimes also sit in a bath made of the decoction of the herb.*"

OTHER COMMON USES: Poultices of the young leaves can be made for minor cuts. Mash some leaves and place under a plaster overnight to really help those garden injuries that our hands suffer regularly.

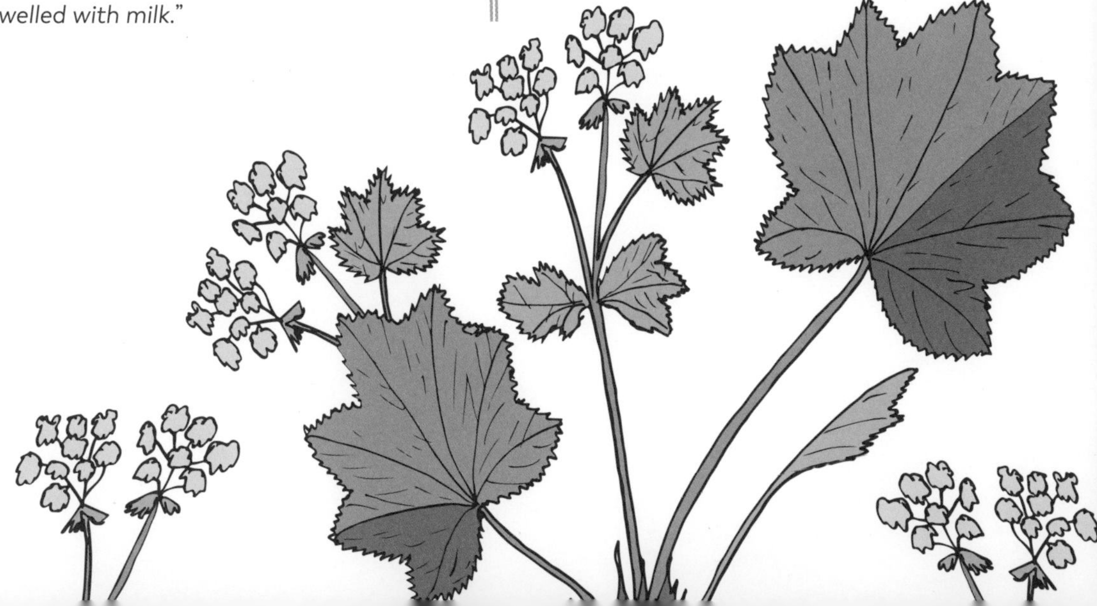

LADY'S MANTLE BREAST BOOSTER

Best done at bath time when you won't get disturbed.

INGREDIENTS

100g lady's mantle leaves and flowers (even better if they have the magical dew on them)

300ml freshly boiled water

Equipment needed

Heatproof bowl

2 flannels or cotton muslins

Clean and sterilized jam jar

METHOD

Place the leaves and flowers in the bowl, pour on the boiled water.

Leave to infuse for 10 minutes and allow to cool. Pop it into the fridge if you're feeling brave.

Soak the flannels in the cold liquid, wring out and place one over each breast.

Lie back and relax for 20 minutes. Repeat daily.

Pour the remaining liquid into a jam jar and keep in the fridge. Keeps for 1 month.

ANTI-ITCH HERBAL BATH TEA

Herbal bath bags can help to clear the skin and re-invigorate the mind and body. Lady's mantle can be used to treat intimate infections and calm eczema and skin rashes as well as speeding up the healing of minor cuts. Calendula is my go-to remedy to soothe irritated skin. Marshmallow root is anti-inflammatory to ease itching, and oats are antioxidant and anti-inflammatory. Add a glug of your homemade apple cider vinegar (see page 34) for its antibacterial properties and you have a lovely healing bath tea.

INGREDIENTS

1 large lady's mantle leaf and flowers

2 calendula flowers

1 tbsp dried marshmallow root

2 tbsp organic oats

Equipment needed

Small cotton drawstring bag

METHOD

Tear up the lady's mantle leaf and flowers, and mix together with the other ingredients.

Fill the drawstring bag and secure tightly.

As you are running a bath tie the bag underneath the hot tap so that the water runs through it.

Pop it in the bath with you squeezing it out several times to release the tea.

Once finished compost the contents and rinse out the bag to use again.

Other bath tea ideas:

For colds: Thyme, lavender and a thumb-sized piece of fresh ginger, grated.

For relaxation: Lemon verbena, lavender, peppermint and camomile.

For aching muscles: 2 tbsp Epsom salts, peppermint, camomile, rosemary, bay.

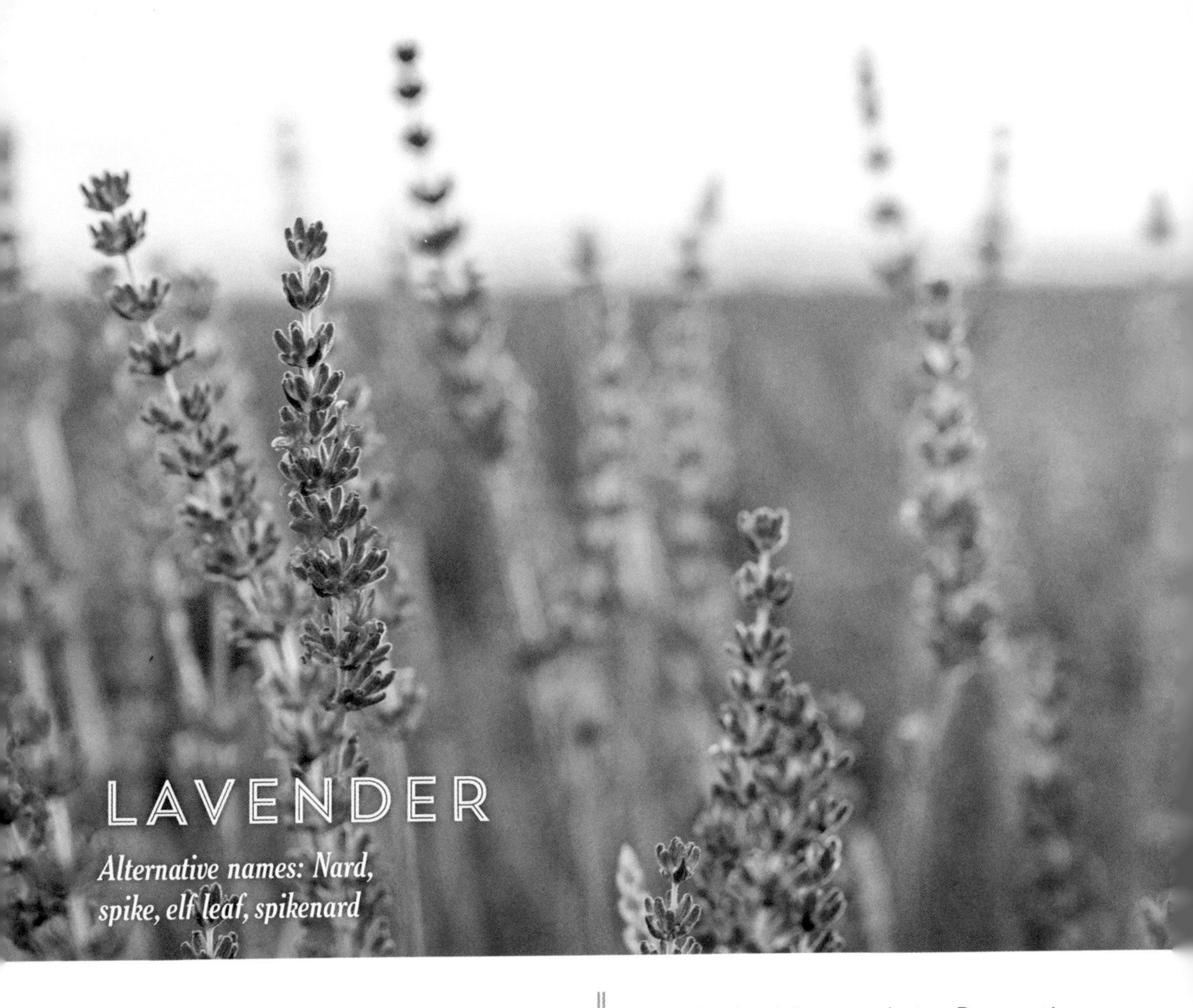

LAVENDER

Alternative names: Nard, spike, elf leaf, spikenard

HOW TO IDENTIFY: Delicate purple lavender flowers sit on top of long skinny stems with characteristic camphor-like scent.

HISTORY: Still-fragrant lavender was found in the tomb of Tutankhamen and it is believed that Cleopatra used the heady scent of lavender to help her seduce Mark Antony.

Used in bath houses during Roman times, *lavare* comes from the Latin meaning "to wash". Lavender gave the bathwater a lovely perfume and helped to restore the skin. The Romans introduced lavender to Britain to ward off the nits and fleas that they discovered were prolific amongst the native population.

FOLKLORE: A bedtime drink of lavender tea on St Luke's Day (18 October) while reciting this charm – "*St Luke, St Luke be kind to me, in my dreams, let me my true love see*" – will reveal a future husband.

Adding lavender to the bathwater of bewitched children will drive out their demons. Hanging lavender above your doorway or burning an incense of lavender, frankincense, basil, rue and lemon balm will protect your home from further unwanted visitors.

Not that long ago, ladies wore small lavender pouches in their cleavage to attract suitors. The lyrics of a well-known lullaby illustrate this:

"Lavender's green dilly dilly,
Lavender's blue,
You must love me, dilly dilly,
'cause I love you."

FOLK MEDICINE: A herb of very many uses, Culpeper recommends:

"A decoction made with the flowers of lavender, hore hound, fennel and asparagus root, and a little cinnamon, is very profitable used to help the falling sickness [epilepsy] and the giddiness or turning of the brain: to gargle the mouth with the decoction thereof is good against the toothache."

Lavender oil was massaged into paralyzed limbs to stimulate movement while oleumspicoe, made by mixing lavender oil with turpentine, was massaged into stiff joints and sprains.

OTHER COMMON USES: Lavender is a well-known aid to restful sleep and can be found in many skin care products for its anti-inflammatory and antibacterial properties that calm and heal acne and eczema.

Use it sparingly in biscuits and cakes – too much will taste soapy – and always buy organic or grow your own to ensure that no pesticides have been used.

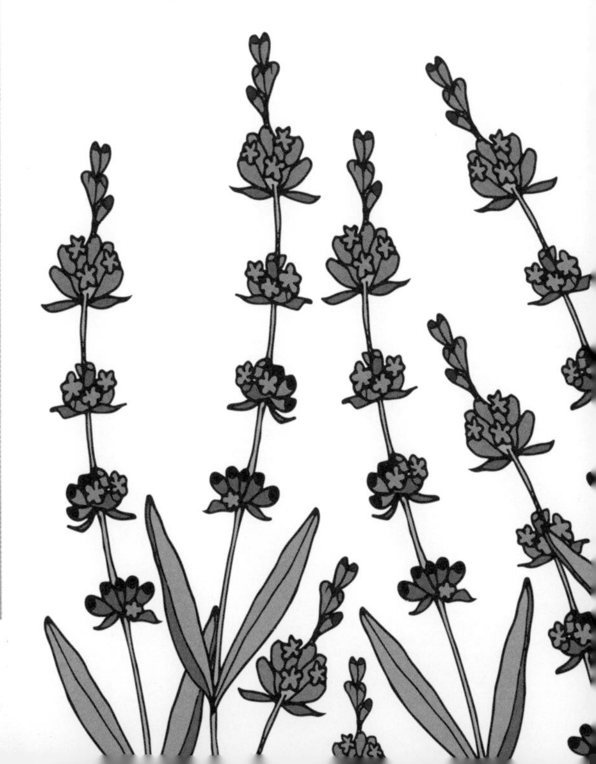

FOUR THIEVES VINEGAR

One of my favourite folkloric tales is that of the Four Thieves who were infamous for stealing from corpses in plague-ridden France during the fourteenth century. They went from infected house to infected house, stealing from the dead and poor souls infected by the plague, yet never becoming ill themselves!

Eventually the authorities caught up with them but promised them leniency if they would share their secret. What they revealed was a concoction of anti-viral and antibacterial herbs that they infused into vinegar; they soaked this into a sponge and wore it in a mask to protect them from the plague.

There are many versions of this online and in books, but as long as you use herbs that have antibacterial and anti-viral properties you can really make it your own.

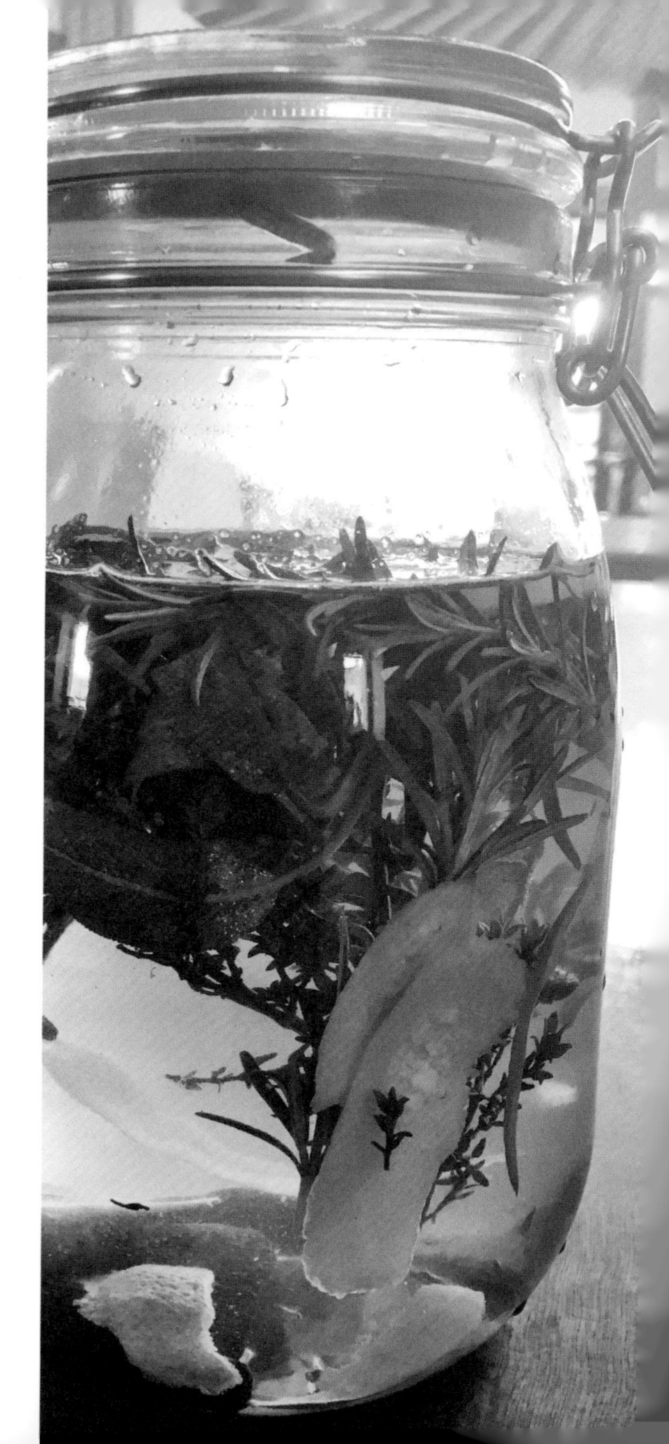

Don't worry if you don't have access to fresh herbs, dried ones will work just as well, but change the quantities to teaspoons instead of tablespoons.

Makes 1 litre

INGREDIENTS

2 tbsp fresh lavender flowers

2 tbsp fresh rosemary

2 tbsp fresh mint

2 tbsp fresh sage

2 tbsp fresh lemon balm

2 tbsp fresh thyme

10 black peppercorns

4 cloves of garlic

1 litre white wine vinegar

Equipment needed

Large clean and sterilized glass jar

Muslin or clean tea towel

Sterilized glass bottles

Spray bottle

METHOD

Chop all the herbs, crush the garlic and peppercorns and put into a large jar that has a non-metallic lid (the vinegar will rust a metal lid).

Gently warm the vinegar in a saucepan, don't let it boil.

Pour the warmed vinegar over the herbs and stir well.

Pop on the lid and place the jar in a cool, dark place for at least four weeks shaking as often as you can remember.

At the end of this time strain your Four Thieves vinegar through a clean tea towel or muslin squeezing the herbs to release as much vinegar into a jug as possible.

Compost the herbs and store the vinegar in sterilized glass bottles. Remember to label the bottles and keep them in a cool dark place.

Four Thieves vinegar can be decanted into a spray bottle for use as a natural cleanser and disinfectant in bathrooms and on kitchen worktops and if you spray it on your doorstep it will keep your enemies away!

Will keep for a couple of years.

LAVENDER LOTION BAR

I recently discovered body lotion bars and now I'm totally obsessed with their convenience, versatility and how beautiful they can be made to look.

Always buy organic ingredients if at all possible as anything that you put onto your skin will be absorbed into your body – we deserve the best. This lavender lotion bar will melt when rubbed over your arms and legs and is especially useful on dry and cracked heels and elbows. There are some gorgeous moulds available online that really turn these bars into something special – pop them into a tin for a lovely natural homemade gift.

Makes approximately 120ml

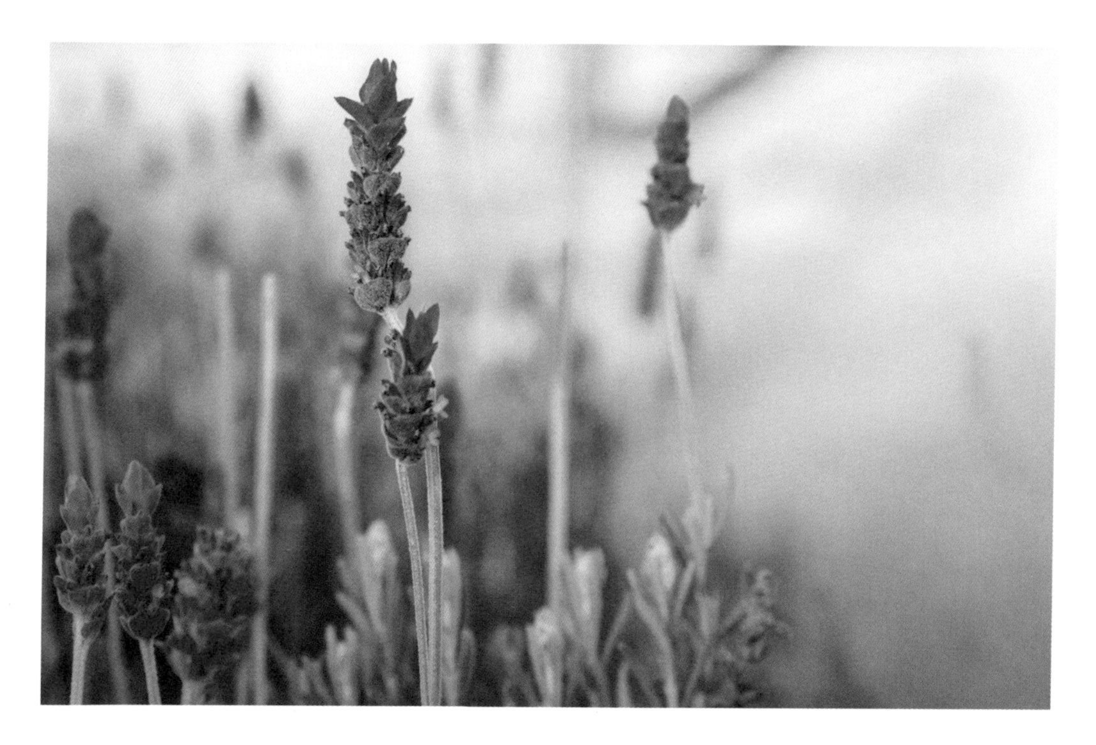

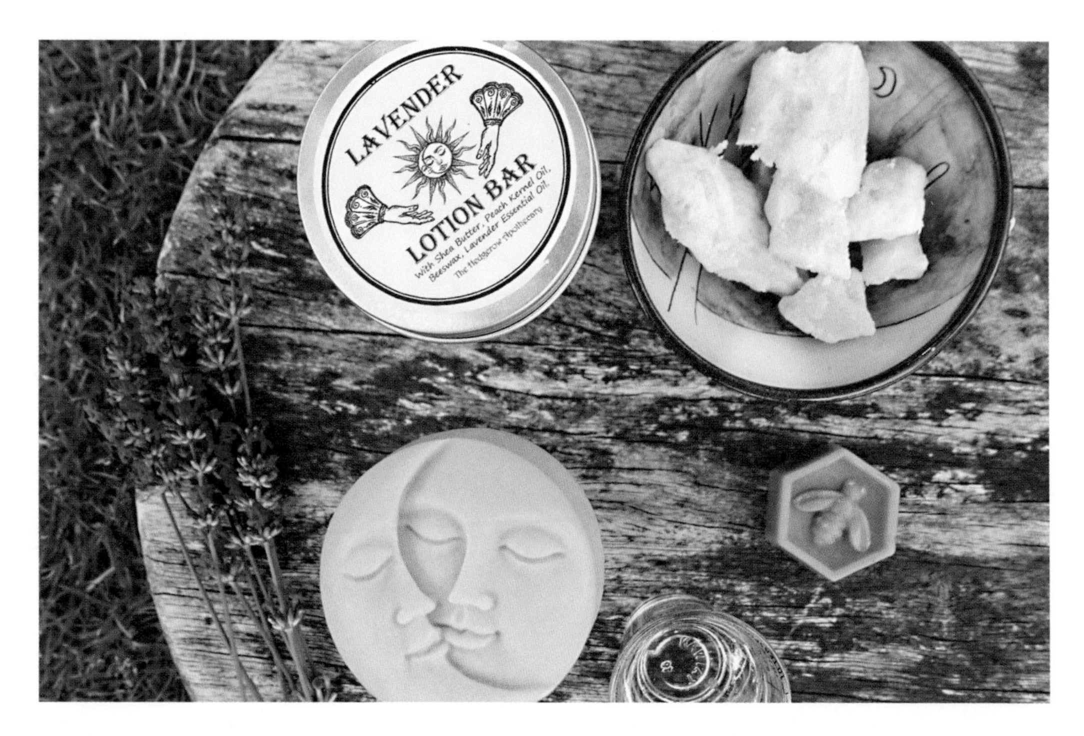

INGREDIENTS

35g organic shea butter

35ml lavender infused carrier oil

45g unrefined beeswax (I source mine from a local beekeeper)

20 drops organic lavender essential oil

Equipment needed

Heatproof bowl

Silicone moulds

METHOD

Melt the beeswax, shea butter and carrier oil in a heatproof bowl placed over a pan of boiling water.

Once melted, take the mixture off the heat, combine and stir in the essential oil, trying not to create any bubbles.

Pour into silicone moulds if you have them, or you can use cupcake cases or any small flexible containers that you have around the kitchen.

Allow to cool completely before popping out of the mould.

Will last for about a year if kept in the fridge.

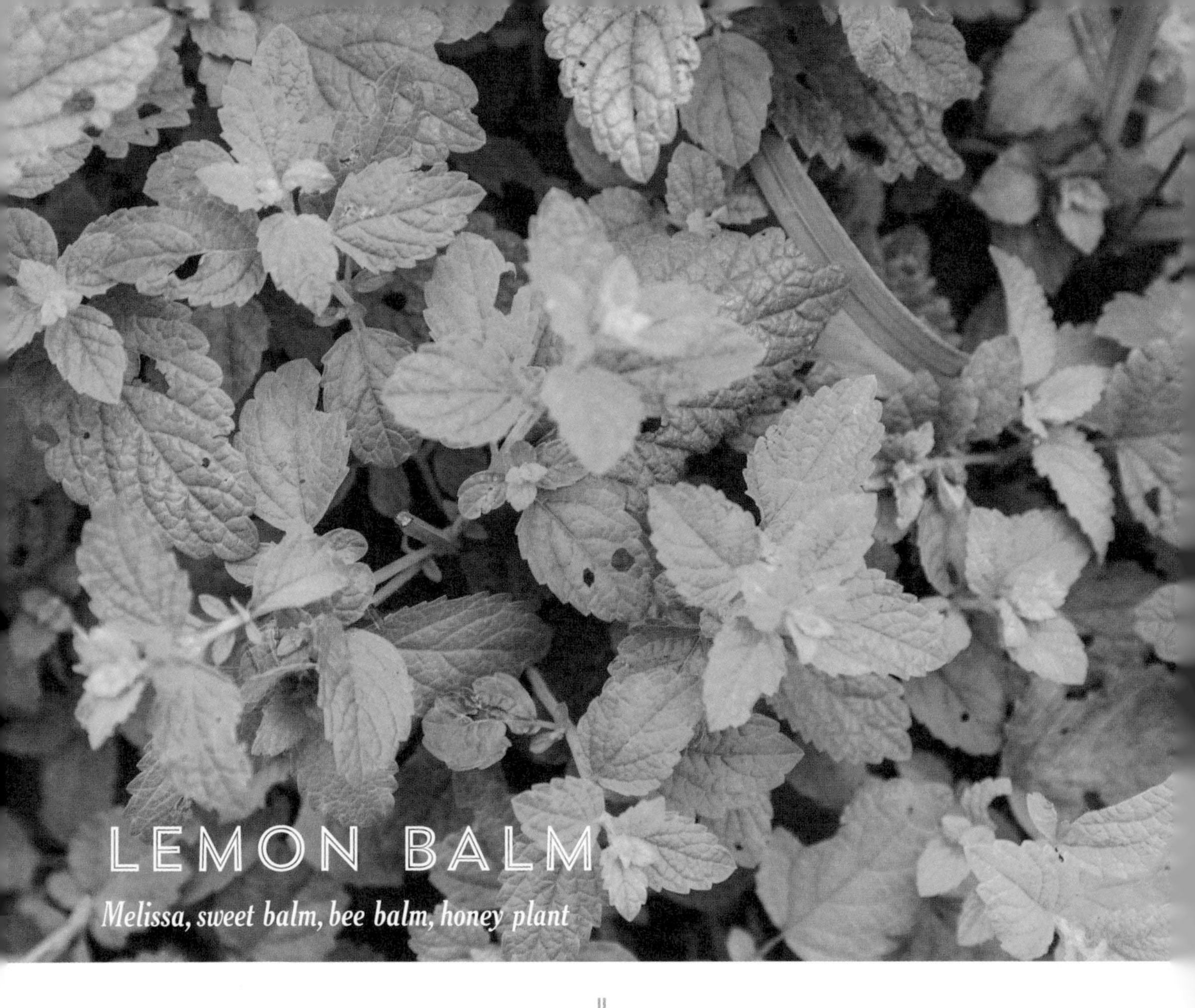

LEMON BALM

Melissa, sweet balm, bee balm, honey plant

HOW TO IDENTIFY: Lemon balm is a characteristically square-stemmed member of the mint family. Run your hands through this herb and you'll get a sharp lemony scent that makes it easily recognizable. Growing to 80 cm (31 inches) it is tall and bushy, and once you have lemon balm in your garden you have it for life.

HISTORY: Lemon balm was planted near beehives in Ancient Turkey and around the Greek temple of Artemis to keep the sacred honeybees happy and to discourage them from swarming.

It was brought to Europe via the Spanish trade routes, where it made its way to monastery gardens to be used medicinally.

According to *The London Dispensary* in 1696 lemon balm was claimed to "*renew youth, strengthen the brain and reduce baldness*" as well as being able to "*revivify a man*".

FOLKLORE: The Knights Templar tied a sprig of lemon balm onto the handle of their swords in the belief that it would heal any wounds that they suffered during battle.

Carry a sprig of lemon balm around with you and you will attract love. If that fails a potent love potion can be made by soaking the herb in wine and sharing it with your prospective partner.

FOLK MEDICINE: In the Middle Ages lemon balm was used among other things as a treatment for a rabid dog bite, for boils and skin eruptions, as a cure for baldness and for easing the pain of toothache.

Nicholas Culpeper, the seventeenth-century herbalist, recommends the use of lemon balm for "*weak stomachs, to cause the heart to become merry, to help digestion, to open obstructions of the brain, and to expel melancholy vapours from the heart and arteries.*"

As the twentieth-century herbalist Maud Grieve tells us in her book *A Modern Herbal* lemon balm steeped in wine "*comforts the heart and drives away melancholy and sadness.*" Monks and nuns famously used lemon balm to make Carmelite water, which oddly enough uses wine not water, as a cure for headaches, digestive complaints and to lift the spirits.

OTHER COMMON USES: An infusion of lemon balm can be sprayed onto plants to repel insects, and keeping a bunch of lemon balm on your kitchen windowsill discourages flies and insects from entering.

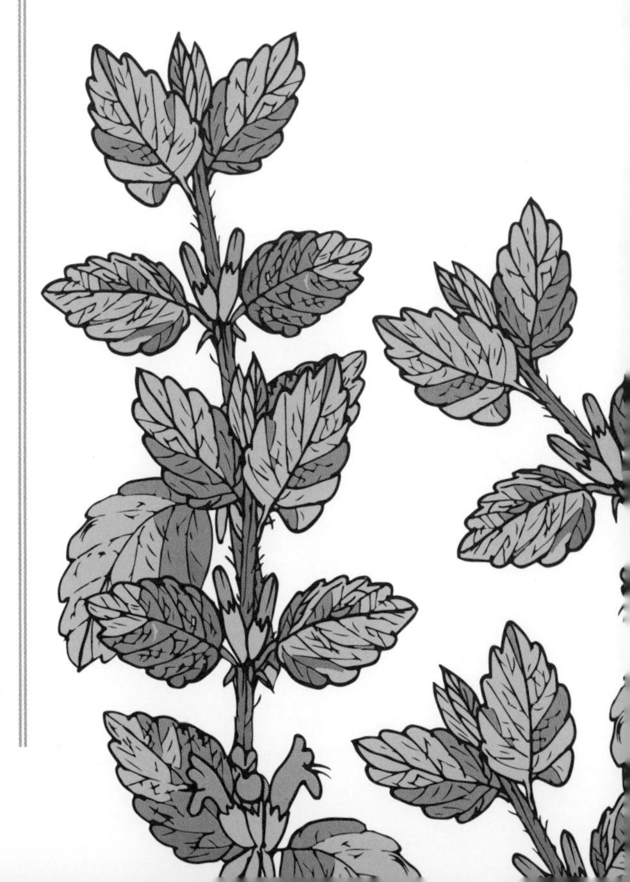

THE QUEEN OF HUNGARY'S FACIAL MIST

Queen Elizabeth of Hungary (1305–1380) was famed for her beauty and incredibly youthful complexion. Legend has it that at the grand old age of 70 she looked so young that the 25-year-old grand duke of Lithuania asked for her hand in marriage! The recipe may have been created for her by an alchemist or a monk, or a band of travelling Romanies – no one really knows.

It's probably best to use dried herbs for this one – choose organic wherever possible. Each of these herbs is known for its beneficial effect on skin.

Makes about 500ml

INGREDIENTS

6 tbsp lemon balm
1 tbsp rosemary
4 tbsp rose petals
3 tbsp calendula
3 tbsp mint
1 tbsp grated lemon peel
1 tbsp sage
4 tbsp camomile
250ml organic apple cider vinegar (see page 34)
250ml distilled witch hazel
Lavender or rose essential oil

Equipment needed

Large clean and sterilized jar
Muslin or fine sieve
Clean spray bottles

METHOD

Pour all of the herbs into a sterilized jar; don't use one with a metal lid as the vinegar will make it rust.

Pour over the vinegar; it should cover all of the herbs. Close the jar tightly and shake.

Place the jar onto a sunny windowsill for 3 weeks, shaking as often as you remember.

Strain the liquid through a muslin or fine sieve into a measuring jug. Compost the used herbs.

Add witch hazel in a ratio of 1:1 and mix in 10 drops of essential oil.

Pour the mixture into clean spray bottles, label and store in a cool dry place.

Shake well and use as a facial toner, an aftershave or a cooling body spritz.

Keeps for up to a year.

CARMELITE WATER

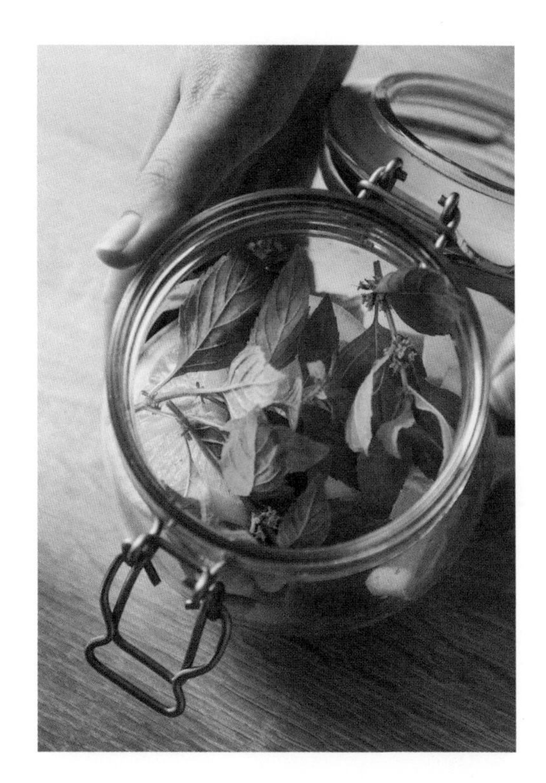

This herbal tonic was created in the Carmelite monasteries in Europe in the fourteenth century. The recipe was closely guarded by the monks and nuns of each abbey, as were many of their herbal remedies. It is said that using Carmelite water regularly will encourage a positive outlook, boost the immune system, aid digestion and allow pleasant dreams.

Nutmeg also helps with indigestion as well as being antioxidant, antibacterial and anti-inflammatory – use freshly grated if possible to maximize the benefits.

Makes 70cl

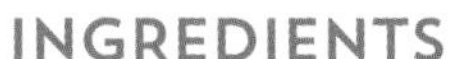

INGREDIENTS

50g fresh lemon balm, roughly chopped

1 tbsp dried angelica

Grated zest of 1 organic lemon

¼ tsp freshly grated nutmeg

70cl white wine

Equipment needed

Large clean jar

Fine sieve or muslin

METHOD

Place all ingredients in a large jar and shake well to combine.

Put in the fridge to steep for 24 hours.

Pour through a fine sieve or muslin, squeezing the herbs to extract all the wine.

Drink a small glass as required, keeps for about a week.

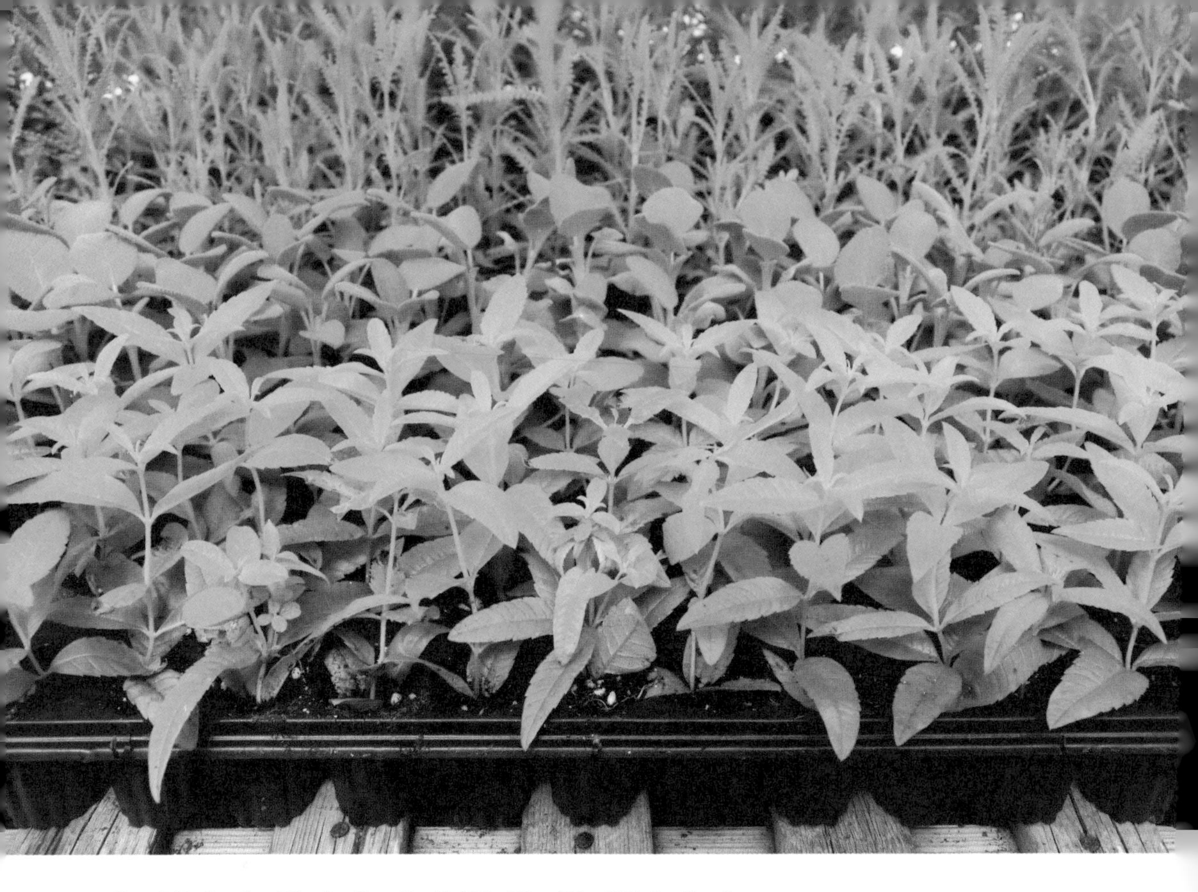

LEMON VERBENA

Alternative names: Verveine citronnelle, lemon bee brush, lemon Louisa

HOW TO IDENTIFY: The pale green spear-like leaves of lemon verbena smell incredibly lemony when crushed, immediately taking me back to my childhood memories of buying a quarter of sherbet lemon sweets from the corner shop after school.

HISTORY: Lemon verbena didn't appear in the UK until the eighteenth century when it was brought over by the Spanish for use in perfumery. By the end of the nineteenth century this tender plant could be found all over Europe in greenhouses and indoor gardens to be used as a flavouring substitute for lemons and distilled into oil for the cosmetic industry.

Victorian ladies placed the leaves in their handkerchiefs and inhaled the scent as smelling salts when overcome by the tightness of their corsets.

FOLKLORE: Wearing a sprig of lemon verbena will make you more attractive to the opposite sex, most probably because you will smell delicious!

The purifying properties of lemon verbena have historically been used to purify altars, while bathing with lemon verbena leaves will cleanse you of any evil influences.

Ancient Greeks slept with lemon verbena under their pillows to give them sweet dreams or drank lemon verbena tea to make them "as strong as Titan".

Lemon verbena is notoriously tricky to propagate from cuttings and it was believed that *"anyone who can make cuttings of lemon verbena grow will not die unmarried"*.

FOLK MEDICINE: The Inca tribes of Peru are believed to be the first people who discovered the wonderful medicinal benefits of lemon verbena using it to help balance the gut bacteria and reduce flatulence as well as harnessing its antioxidant, anti-inflammatory and anti-anxiety properties.

As lemon verbena didn't reach our shores until the eighteenth century it wasn't known to the seventeenth-century herbalist Culpeper meaning that little historical medicinal use from that period is available.

Lemon verbena tea helps with digestion, trapped wind, insomnia and gout, and is drunk to relieve colds and fevers. The scent of lemon verbena can be uplifting, calm the nerves and help to release muscle tension.

OTHER COMMON USES: Still used for its incredible scent by one famous French cosmetic producer in their lemon verbena range of shower gels, eau de toilette and many other products. Leaves can be placed amongst linens to keep them smelling fresh and repel midges, moths and flies.

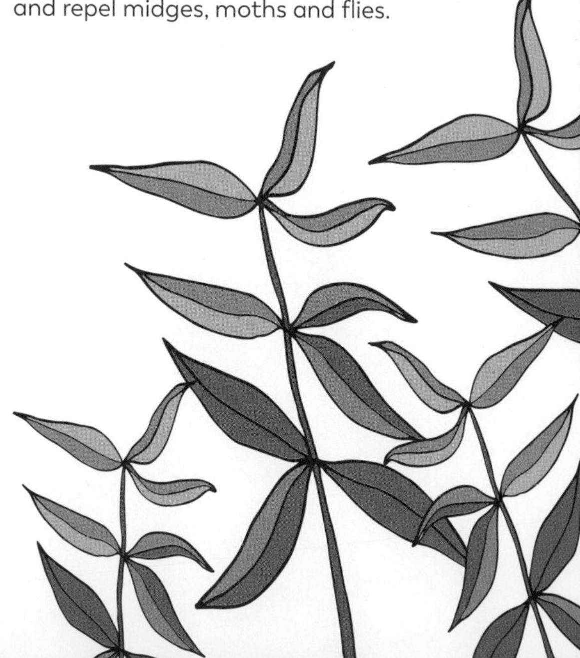

HERBAL CAR AIR FRESHENER

Just the scent of lemon verbena makes me smile and I often walk through the garden just so that I can pull my hands through the lemon verbena and inhale deeply – instant happy!

I have a deep loathing of mass-produced air fresheners in my home and car – they just don't smell pleasant and are full of chemicals. This little sachet of loveliness can be made in minutes and hung over the air inlets in your car to make your journey calmer and more enjoyable.

INGREDIENTS

Lemon verbena leaves

Equipment needed

Small drawstring muslin bag

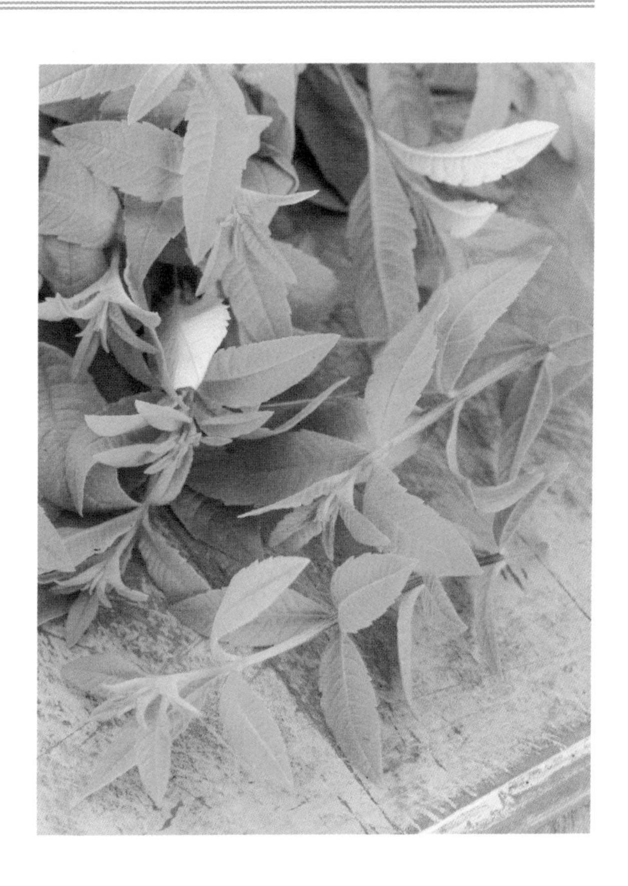

METHOD

Fill the drawstring bag with the lemon verbena leaves and tie the drawstring securely. Hang over an air vent; gently crush the leaves to release the scent into the car as you drive.

The herbs will dry out and lose their scent after a while, so refresh regularly either with lemon verbena or use your favourite herb. Rosemary, thyme and lavender flowers work well, or try a combination.

LEMON VERBENA AND CUCUMBER WATER

Lemon verbena helps to release the happy hormones of dopamine and serotonin, a burst of vitamin C from the lemon to support your immune system and potassium-rich cucumber to lower blood pressure. Tastes good too!

Makes 1 litre

INGREDIENTS

Handful of fresh lemon verbena leaves

½ organic cucumber, sliced

1 organic lemon, sliced

250ml boiling water

750ml cold water

Equipment needed

Large heatproof jug or jar

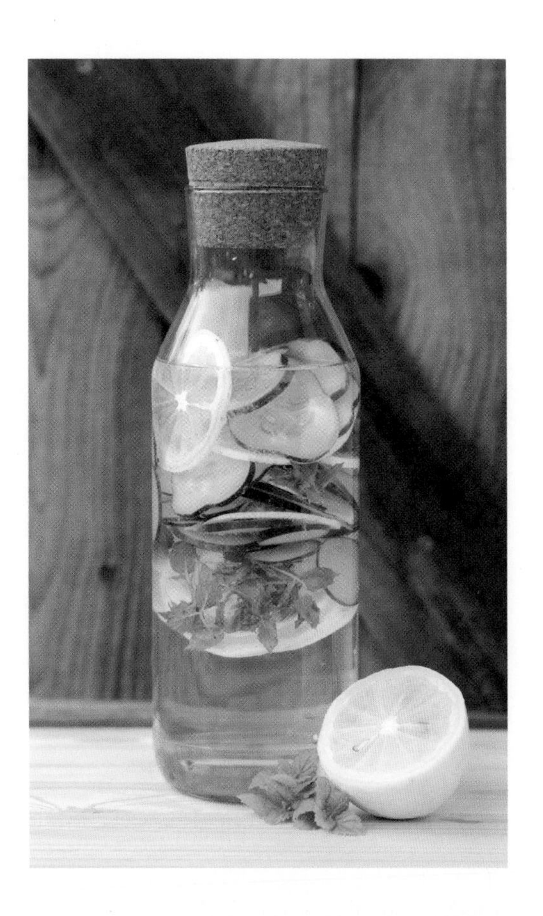

METHOD

Put the lemon verbena leaves into the jug and pour over the boiling water. Allow to cool.

Add the sliced lemon and cucumber and the cold water. Pop into the fridge for a couple of hours.

Serve in tall glasses over ice while sitting in a sunny garden.

Drink immediately.

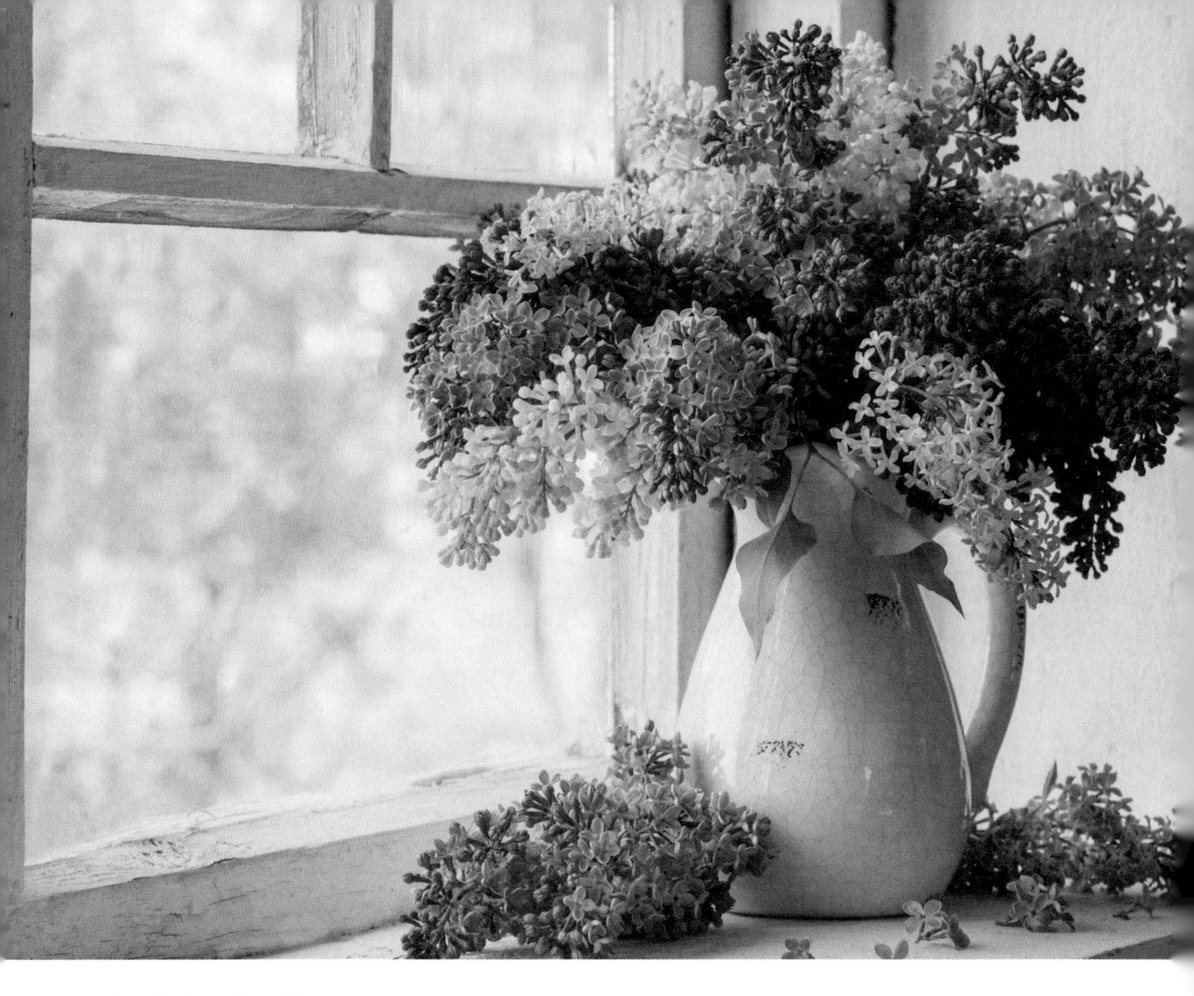

LILAC

Alternative names: Syringa, lily oak, tree lilac

HOW TO IDENTIFY: Lilac is a tall slow-growing shrub, most identifiable by its long fragrant clusters of purple through to white flowers that appear in May.

HISTORY: The name *syringa* comes from the Greek word meaning "pipe" – the soft pulp is easily removed from inside the stems to form a long thin hollow pipe.

Greek mythology tells us that Pan made his famous pipes from lilac when he failed to win the affection of the nymph Syringa.

Lilac became prevalent in cottage gardens in the sixteenth century, having been brought back from the mountains of south-eastern Europe by explorers. The herbalist John Gerard had lilac growing "in very great plenty" in his garden in 1597.

FOLKLORE: With their intoxicating fragrance, lilac flowers were regarded as magical by the Celts. Their scent was considered unlucky by others, as they feared it would make them sleepy and vulnerable to being kidnapped by faeries.

Lilac flowers also come in white and these were regarded as very unlucky and should never be brought into the house, and definitely under no circumstances put in the bedroom of a sick person.

Fragrant lilac flowers were often used to mask the scent of death by placing them in the open coffin – not surprising, then, that they have gained such morbid associations.

Lilac planted outside around the home will keep away those who intend to do you harm, some blooms kept indoors will drive away any unwelcome spirits. Lilac flowers have a reputation for increasing psychic powers, aiding divination (fortune telling) and giving you blessings on your life's journey.

FOLK MEDICINE: Sixteenth-century colonists in the USA used lilac as a "vermifuge" to treat intestinal worms, lower fevers, and as a treatment for malaria.

Lilac tea has been used as a hair and facial tonic since the sixteenth century.

OTHER COMMON USES: Pop a few blossoms in a jug of cold water for a calming drink infused with the taste of spring. Lilac blossom tea is good for the digestion.

The flowers are edible and can be crystallized to decorate cakes.

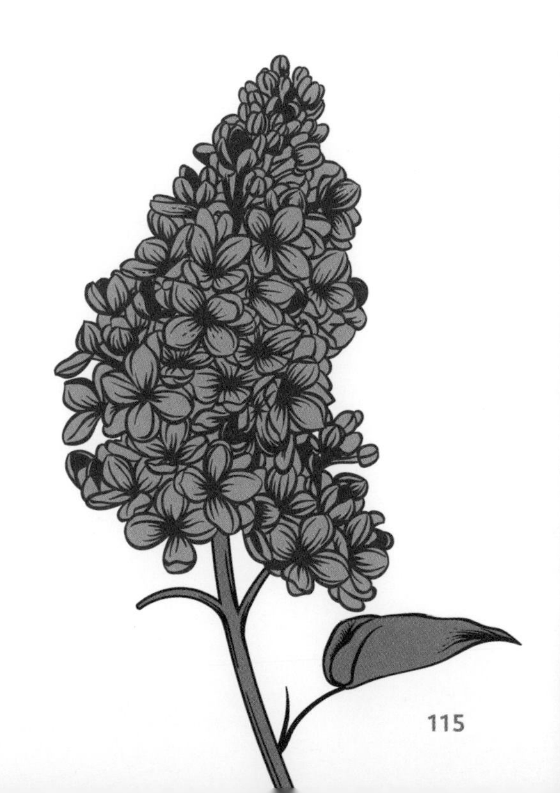

LILAC BLOSSOM FACIAL SPRITZ

The anti-inflammatory and antioxidant properties of lilac flowers and witch hazel will help to soothe minor sunburn and ease minor skin conditions.

If you don't have lilac growing in your own garden keep an eye out for lilac blossoms in your neighbours' gardens between May and June. Pick the freshest flowers that you can find.

Makes 400ml

INGREDIENTS

Two or three lilac blossoms should fill a standard jam jar

400ml organic witch hazel

Equipment needed

Large clean and sterilized jam jar

Cotton pads

Spray bottle

METHOD

Lay the lilac blossoms on kitchen paper and allow to wilt overnight.

Chop the blossoms, stems and leaves and put them into your clean and sterilized jam jar.

Pour over enough witch hazel to completely cover the plant matter.

Put on the lid, stir, label and keep in a cool dry place for two weeks, shaking it occasionally.

After 2 weeks, strain out the flowers and put them on the compost.

You can either soak cotton pads in facial spritz and gently apply to skin or put the toner into a bottle with a spritz attachment and spray directly onto your face.

Keep in the fridge if you wish and use within 6 months.

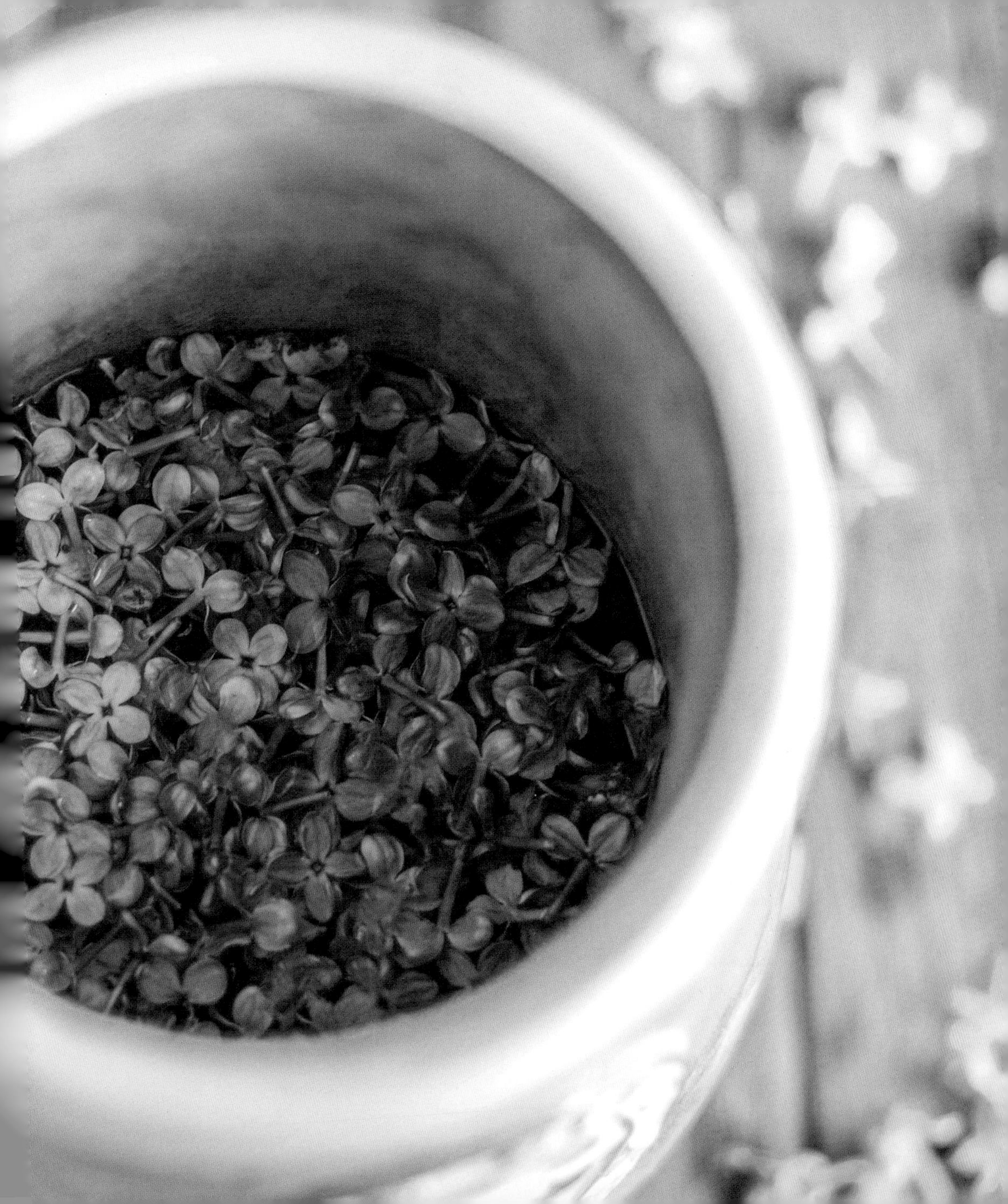

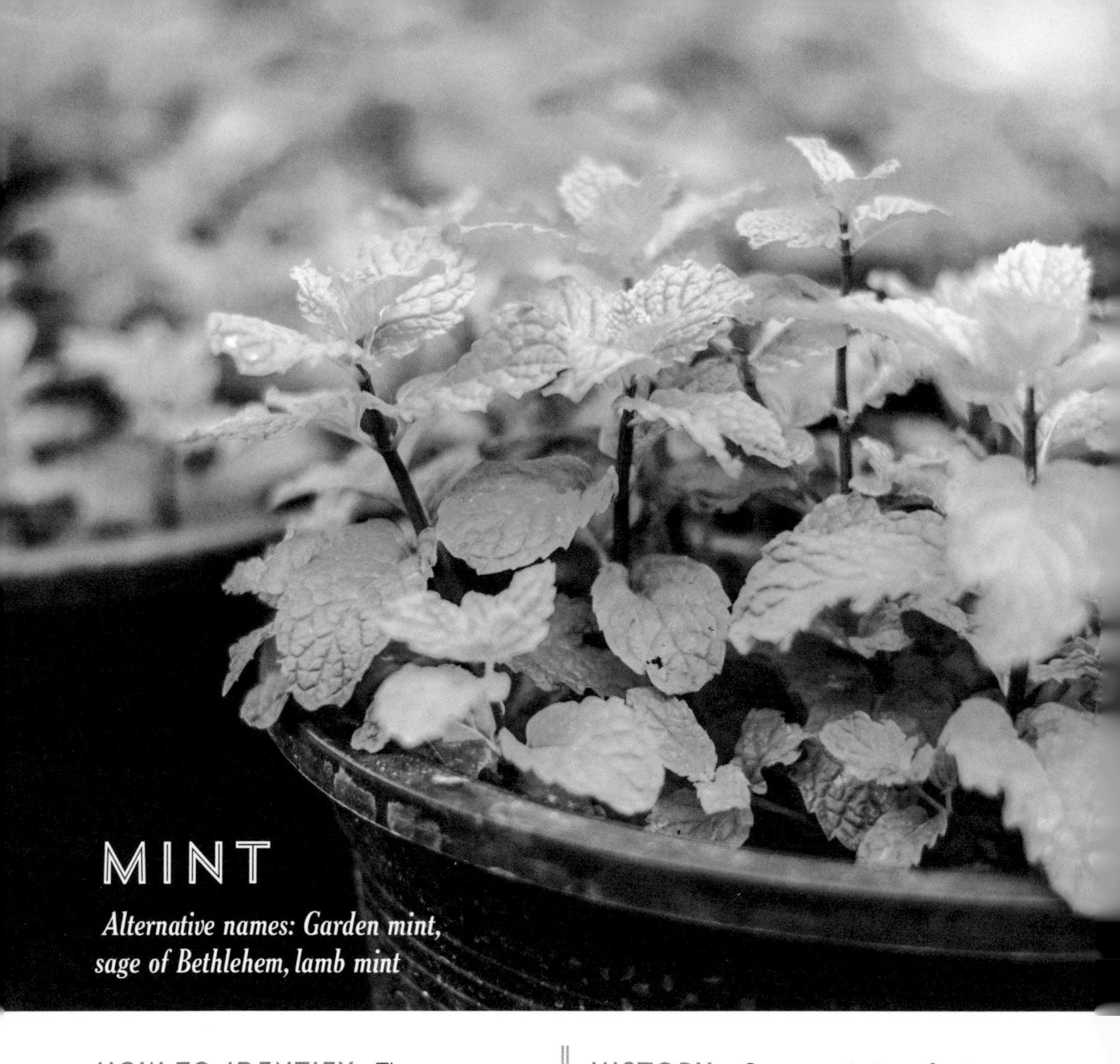

MINT

Alternative names: Garden mint, sage of Bethlehem, lamb mint

HOW TO IDENTIFY: There are many different varieties of mint available in garden centres, most of which will have square stems, jagged-edged leaves and a distinctive minty smell.

HISTORY: Some varieties of mint are native to Europe and have been used in medicine and cooking for centuries but of course the Romans introduced us to many more.

The Ancient Greeks rubbed mint under their arms as a deodorant as well as using it in funeral rituals to disguise the smell of death.

The aroma of fresh mint in Roman houses signified hospitality. It was added to baths for the scent, enjoyed as a culinary and medicinal herb and used in teeth-cleaning for fresh breath.

Mint was strewn on the floors of homes, hospitals, churches and synagogues, releasing its fresh smell when it was trodden underfoot. This also served to repel insects and deter mice, which apparently detest the smell of mint.

FOLKLORE: Mint infused in hot water and used as a floor wash will keep away troublesome visitors and help to return the household back to harmony after arguments.

A couple of mint leaves in your purse or wallet will make sure that money comes your way, while mint leaves in your shoes will bring good luck and remove any perceived obstacles in your way. Mint under your pillow encourages dreams of the future and will also help to ease hay fever symptoms, while wearing a crown of mint can sharpen the brain and aid concentration.

Mint is believed to be "shy" – if you plant some it's important that you don't look at it for a month as it will not thrive.

FOLK MEDICINE: Gilbert of England in his thirteenth-century *Compendium of Medicine* recommends that for the:

> *"... stinking of the mouth, if there be no rotten flesh, let the mouth be washed with wine that birch or mint has been soaked in. And let the gums be well rubbed with a rough linen cloth until they bleed. And let him eat marjoram, mint and parsley til they be well chewed. And let him rub well his teeth with the herbs he chewed and also his gums."*

The Roman author Pliny the Elder writes of mint, "*it prevents the recurrence of lascivious dreams*". This differs from the view of Alexander the Great who forbade his soldiers to diffuse peppermint oil before battle fearing that it would stir erotic thoughts and thus lessen their desire to fight. This was echoed by Culpeper who wrote that mint "*stirs up venery [the pursuit of sexual pleasure], or bodily lust*".

OTHER COMMON USES: It's commonly used in the kitchen for both sweet and savoury dishes and tea. However, a vase of mint placed by an open window will help to deter flies and insects and smell lovely, too.

MINT AND ROSEMARY SALT SCRUB

Salt scrubs are so easy to make with just a few store cupboard ingredients. Choose a natural sea salt but not one with large grains as this can be too abrasive on your skin. Not enough salt? No problem, just use granulated or caster sugar instead.

Mint is antibacterial and antioxidant and will brighten your skin tone, while rosemary's anti-inflammatory properties will reduce redness and calm any skin breakouts. Coconut oil is naturally moisturizing and hydrating, and when combined with salt to gently exfoliate, it will leave your skin baby-soft. Using a salt scrub stimulates your circulatory system, making you feel good inside and out.

Makes 225g

INGREDIENTS

2 tbsp fresh mint, finely chopped (if garden mint or peppermint isn't readily available any variety can be used)

2 tbsp fresh rosemary, finely chopped

150g natural salt

75g organic coconut oil at room temperature

Equipment needed

Clean sterilized jars

METHOD

Place all the ingredients into a bowl. Combine using your hands until thoroughly mixed.

Scoop it into clean, sterilized jars.

Massage into your hands, feet and legs for 30 seconds while sitting on the side of the bath, rinse and pat dry.

Never use on your feet while in the shower as the coconut oil will make them very slippery!

Use within 1 month.

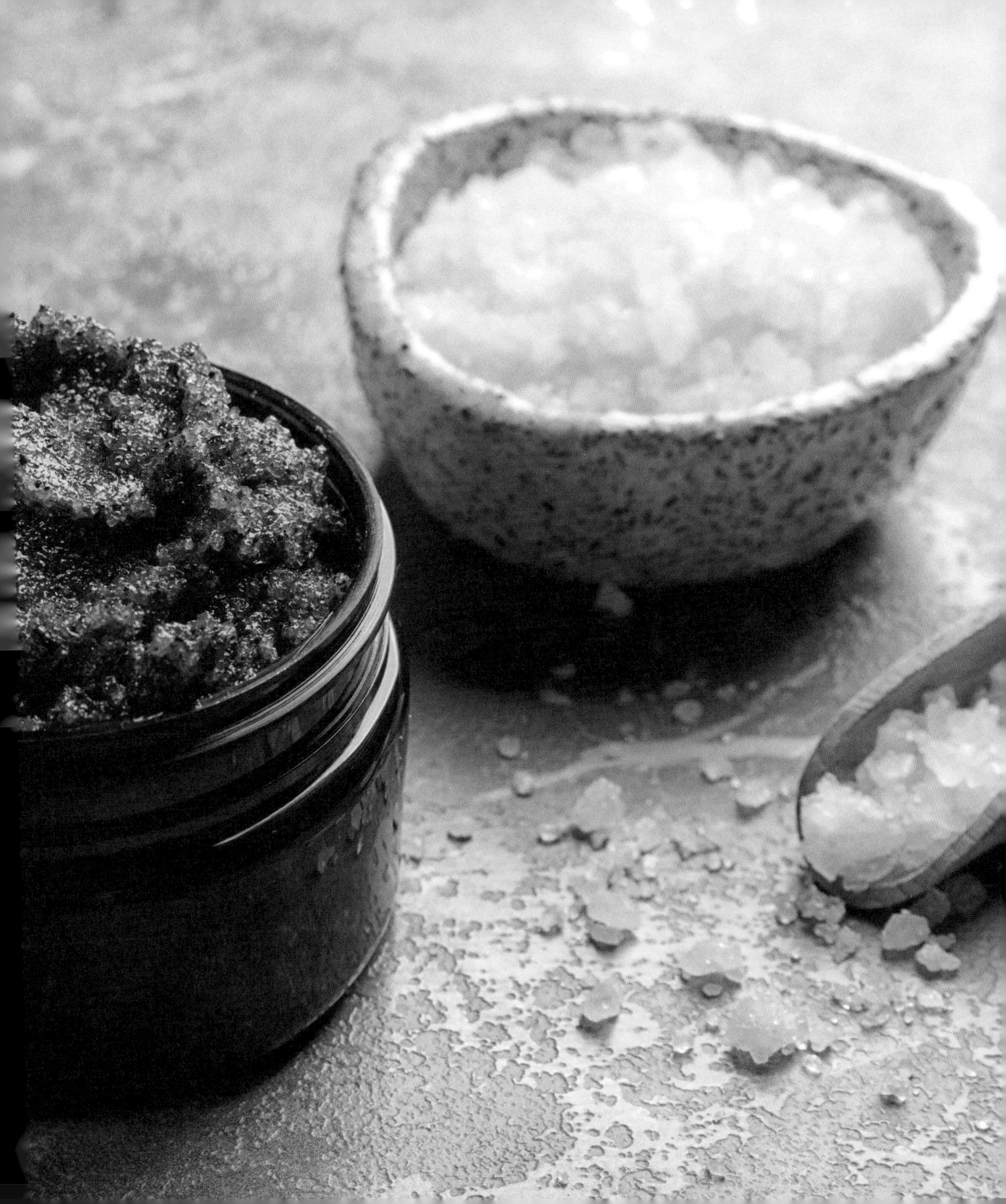

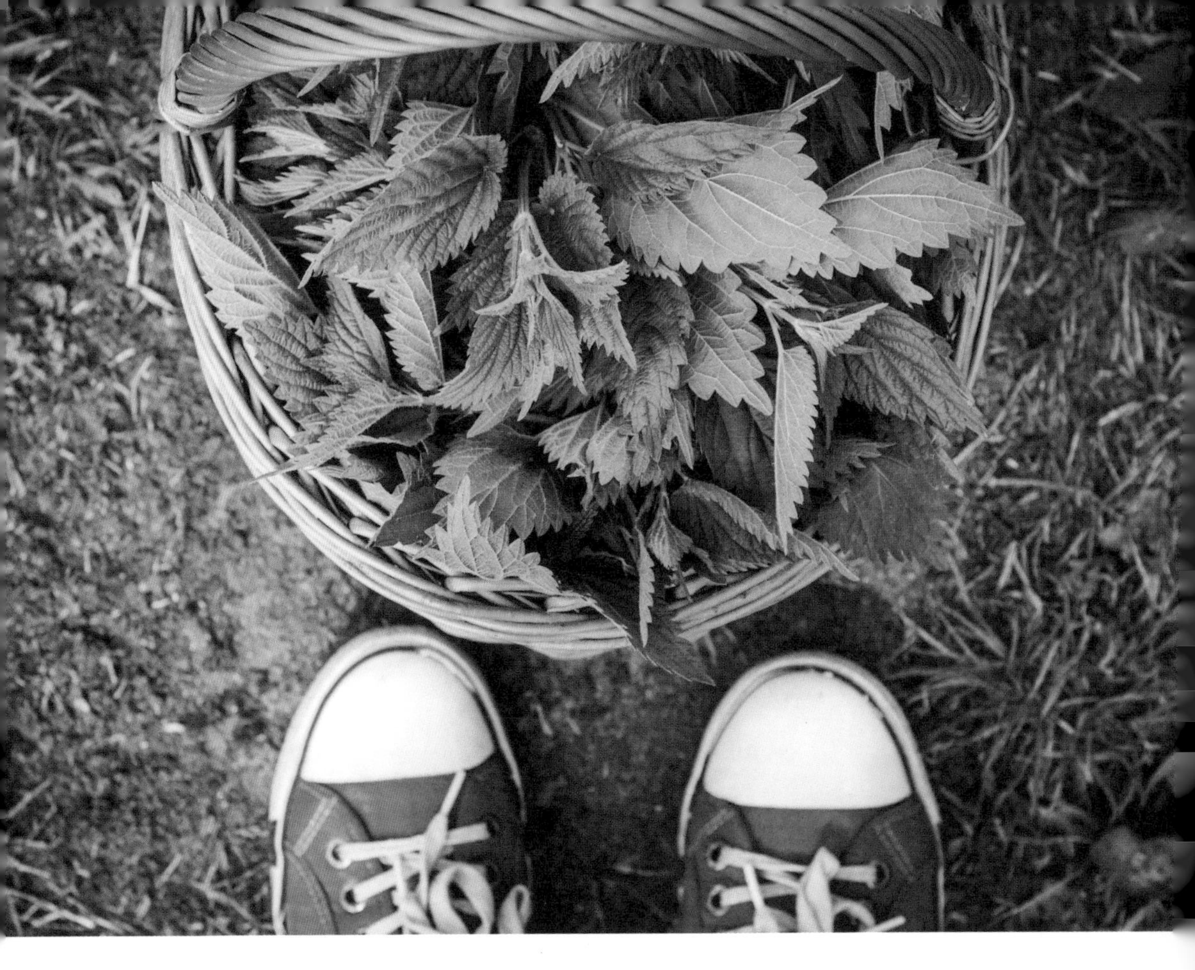

NETTLE

Alternative names: Stinging nettles, devil's plaything, burn nettle, hoky-poky

HOW TO IDENTIFY: Growing everywhere it would seem where there might be vulnerable bare arms and legs, nettles are usually felt before they are seen! Dark green, hairy, heart-shaped stingy leaves are arranged set opposite each other in pairs along a tall, straight stem. The flowers form at the base of the leaves and are greenish-white with yellow anthers.

HISTORY: The nettle plant contains strong fibres that have been spun since the Bronze Age for making cloth and cord.

During World War One, when cotton was scarce, nettle fibre was cultivated on a huge scale to make into uniforms for German and Austrian soldiers. Green dye made from the nettles helped to make camouflage uniforms for the British army during World War Two, and there were even plans to construct aircraft wings from nettle fibres. During rationing, many people used nettles in their cooking as they were a good source of vitamin C and iron.

FOLKLORE: Nettles were used to thrash the devil out of poor souls believed to be possessed. Holding a nettle during a thunder-storm – if you can bear the stings – will prevent you from getting struck by lightning. Carry yarrow with it and it will help you become fearless – very useful during a thunderstorm!

To stimulate hair growth, try combing nettle juice into your hair; this will make hair soft and glossy, and prevent it from falling out.

FOLK MEDICINE: It was believed that a fever could be cured by picking a nettle up by its roots while reciting the name of the sick person and also the names of their parents. An old remedy for rheumatism and arthritis involved whipping the affected joints with fresh nettles and rolling naked in a nettle patch was said to cure hay fever – despite a nasty nettle rash!

In the seventeenth century, earache was soothed by dripping nettle juice into ears. Mix nettle juice with egg white and rub onto temples to cure insomnia or use it to ease burns and rashes.

OTHER COMMON USES: Full of vitamins, protein and iron, nettles make a useful substitute for spinach.

Today, the chlorophyll of nettles is used as a green dye and is known as the food colourant E140.

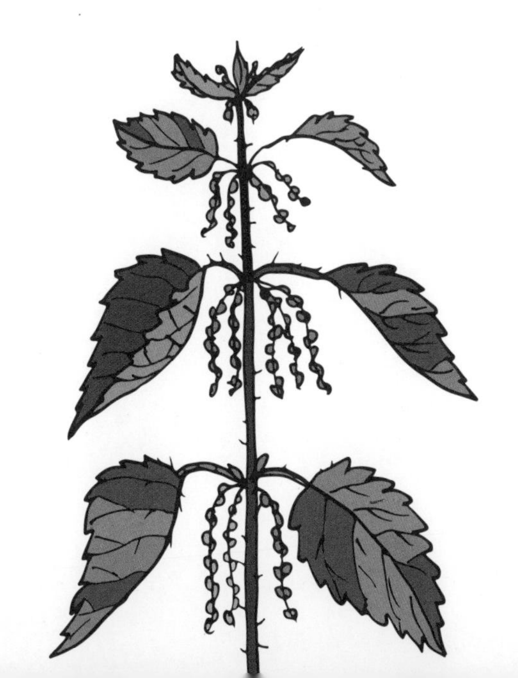

STINGING NETTLE AND LEMON CAKE

This is one of my favourite cake recipes, combining my own wonderful free-range eggs with humble stinging nettles foraged from the garden. Don't worry, cooking the nettles will make the stings completely disappear.

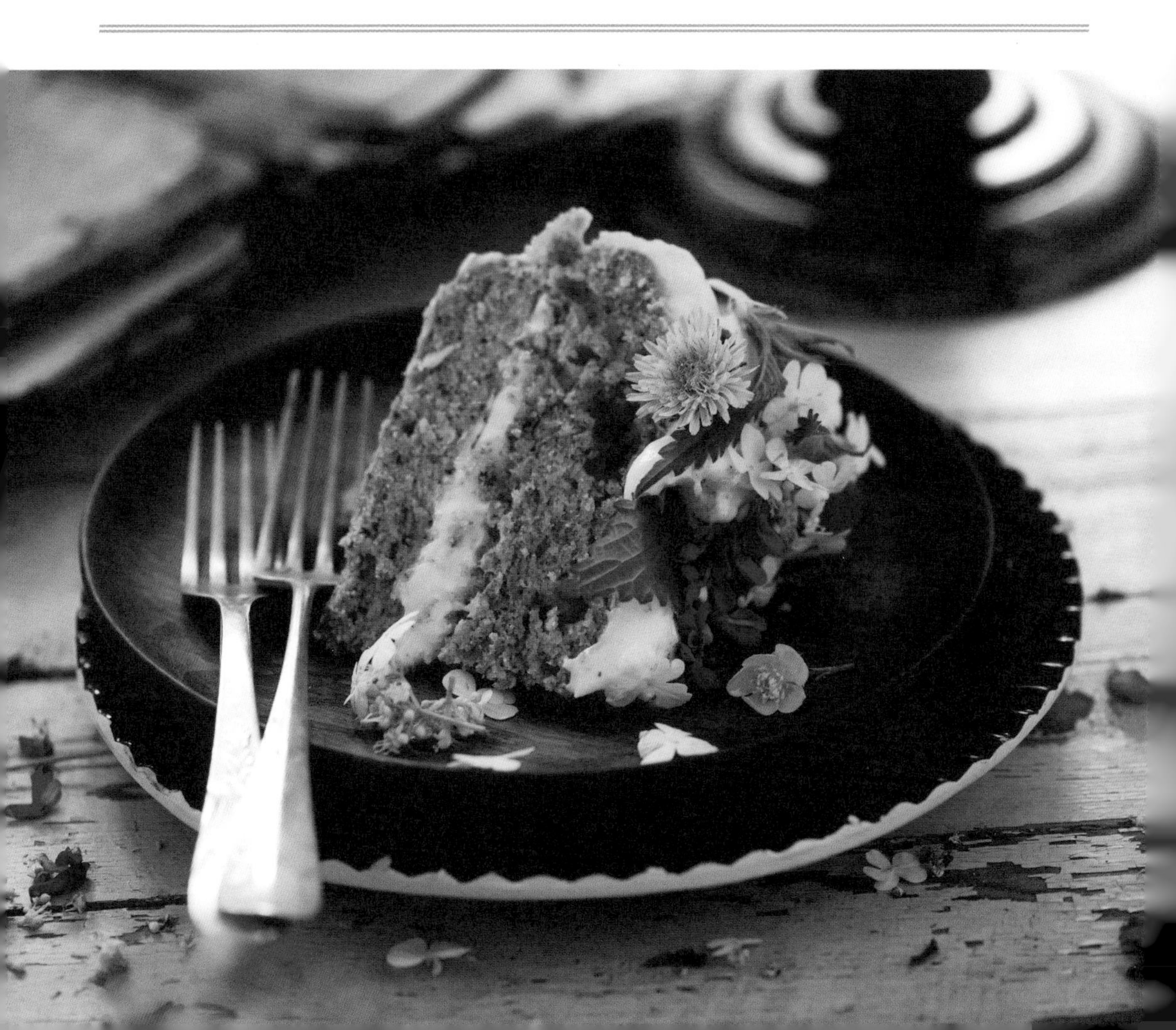

INGREDIENTS

For the cake:

100g young nettle leaves (only pick the top four leaves and use gloves!)

Zest and juice of 1 organic lemon

200g softened butter

150g caster sugar

3 large organic free-range eggs

2 tsp vanilla extract

250g plain flour

2 tsp baking powder

½ tsp salt

For the filling and topping:

250g mascarpone cheese

3 tbsp sifted icing sugar

Zest and juice of 1 organic lemon

Equipment needed

Rubber gloves

Two 18cm round cake tins

METHOD

Preheat oven to 170°C (325°F), grease and line two 18cm round cake tins.

Wearing rubber gloves, wash the nettles discarding any stems.

Put the nettles in a colander and steam over a pan of boiling water for 5 minutes. Allow the nettles to cool then add the lemon juice and puree using a stick blender. Set aside.

In a large bowl cream together the butter and sugar until light and fluffy. Gradually beat in the eggs, nettles, lemon zest and vanilla extract.

Sift in the flour, baking powder and salt and carefully combine.

Spoon the mixture into the prepared tins and bake for 25 minutes until a skewer comes out clean.

Cool for 10 minutes before turning out onto a wire rack to cool completely.

For the icing:

Gently stir the mascarpone to loosen, sift in the icing sugar then add the lemon juice and finely grated zest. Don't over work the filling or it will become too runny.

Spread one third of the mixture over one of the nettle sponges and sandwich together.

Cover the cake completely with the rest of the icing to hide the green surprise inside.

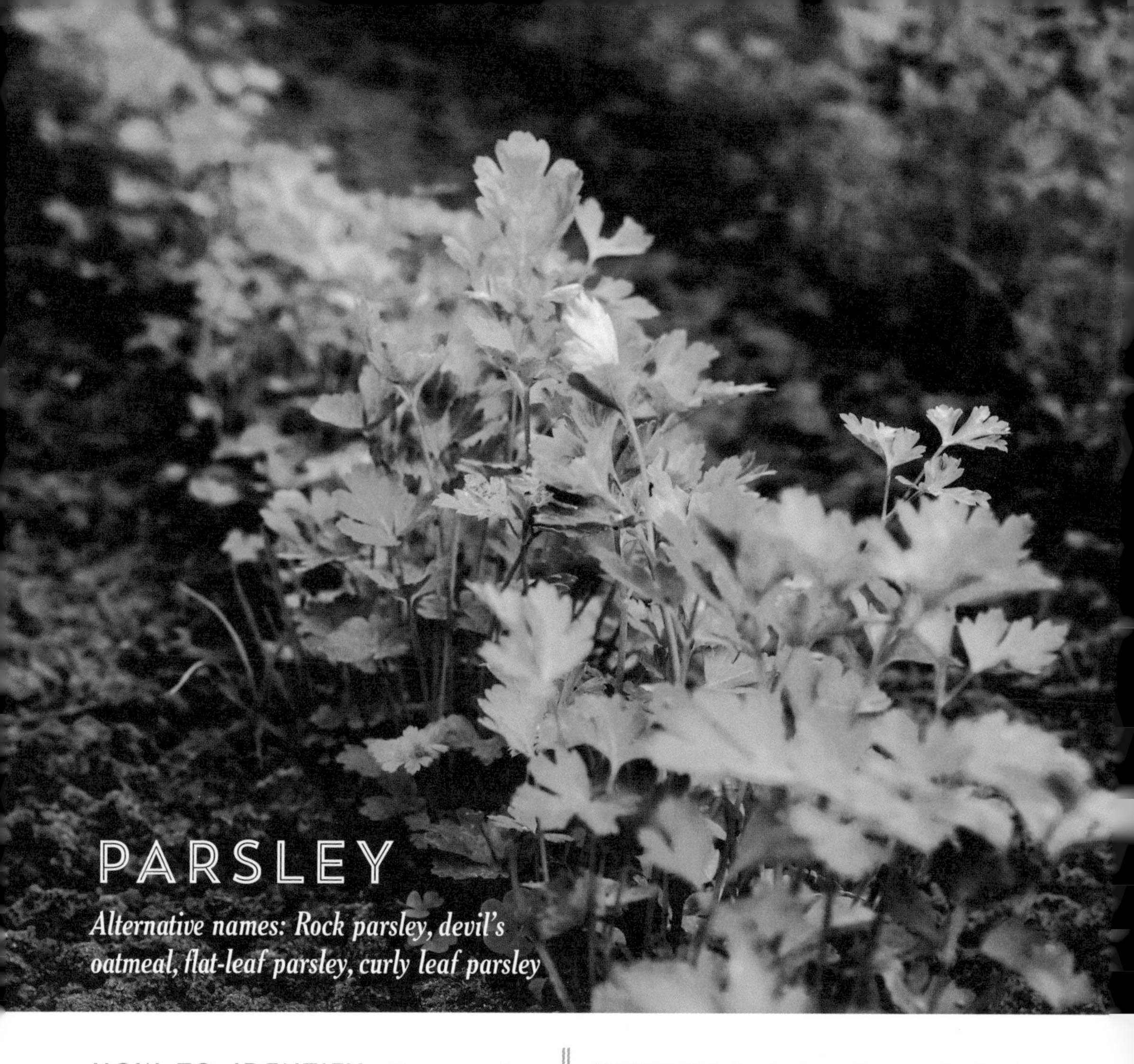

PARSLEY

Alternative names: Rock parsley, devil's oatmeal, flat-leaf parsley, curly leaf parsley

HOW TO IDENTIFY: There are two varieties of parsley in common use: curly parsley, with its ruffled curled leaves, and flat-leaf parsley, with broad leaves not dissimilar to coriander.

HISTORY: In Ancient Greece the bodies of dead heroes were prepared for their journey to Elysium by being adorned with sweet-smelling flowers and herbs, parsley being among them as it was believed to be a particular favourite of Persephone, queen of the underworld.

Greeks often used parsley at funerals and planted parsley on graves – when nearing death, someone would be described as being "in need of parsley".

The Romans did not commonly eat parsley in cooking, though; it was served as a breath freshener at the end of the meal and grown as fodder for chariot horses. Although probably introduced to Britain by the Romans and grown in physic gardens, parsley wasn't universally accepted as a culinary herb until the Middle Ages.

FOLKLORE: Parsley seeds are notoriously difficult to germinate, and for this reason they should be sown before midday on Good Friday by the lady of the house. Parsley seeds should thrive on Good Friday as it is believed to be the only day when the devil has no control over the living things on earth. Parsley should never be transplanted or you risk opening up the ground for the devil; *"transplant parsley, transplant sorrow"*.

It is also generally considered very unlucky to give a parsley plant to anyone as a gift, unless they are trying to conceive, in which case she will fall pregnant within a year.

FOLK MEDICINE: Culpeper tells us that:

"The leaves of parsley laid to the eyes that are inflamed with heat, or swollen, doth much help them, if it be used with bread or meal, and being fried with butter, and applied to women's breasts that are hard through the curdling of their milk, it abates the hardness quickly, and also takes away black and blue marks coming of bruises or falls."

It is said that *"if parsley is thrown into fishponds it will heal the fish therein."*

Sheep absolutely love to eat parsley and it also increases their milk yield.

Known to freshen breath, parsley can be included in my dog biscuit recipe (see page 88) and also chewed to aid digestion after garlic-heavy meals.

OTHER COMMON USES: Parsley is a great companion to plant with crops such as asparagus, tomatoes, peppers and onions as it encourages them to grow. Keep away from lettuce and mint though as it will inhibit their growth.

PARSLEY UNDER-EYE MASK FOR DARK CIRCLES

Parsley is anti-inflammatory, rich in collagen-making vitamin C and abundant in soothing and firming vitamin K and chlorophyll, which helps to reduce puffiness and lighten dark circles. Lemon juice is included to brighten the skin and raw honey for its antibacterial and skin-softening properties. Sounds good enough to eat!

Makes enough for 2–3 applications

INGREDIENTS

8 tbsp fresh parsley, chopped

1 tsp lemon juice

1 tbsp raw honey

Equipment needed

Pestle and mortar

METHOD

Put all the ingredients into a mortar and grind to a liquid paste with the pestle.

Carefully apply the paste under the eyes where needed.

Lay back and relax for 20 minutes.

Splash off with cold water.

Dab a little on any spots to help them heal, too.

Keeps in the fridge for a couple of days.

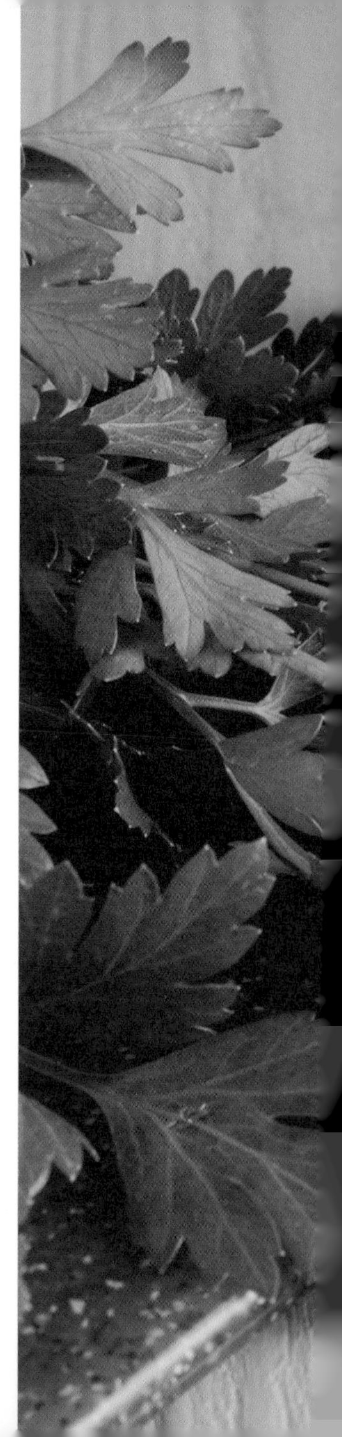

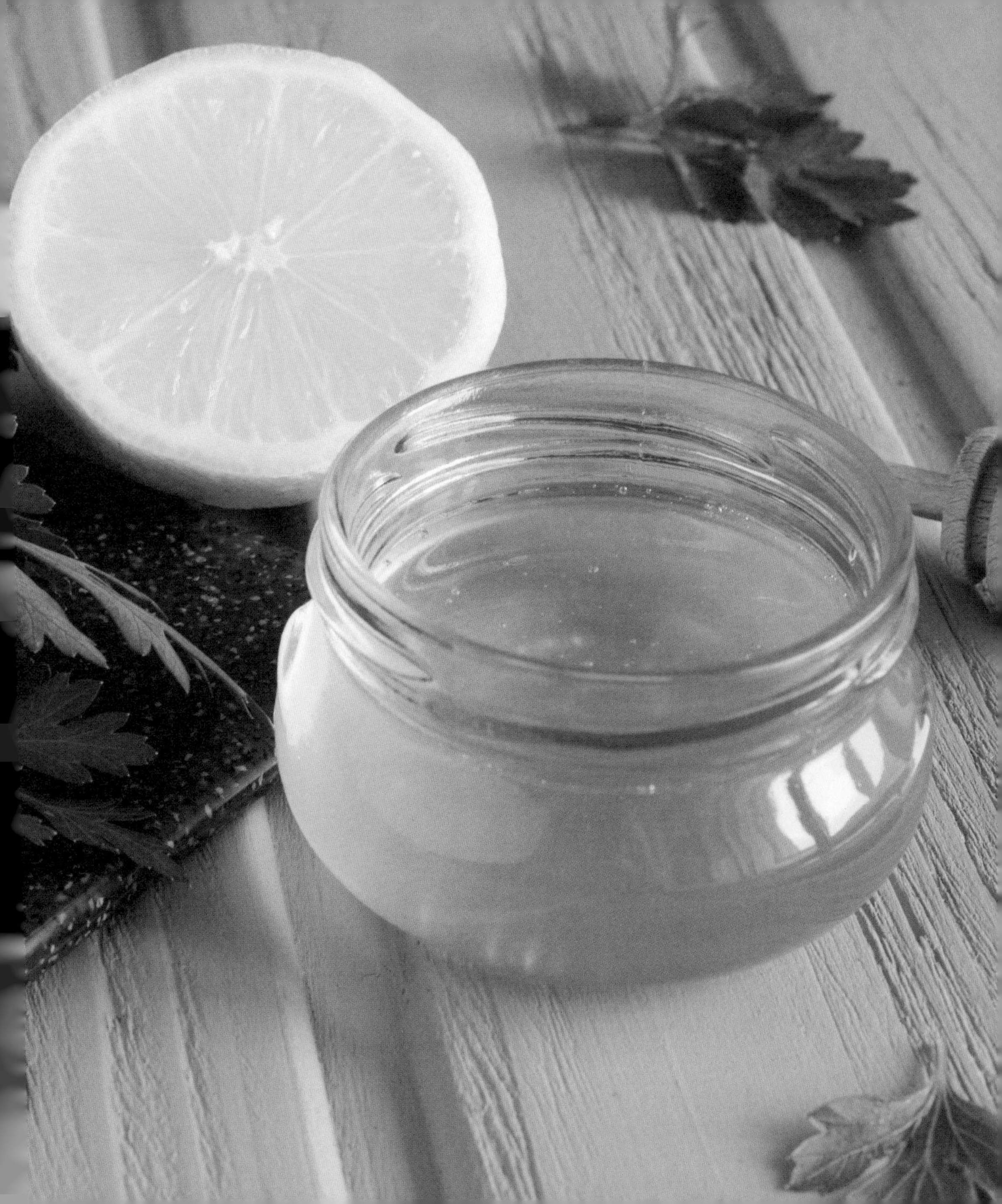

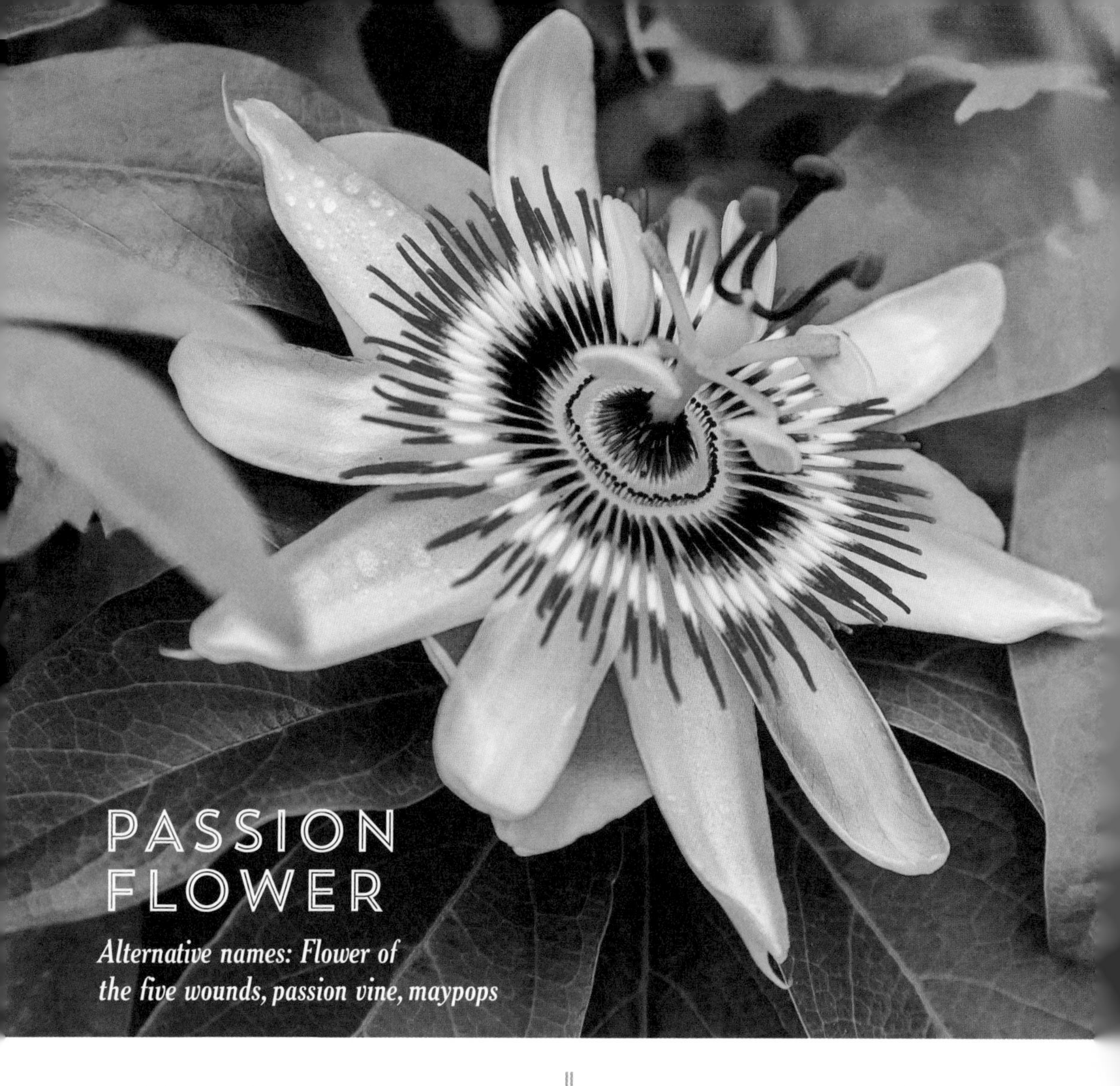

PASSION FLOWER

Alternative names: Flower of the five wounds, passion vine, maypops

HOW TO IDENTIFY: An evergreen climber with stunning white flowers tinted with purple, which produce orange egg-shaped fruits in late summer. Passion flower fruits can be eaten when fully ripe and allowed to drop from the plant BUT be warned that unripe fruit can cause severe stomach upsets!

HISTORY: Jesuit missionaries saw the flower as a "gift from God" helping them to explain the passion of Christ and the crucifixion to the indigenous South American population. Catholic missionaries were believed to be responsible for the naming of this exotic plant, each part representing the story of Christ:

Ten petals – the apostles who were present at the crucifixion.

Five anthers – the wounds of Christ.

Circle of filaments – the crown of thorns.

Blade-shaped leaves – the spear that pierced His side.

Purple tint on petals – heaven.

White petals – purity.

Brought to Britain from the Americas this stunning plant became very popular in the blousy gardens of Victorians. They embraced the associated symbolism by adorning local churches with passion flowers in stained glass windows, on ecclesiastic objects and on lecterns.

FOLKLORE: Plants that climb and cling like passion flower are often used in love charms: historically in Mexico, passion flower leaves or roots were carried in a red bag containing the dried heart of a hummingbird and anointed with "love me" oil to attract love and friendship; thankfully nowadays a hummingbird-shaped charm is used instead.

Bathing in passion flowers for five consecutive days will bring a lover of the opposite sex into your life and it will also rekindle the passion in existing relationships.

Passion flower grown around the front gate or fence will bring peace and blessings to the home.

Wear a passion flower to strengthen the bonds between old friends and attract new ones.

FOLK MEDICINE: Tea made from leaves and roots of the passion flower was used in South America to calm the nerves and treat insomnia and epilepsy.

During World War Two the Nazis attempted to develop a "truth serum" using flavonoids extracted from passion flowers to induce a "euphoria-like" state to encourage prisoners of war to reveal military secrets.

OTHER COMMON USES: The open blooms of the passion flower are perfect for attracting a multitude of pollinators into the garden.

PASSION FLOWER DEEP SLEEP PILLOW

Passion flower is commonly used to aid relaxation and calm anxiety so it makes sense to use it with other soporific herbs to make a sleep pillow.

Hops are a natural sedative. Combine these with lavender which has long been used to help to relax and unwind and you have created a recipe for a good night's sleep.

If you don't have drawstring pouches just use any scrap of natural fabric that can easily be turned into a simple pillow.

Makes one sleep pillow

INGREDIENTS

2 tbsp dried passion flowers

2 tbsp dried hops

2 tbsp dried lavender

6 drops lavender essential oil

Equipment needed

Small natural fabric drawstring bag about 8 x 5cm (3 x 2 inches)

METHOD

Mix together the herbs and put them into the drawstring bag.

Add six drops of lavender essential oil and close the bag.

Place under your pillowcase and enjoy the pleasant herbal aromas as you drift off to sleep.

Not recommended during pregnancy.

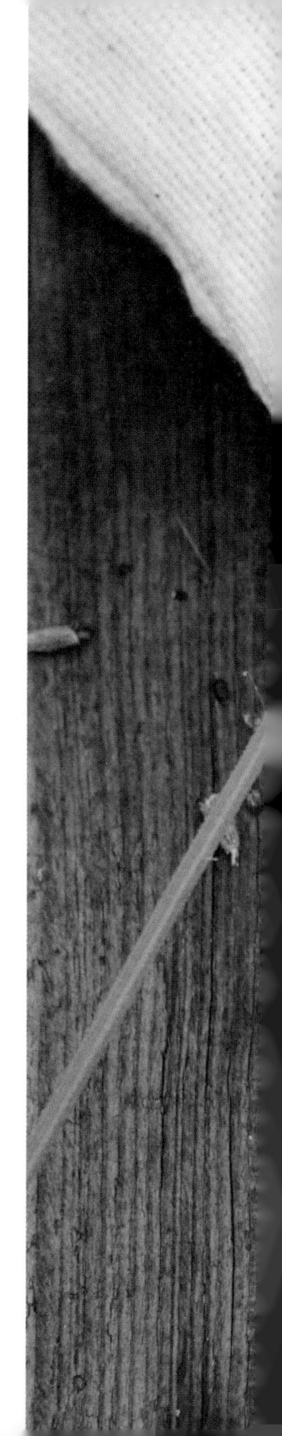

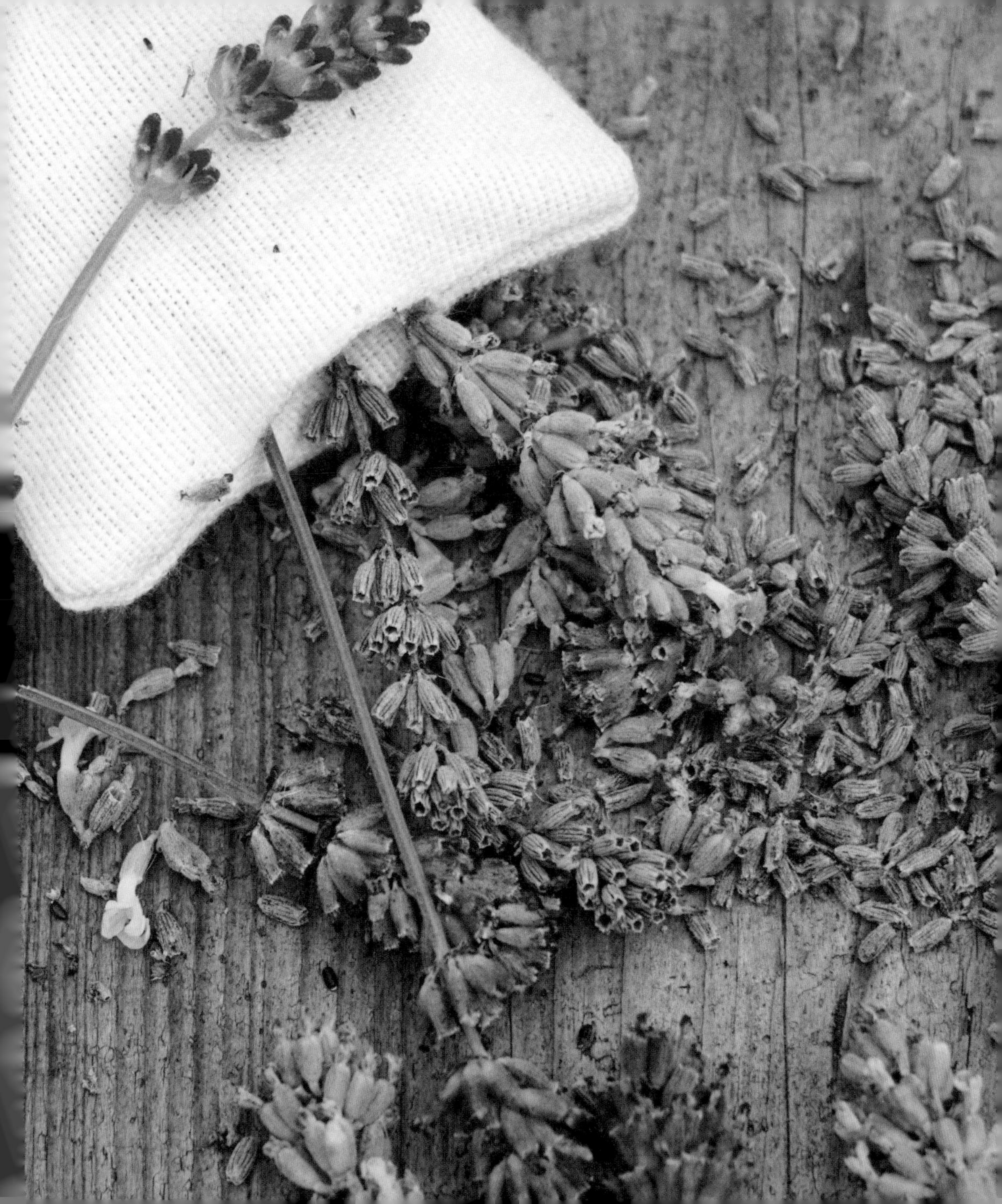

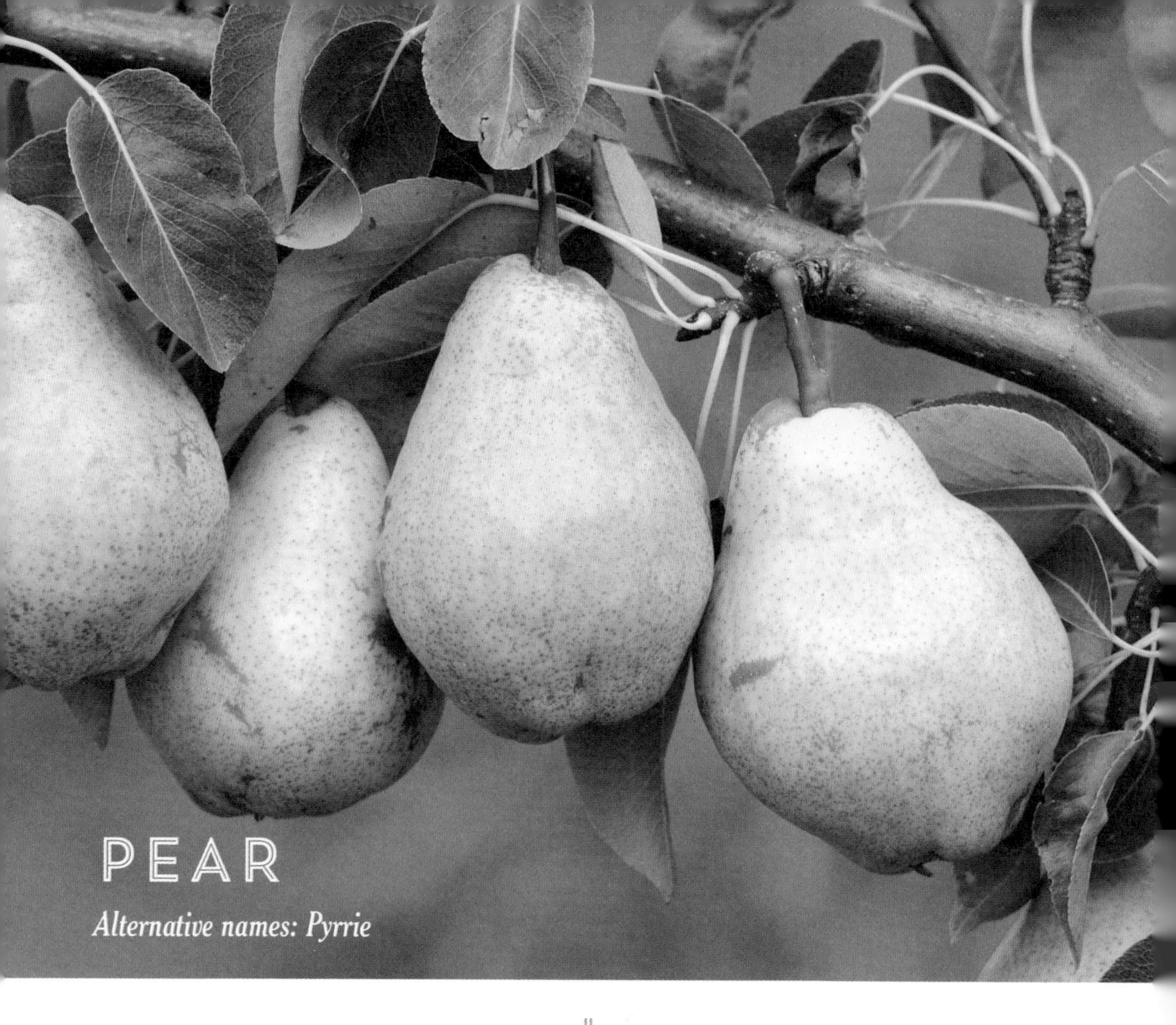

PEAR

Alternative names: Pyrrie

HOW TO IDENTIFY: With over 5,000 varieties to choose from worldwide pears have become a favourite fruit for many. Pear tree bark is grey/brown and broken into distinctive scaly crocodile-skin squares. White blossoms in the spring are followed by easily recognizable fruit in autumn.

HISTORY: First cultivated the UK in about AD 995 during the Roman occupation, pear trees became most popular in the Middle Ages when many varieties were imported from France. The Domesday Book of 1086 makes reference to pear trees being used as boundary markers by the Anglo Saxons suggesting that they were being grown widely at that time.

Cistercian monks in Warden in Bedfordshire were famed for growing the "Warden" cooking pear, which was even mentioned by the clown in *A Winter's Tale* by William Shakespeare:

"*I must have saffron to colour the Warden pies, mace, dates... nutmegs seven, a race or two of ginger... four pounds of prunes, and as many of raisins o' the sun.*" Sounds like an interesting recipe but maybe with rather too many prunes!

FOLKLORE: A pear tree bearing fruit for the first time should only be picked by adults and never children as it will bring them bad luck. Fruit trees that blossom out of season are nearly always regarded as omens of death or bad fortune: "*If the blooms of a pear tree come at undue season, they portend the shroud of someone who will walk under their white flowers.*"

Up until the nineteenth century, pear trees were planted for protection at the north-east gate to a property. This was considered to be "the devil's quarter" and the pear tree would keep the family safe.

On Christmas Eve, unmarried ladies walked backward towards a pear tree and circled it backward nine times to see a vision of their future spouses.

In Europe it was customary to plant a fruit tree in celebration of a wedding to symbolize fruitfulness and longevity; a pear tree was then planted for every daughter and an apple tree for every son.

FOLK MEDICINE: Pears were used as a natural remedy for nausea in ancient Greece and Culpeper says of pears: "*All the sweet and luscious sorts, whether manured or wild, do help to move the belly downwards... those that are hard and sour, do on the contrary, bind the belly as much, and the leaves do so also.*"

OTHER COMMON USES: Pear wood is much sought after and is used to make musical instruments, kitchen utensils, furniture and wood carvings.

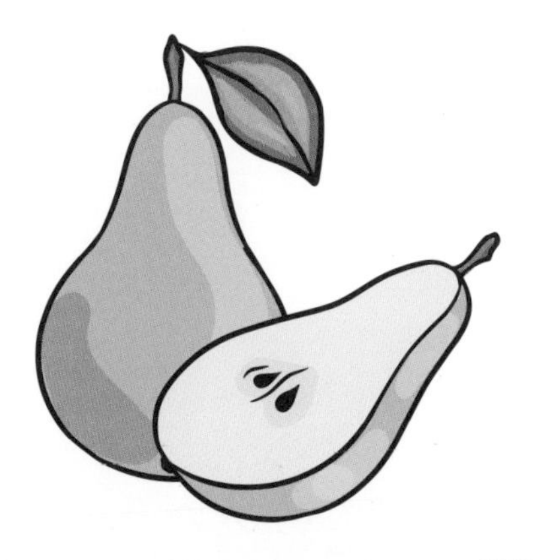

HIGH DUMPSY DEARIE JAM

I've been making this intriguingly named jam for many years now and it's a real favourite amongst family and friends.

The story to this delightfully named jam goes like this: a farmer's wife went around the orchard gathering up all the windfalls to make jam. When asked how she made it, she replied, "*I just dumpsie it in dearie, whatever fruits to hand*"– just wonderful, I so want it to be true.

If you don't have enough of one particular fruit just add more of another, as long as the total comes to 3kg (6lb 10oz), it really doesn't matter. Look out around your neighbourhood for boxes of fruit outside houses in autumn for free; I like to gift a jar of jam to whoever I got the fruit from as a little thank you. Under-ripe fruit works particularly well for jam as it contains more pectin to help it set.

Makes six jars of jam

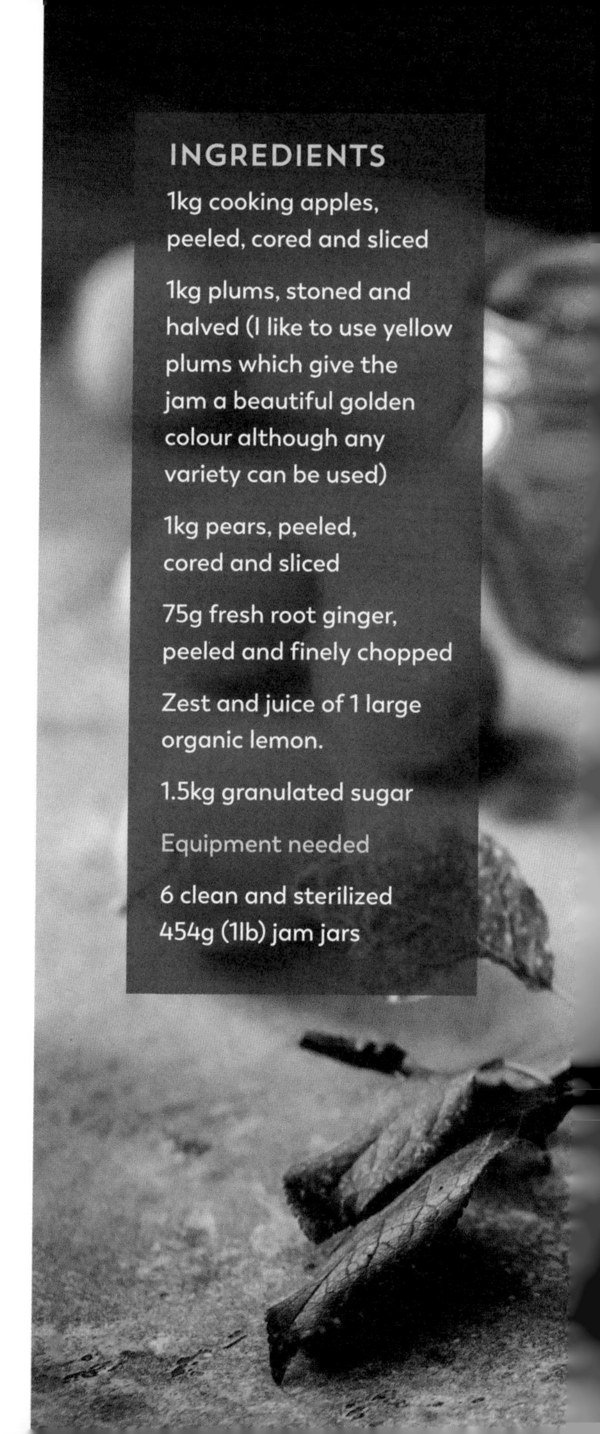

INGREDIENTS

1kg cooking apples, peeled, cored and sliced

1kg plums, stoned and halved (I like to use yellow plums which give the jam a beautiful golden colour although any variety can be used)

1kg pears, peeled, cored and sliced

75g fresh root ginger, peeled and finely chopped

Zest and juice of 1 large organic lemon.

1.5kg granulated sugar

Equipment needed

6 clean and sterilized 454g (1lb) jam jars

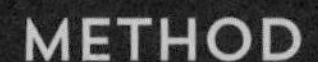

METHOD

Place the prepared apples, pears, plums and ginger in a preserving pan or large heavy bottomed pan with just enough water to cover the base.

Simmer until all the fruit is soft, about 45 minutes.

Off the heat carefully stir in the sugar until dissolved, add the lemon zest and juice.

Boil hard for about 15 minutes without stirring until the setting point is reached (see page 16).

Pour into warm sterilized jars, seal and allow to cool before labelling.

I always reduce the amount of sugar when I make jam as it tastes better and is slightly healthier.

It will keep for a year, once open keep it in the fridge.

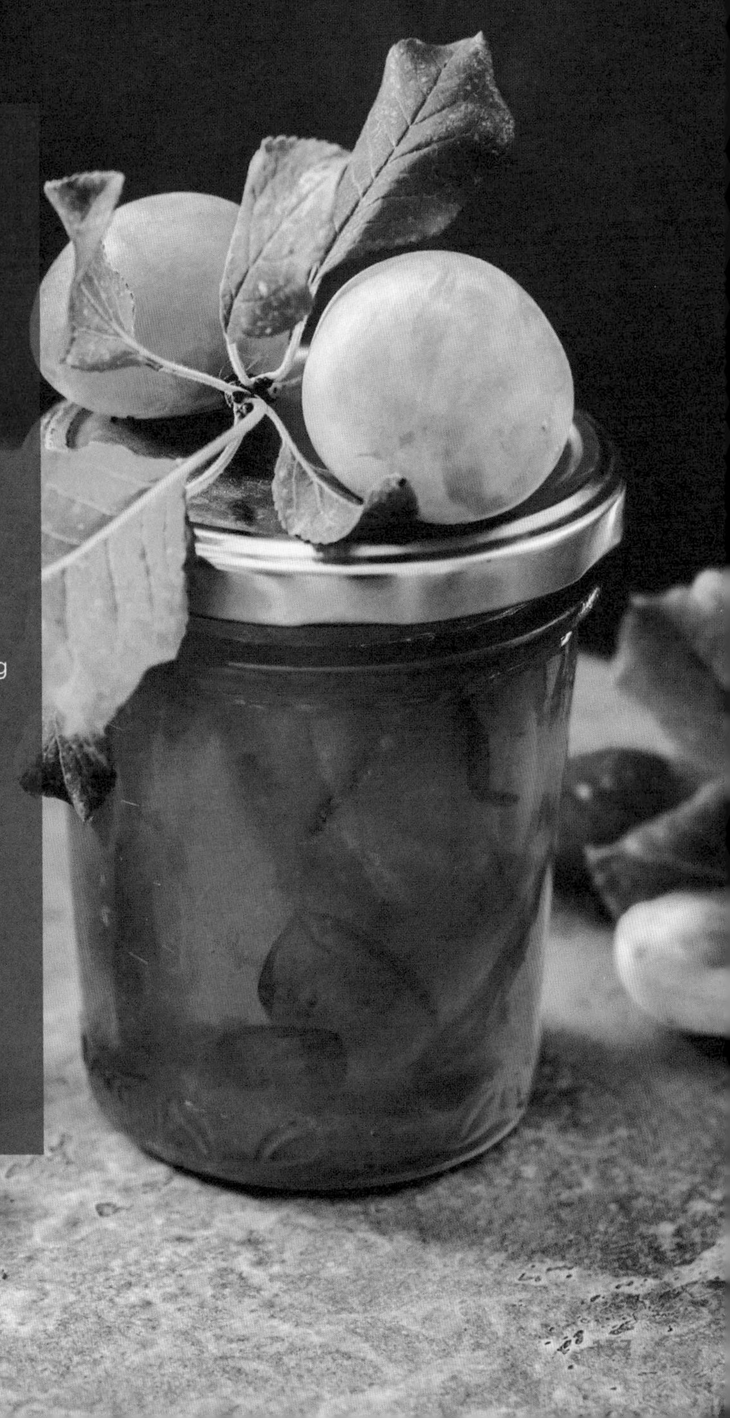

GINGER POACHED PEAR COLD REMEDY

Pears are high in vitamin C and contain powerful antioxidants to combat free radicals and support the immune system.

Ginger can reduce inflammation and congestion as well as being anti-viral, antibacterial and antioxidant. Indulge yourself with this remedy at the first sign of a cold – what a delicious way to take your medicine!

Makes one mug

INGREDIENTS

1 pesticide-free pear quartered and core removed

A large thumb-sized piece of ginger, sliced

200ml water

Cloves and cinnamon to taste

METHOD

Put all ingredients in a pan; simmer until the pear is cooked.

Eat the poached pear while warm.

Drink the juice sweetened with a little raw honey or maple syrup if needed.

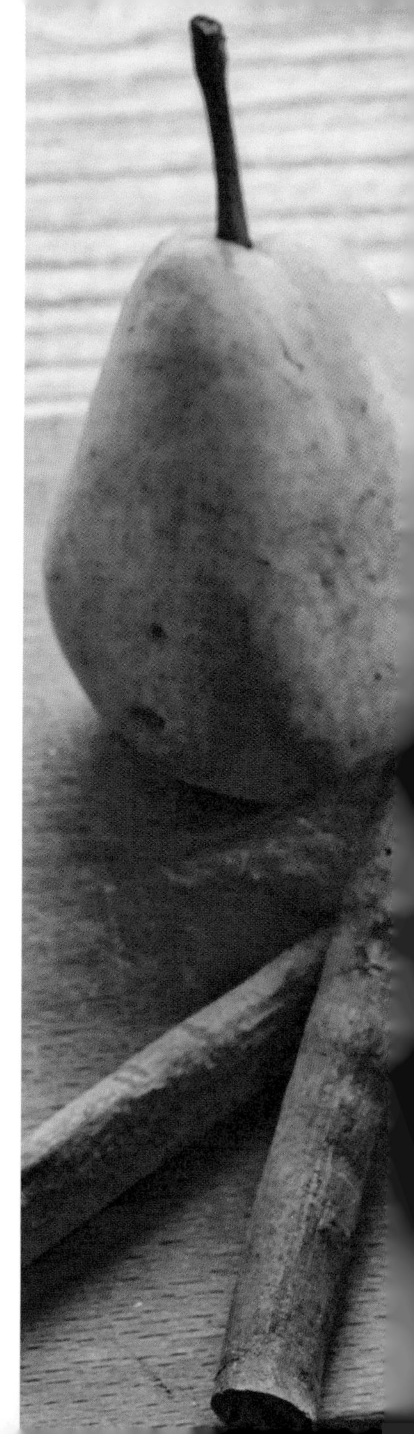

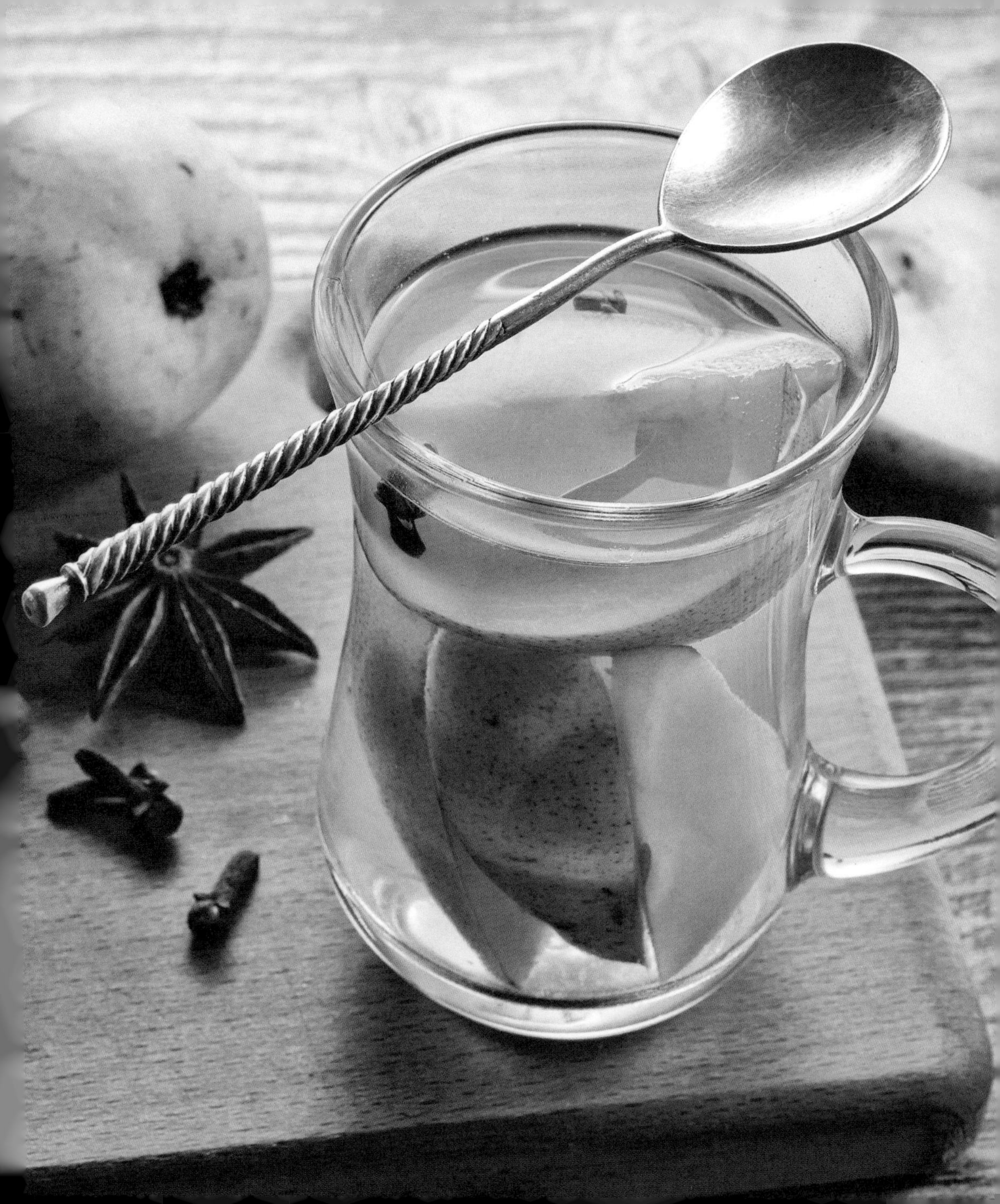

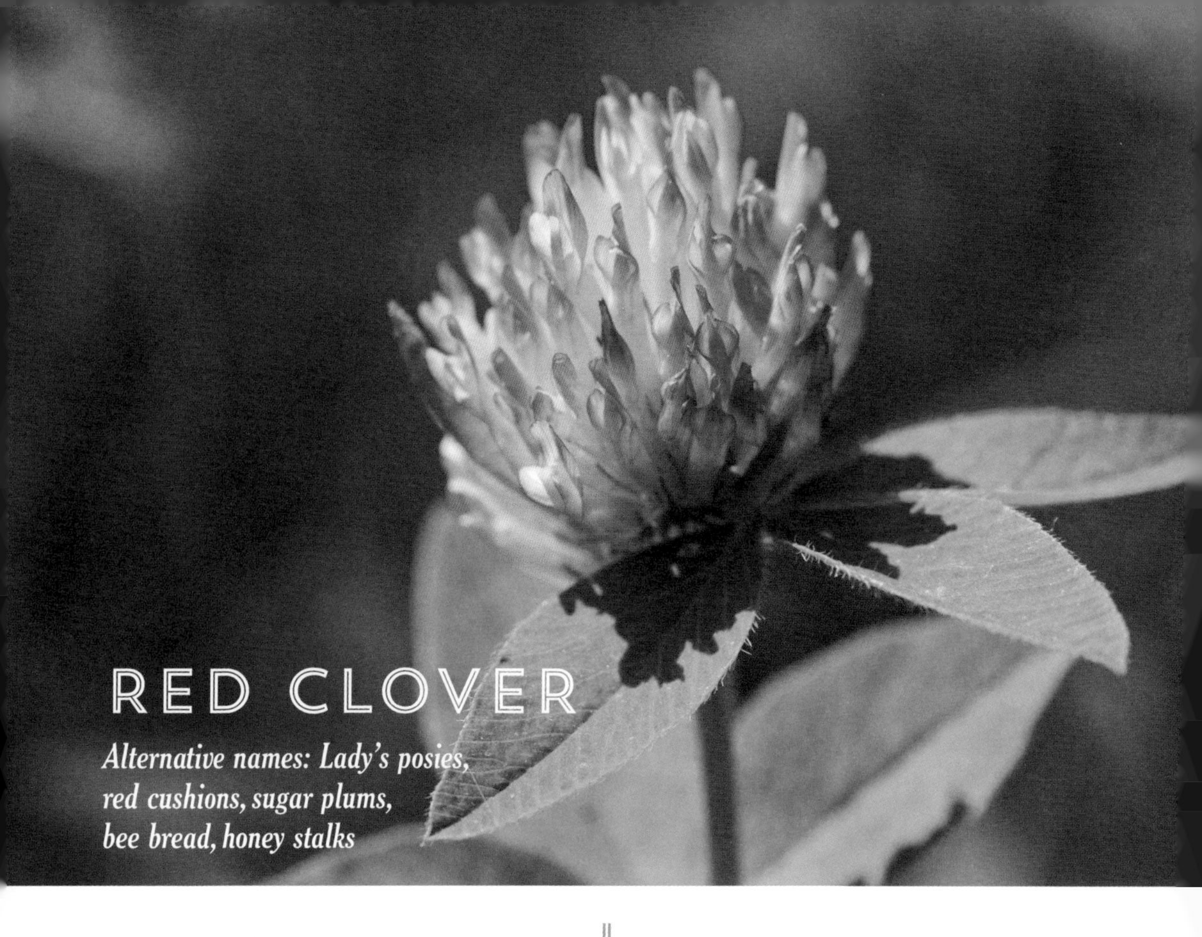

RED CLOVER

Alternative names: Lady's posies, red cushions, sugar plums, bee bread, honey stalks

HOW TO IDENTIFY: This three-leaf clover is commonly found growing in grassy areas and lawns all over Europe. The petite bobble-topped magenta wild flower is a constant irritant to "stripy lawn" gardeners, but a firm favourite with bees, rabbits and cattle.

HISTORY: Introduced from Europe in the seventeenth century as an important pasture crop for cattle, red clover's nitrogen producing roots make it an extremely useful plant for crop rotation.

FOLKLORE: Having three leaves, clover has always been associated with the holy trinity, giving it the ability to keep away evil spirits. Witches become more powerful if they manage to find a five-leaf clover and maidens hope to find a two-leafed clover as they will be able to see their future spouse. Medieval children believed that carrying a four-leaf clover would allow them to see faeries.

Washing with an infusion of red clover made with the morning dew will make freckles disappear, or bathe surrounded by clover if you wish to become rich. Mopping the floor with clover water will chase away any unwelcome spirits in the home.

FOLK MEDICINE: Pliny the Elder recommended that red clover be used to treat bladder stones and dropsy (swellings under the skin), and also as a diuretic as well as for cleansing the liver and improving the circulation.

Honey infused with red clover flowers was considered to be an effective treatment for coughs, bronchitis, asthma and whooping cough. The flowers can be rubbed onto insect bites and stings for instant relief from itching.

Bathing irritated skin in a solution of red clover can give relief from eczema and psoriasis, help soothe itchy scalps and speed up the healing of wounds.

OTHER COMMON USES: More recently red clover has been used by menopausal women to help treat hot flushes and night sweats, and to balance hormones.

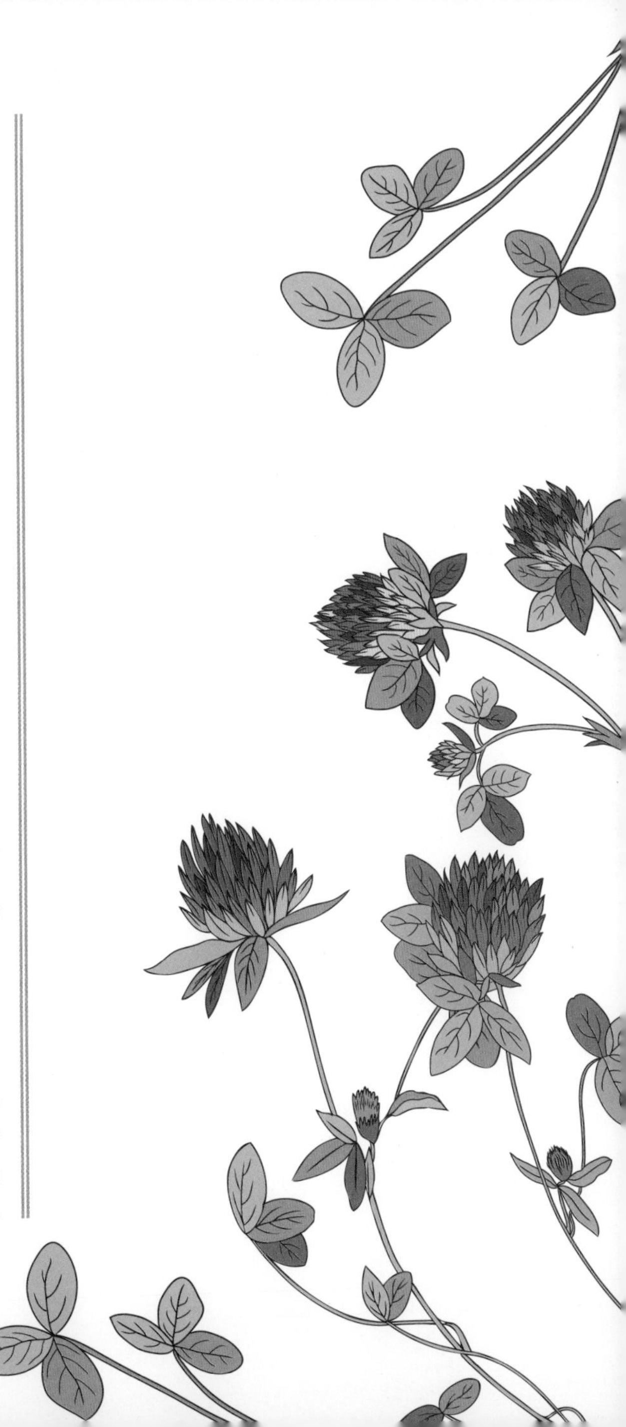

RED CLOVER LEMONADE

Pull off a tiny floret of red clover and you'll be able to suck out its beautiful sweet nectar – no wonder cattle love it so much! Try to pick your red clover flowers as soon as they bloom, keeping away from dog-walking areas and places that may have been sprayed with pesticides.

You would have to eat a lot of red clover blossoms to gain any medicinal benefit; this lemonade is intended as a refreshing and fun summer drink.

Some blossoms frozen in ice cubes in boiled water (to make them clear) would be a really pretty addition to this lemonade.

Makes 500ml

INGREDIENTS

30 fresh red clover blossoms

500ml water

Juice of 1 large organic lemon

Raw honey or maple syrup, to taste

METHOD

Place the blossoms and water in a saucepan and simmer gently for 15 minutes.

Strain the liquid into a jug, compost the blossoms.

Stir in the lemon juice and honey or maple syrup until well mixed.

Chill in the fridge before serving.

Not recommended during pregnancy.

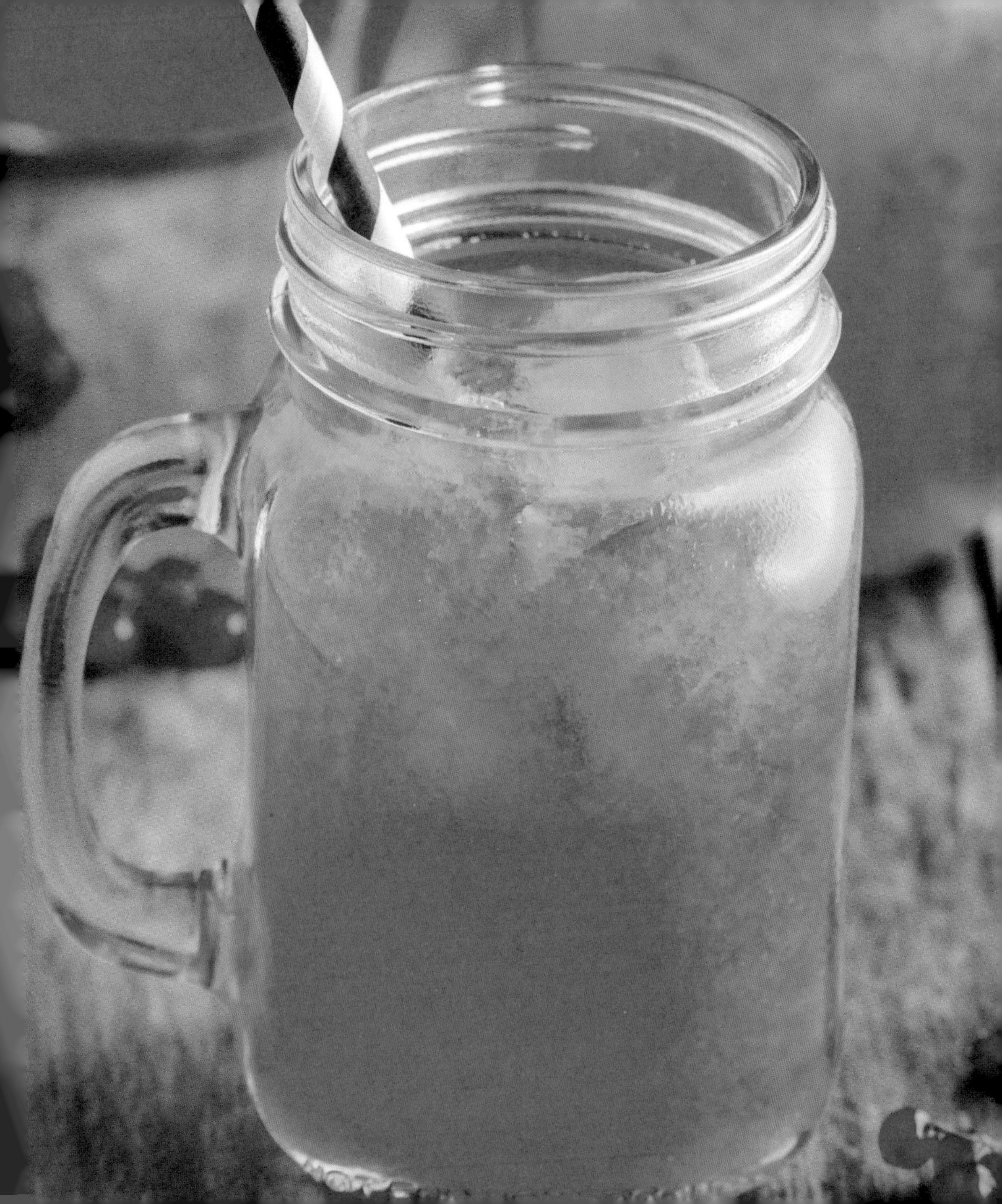

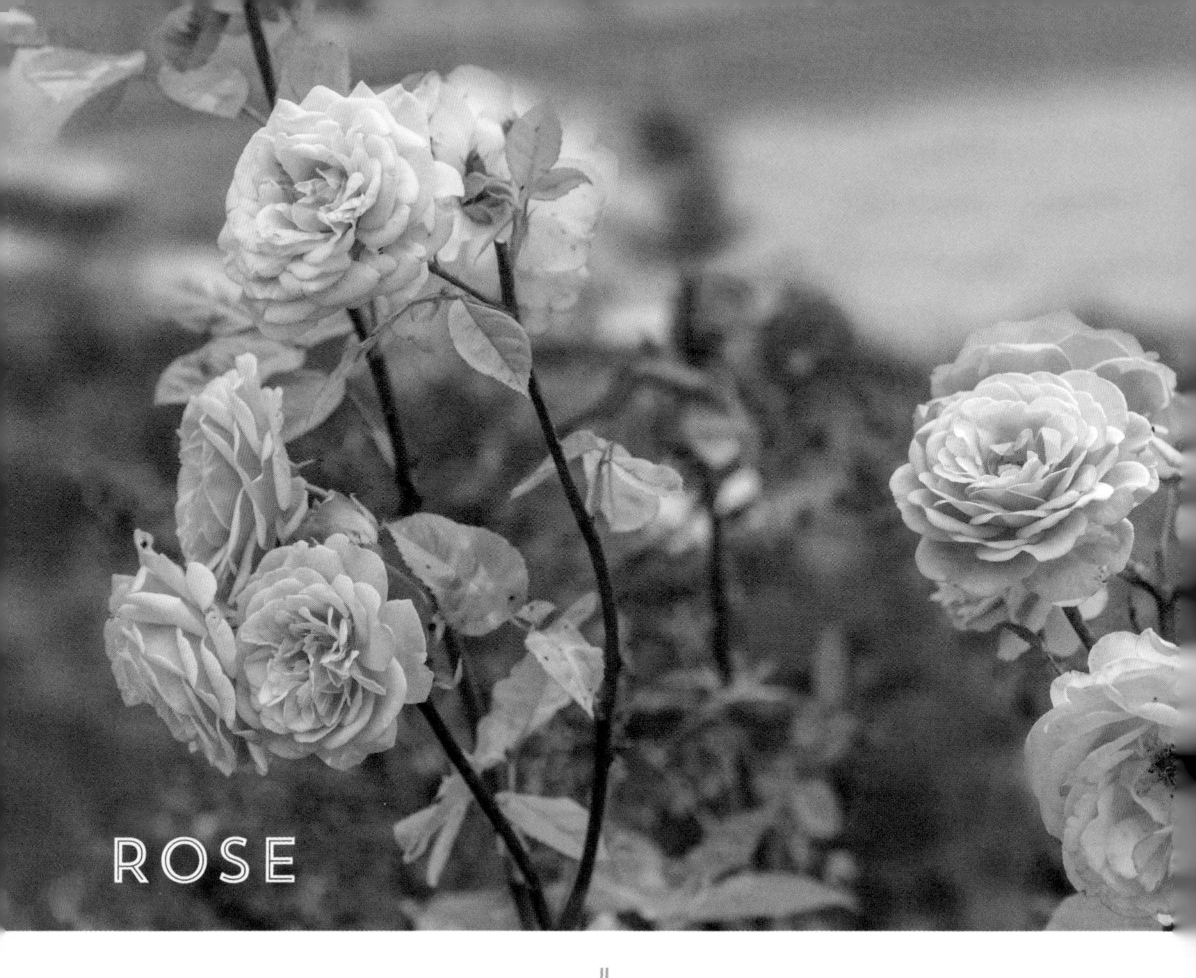

ROSE

HOW TO IDENTIFY: Roses are easily recognized by their prickly stems and fragrant sweet perfume. Pale pink dog roses can be found climbing through hedgerows in the spring to be followed by bright red hips in the autumn. Cultivated garden roses have been grown for their perfume and appearance and have many more petals and colours than wild roses.

HISTORY: Roses were first cultivated in Iran where there was a thriving trade in roses for use in medicine and perfume.

Rosa gallica "Officinalis" or "The Apothecary Rose" was the first species to be cultivated in Europe and was much painted by Renaissance artists. Dried petals were rolled into beads and strung together into "rosaries", as the flower's deep pink colour was said to represent the blood of the Christian martyrs.

FOLKLORE: Midsummer's Eve has traditionally been a popular time for casting love spells; young girls in Somerset would go to the churchyard at midnight and scatter rose petals around them saying: "*Rose leaves, rose leaves, rose leaves I strew. He that will love me, come for me now.*" A vision of their future love would purportedly appear behind them.

A rose picked at midnight on Midsummer's Eve would be wrapped in white tissue and safely stored away until Christmas Day. If the rose was still in bloom, it would be worn by the maiden to be admired at the festivities by her future husband.

Rose magic is not just for girls; a young man will have luck with the ladies he meets if he wears a rose in his buttonhole.

White roses, along with many other white flowers, were once believed to be unlucky and often an omen of death, their scent understood to be "bad for the brain". In more recent times, white roses have been traditional at weddings to symbolize innocence, loyalty and everlasting love.

Throwing rose leaves into the fire will attract good luck; planting roses beside a loved one's grave protects them from evil spirits; a white rose was used to mark a virgin's grave, and a red rose to signify a person who had shown kindness and charity. Only give tightly closed rosebuds as gifts, as any petals that fall off could bring certain death to the recipient.

In Transylvania, witches will ride on the backs of cattle unless the farmer plants wild roses by the gate to their fields.

FOLK MEDICINE: Culpeper recommends syrup of dried roses as it "*strengthens the heart, comforts the spirits, binds the body, helps fluxes and corrosions or gnawing of the bowels, it strengthens the stomach and stays vomiting.*"

Rosehip syrup is bursting with vitamin C and has long been made by country people as a powerful remedy for colds and flu.

Rose water was used to fade scars, reduce redness, and as a soothing compress for headaches.

Rose petal tea is a gentle diuretic with the added benefit of being an aphrodisiac.

OTHER COMMON USES: Dried rose petals thrown at weddings are an eco-friendly alternative to commercially produced confetti. Rose petals are edible and can be made into jams and vinegars or crystallized to decorate cakes.

ROSE AND LAVENDER BODY DUST

A silky homemade "talcum powder" this rose and lavender body dust will help to keep skin dry and prevent soreness through chafing. Making your own cooling dusting powder means you can choose which ingredients will benefit your skin type: pick from rose, lavender, calendula, sage, peppermint, violets and many more.

Rose petals are hydrating and nourishing with antioxidant, antiseptic and antibacterial properties to soothe the skin. Lavender is anti-fungal and anti-inflammatory making it a perfect partner for rose. This body dust uses ingredients that you probably have in your kitchen cupboard and flowers from your garden – what could be easier?

Makes 200g

INGREDIENTS

100g cornflour

50g bicarbonate of soda

25g dried rose petals

25g dried lavender flowers

2 drops rose essential oil

2 drops lavender essential oil

Equipment needed

Food processor

Fine sieve

Powder puff or empty talc container

METHOD

Put the cornflour, bicarbonate of soda, rose petals and lavender flowers in a food processor and pulse until you have a fine powder.

Add the essential oils and pulse again to mix.

Use a sieve to create a fine, soft powder.

Dust liberally onto dry skin after a bath using a powder puff or shaker.

To be used sparingly on intimate areas.

SOOTHING ROSE LIP BALM

Make sure that you use pesticide-free roses with a good scent for this remedy or they may not contain the beneficial properties that you need. The raw honey is antibacterial and antioxidant for healing, aloe vera adds moisture to dry lips and vitamin E oil promotes cell generation.

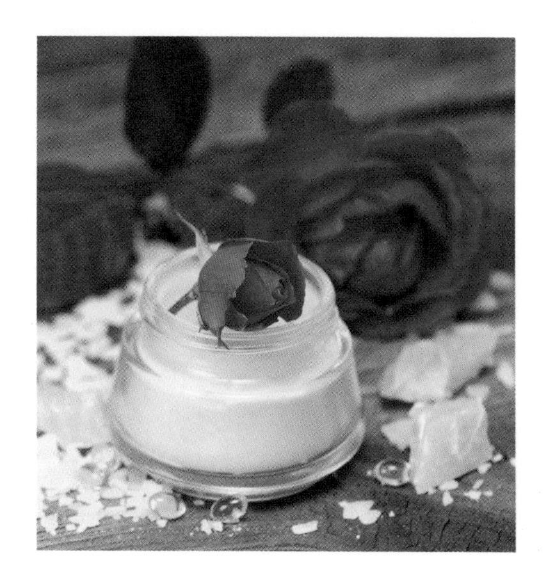

Makes about 110ml

INGREDIENTS

100ml rose infused carrier oil

10g unrefined beeswax, or soya wax for a vegan alternative

1 tsp raw runny honey, or use maple syrup for a vegan alternative

½ tsp aloe vera gel

½ tsp vitamin E oil

Equipment needed

Heatproof bowl

Small jars or tins

METHOD

Melt the rose oil with the beeswax in a heatproof bowl over a pan of boiling water.

When the wax has dissolved take off the heat, add the honey, aloe vera and vitamin E oil stirring all the time.

Pour into small sterilized jars or tins; allow to cool completely before covering with a lid.

For a tinted lip balm, rose petal or beetroot powder can be added to the melted mixture.

Keeps in the fridge for 6 months.

Apply as needed.

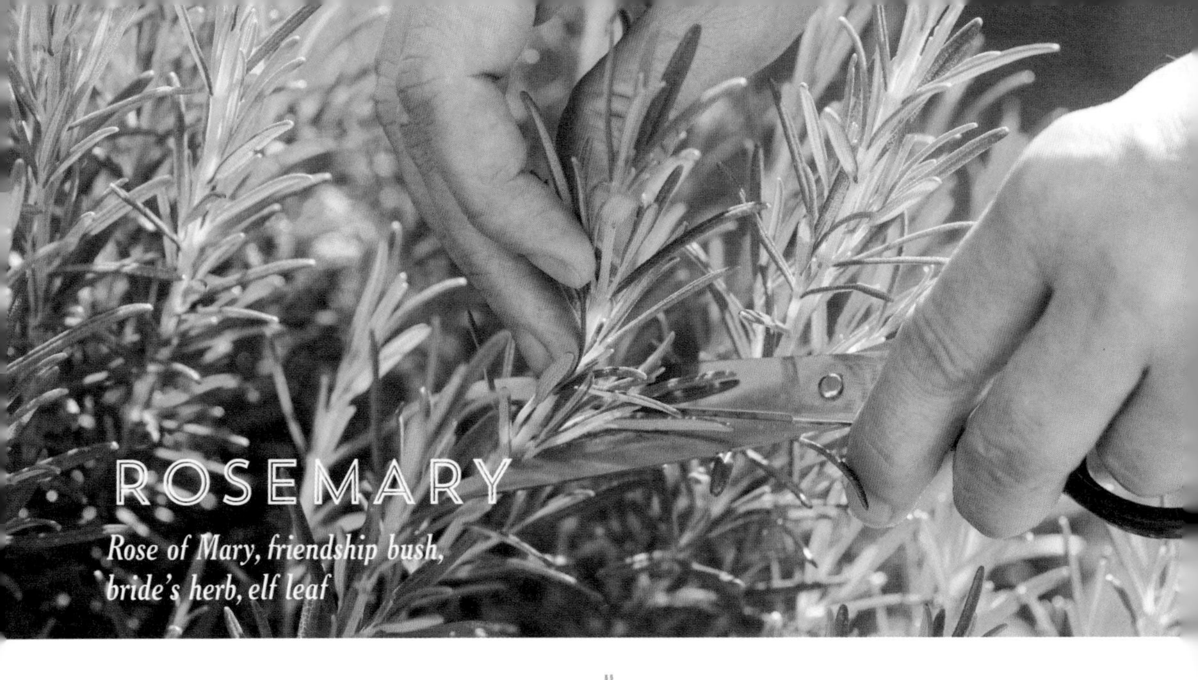

ROSEMARY

Rose of Mary, friendship bush, bride's herb, elf leaf

HOW TO IDENTIFY: Rosemary is a tall fragrant bluish grey herb with needle-like leaves and tiny blue flowers.

HISTORY: Queen Philippa, the wife of King Edward III, received the first rosemary cuttings from her mother from Belgium in the fourteenth century. These were planted in the garden of their royal residence in the old palace of Westminster.

By the sixteenth century its popularity had spread and rosemary had become common in many gardens. John Parkinson, herbalist to Charles I, noted: "*not only that rosemary grew in every Englishwoman's garden, but that it was commonly used as a token at both weddings and funerals.*"

Anne of Cleves carried rosemary in her wedding bouquet when she married Henry VIII to symbolize love and fidelity. Unfortunately, it didn't really work for her and she was queen for just six months.

The rosemary in a bridal bouquet should then be planted in the garden to be used at the weddings of daughters and granddaughters.

Rosemary is frequently referenced by William Shakespeare, for example, in Hamlet, Ophelia says: "*There's rosemary, that's for remembrance. Pray you love remember.*" While in *A Winter's Tale* Perdita welcomes the disguised king with a posy of herbs: "*there's rosemary and rue... grace and remembrance to you both.*"

Rosemary was laid with the dead to disguise bad smells and each mourner would throw a sprig onto the coffin as it was interred as a symbol of remembrance.

FOLKLORE: While fleeing from Egypt the Virgin Mary laid her blue cloak over a white flowering rosemary bush to let it dry, turning the flowers blue forever.

It is also believed that rosemary can only grow to the height of Jesus and will only live to 33 years, which was Jesus' age at the time of his crucifixion.

Growing rosemary in your garden not only protects your family from witches but also ensures that you will never be short of friends. It grows particularly well in the garden of a dominant wife!

In the fourteenth century the feet of thieves were washed in rosemary vinegar, supposedly to sap their energy and stop them from committing further crimes.

Hung over cradles, rosemary was said to protect babies from being stolen by faeries, sniffed regularly this herb will help you age gracefully and a man that doesn't love the smell of rosemary will never find true love.

FOLK MEDICINE: During the plague in the seventeenth century, rosemary was hung in houses and worn around the neck for protection from contagion. In London alone, 75,000 people died from the plague making rosemary a very valuable commodity. In 1625 the price rose from 1 shilling (5p) for an armful of rosemary branches to a whopping 6 shillings (30p) for just a handful, bearing in mind that you could buy a whole pig for just 1 shilling (5p) that does seem hugely expensive!

Culpeper recommended many uses of rosemary:

"It helps a weak memory and quickens the senses... It is a remedy for the windiness of the stomach, bowels and spleen, and expels it powerfully... It helps dim eyes, and procures a clear sight, the flowers thereof being taken all the while it is flowering every morning fasting, with bread and salt."

Rosemary was burned with juniper in hospitals and sick rooms to cleanse the air and stop the spread of infection. It was often hung over the bed in a green cloth bag with some pennies as this was believed to boost fertility.

OTHER COMMON USES: Recent studies suggest that the scent of rosemary essential oil can improve performance in exams by stimulating the memory quite significantly – one for those of you with teenage children to remember.

ROSEMARY MOUTHWASH

Homemade mouthwash allows you to be in control of the ingredients – there are no hidden chemicals or nasties in here and it works out cheaper too!

Rosemary's antibacterial properties help to fight bad breath and plaque build up, mint is antibacterial and anti-inflammatory, and cloves have long been used in oral products for gingivitis and as a mild anaesthetic for toothache.

Make a fresh batch of mouthwash every week. Swoosh after brushing but don't swallow.

Makes 500ml

INGREDIENTS

500ml boiling water

1 tsp fresh pesticide-free rosemary leaves, chopped

1 tsp fresh pesticide-free mint or peppermint leaves, chopped

1 tsp cloves

Equipment needed

Clean 500ml glass bottle

METHOD

Add the boiling water to a saucepan along with all the other ingredients.

Simmer for 20 minutes then allow to cool.

Strain the liquid into a clean bottle.

Pour a shot-sized amount of the mouthwash into a glass.

Swoosh around the mouth thoroughly then spit out.

Large amounts of rosemary are not recommended during pregnancy.

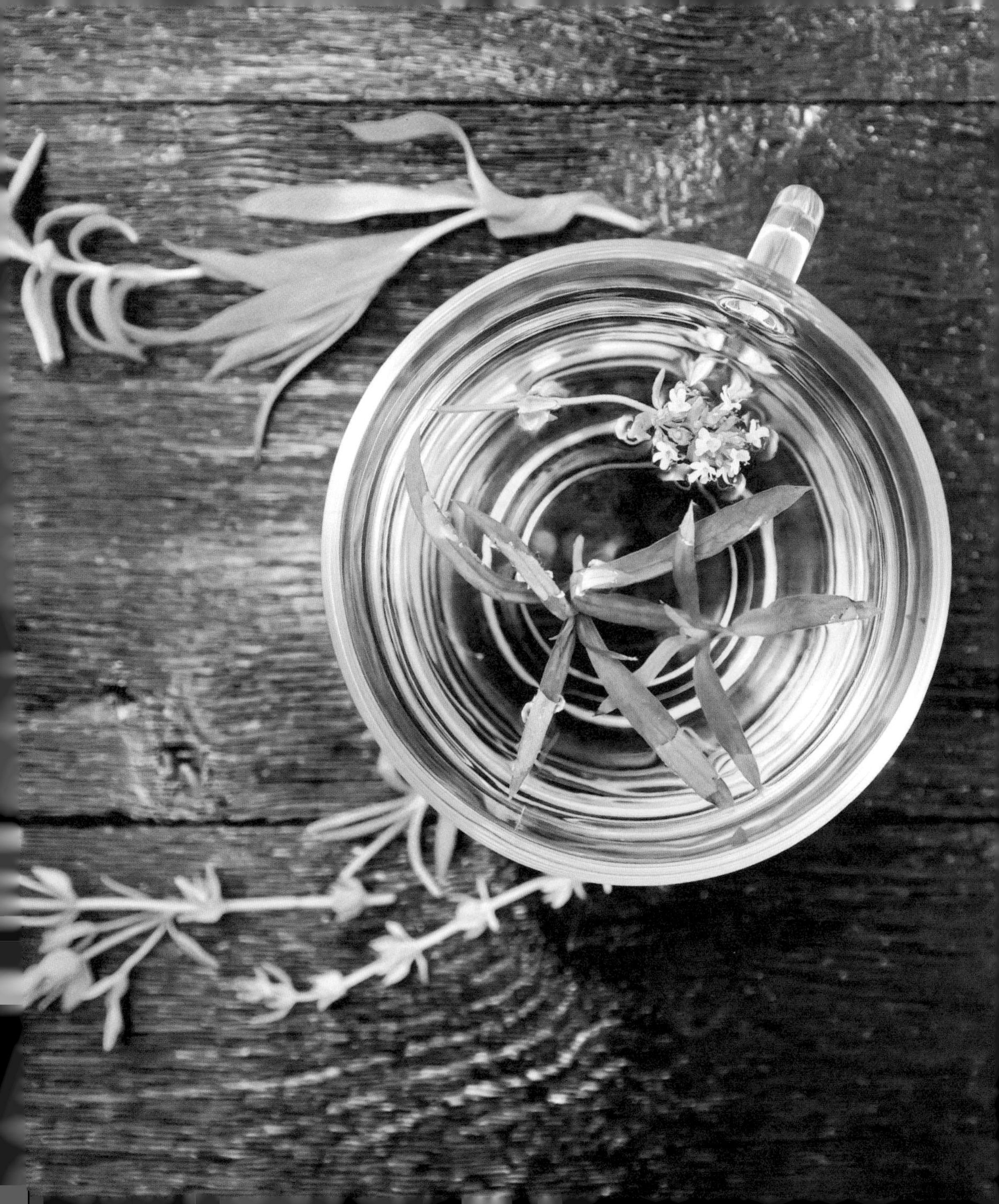

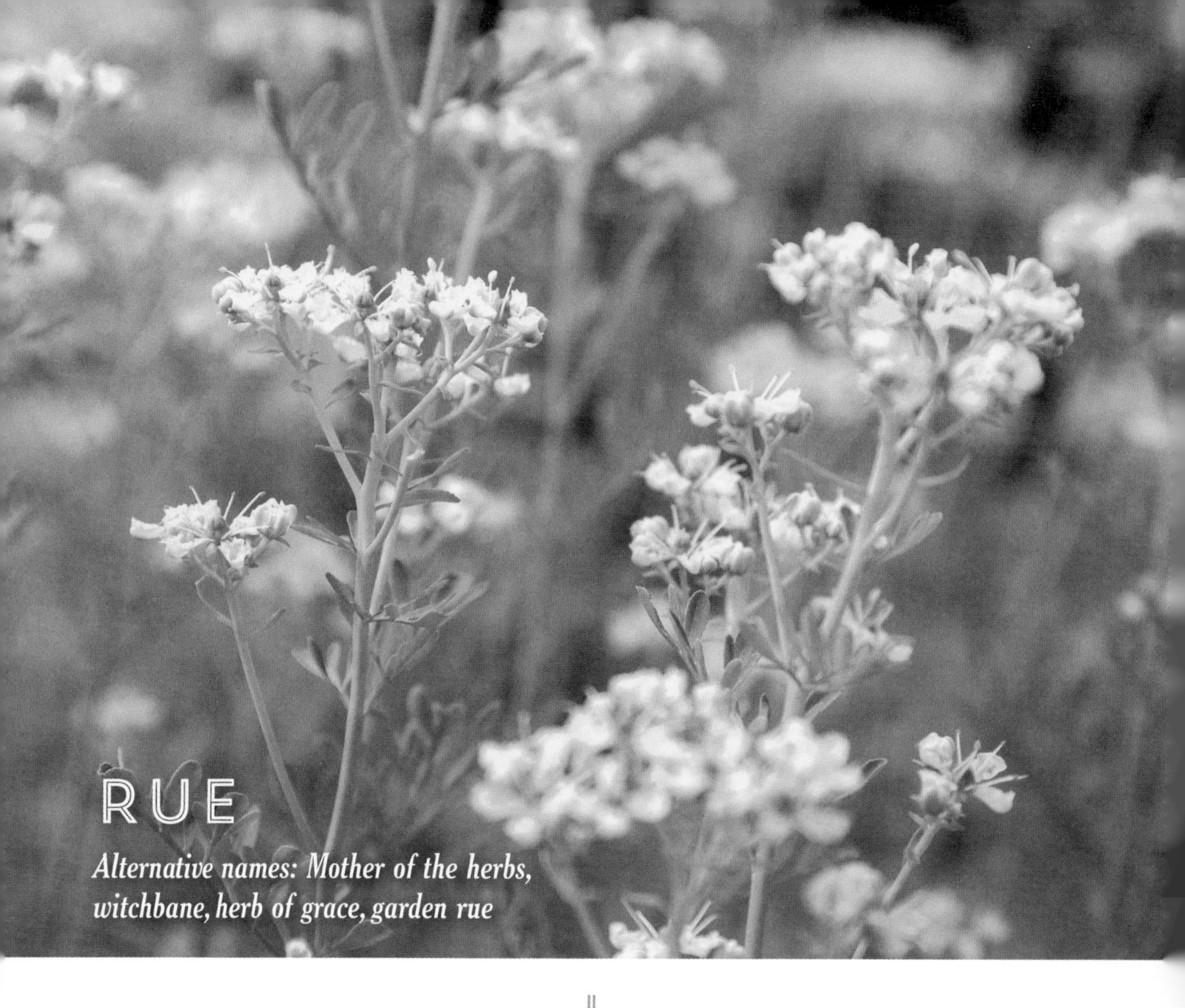

RUE

Alternative names: Mother of the herbs, witchbane, herb of grace, garden rue

HOW TO IDENTIFY: Rue has bluish green fern-like leaves and four-petalled yellow flowers.

HISTORY: Rue is one of the oldest garden plants, grown for its medicinal and domestic uses, in Europe. Regarded by the Romans and Greeks as protective against the "evil eye" rue was brought to our shores by the Roman invaders.

The Catholic Church used sprigs of rue to sprinkle holy water onto the congregation before high mass and exorcisms, and sprigs of rue were placed on coffins to protect the dead in the afterlife leading to its moniker "herb of grace".

FOLKLORE: Be careful where you plant rue; it is beneficial if grown next to fig trees, however it can alter the soil around its roots killing off or inhibiting the growth of sage, cabbages, peas, beans and strawberries.

Plants or cuttings of rue that have been stolen are believed to grow much better than bought ones; this is apparently true of roses, too.

Bunches of rue were hung around the waist and over doors and windows to deter witches, giving rise to one of its alternative names, witchbane.

In Italy silver charms in the form of a rue stem were hung above babies' cots and worn around the neck of adults as protection from witches. The charm consisted of a rue stem hung with several apotropaic talismans (charms that repel evil) – these could be a rose, a wand, a crescent moon, a snake; the charms can vary from region to region and often include Catholic symbolism.

FOLK MEDICINE: Houses facing east were believed to be particularly at risk from the plague as they could be infected by the "air blows from France". Our ancestors believed that the infection was airborne and hung rue above windows and doors as well as strewing the herb on the floor – much more effective as rats and fleas detest rue!

Culpeper had much to say about rue:

"An ointment made of the juice thereof with oil of roses, ceruse, and a little vinegar, and anointed cures St. Anthony's fire [poisoning from fungus on rye bread] and all running sores in the head: and the stinking ulcers of the nose or other parts... The juice thereof warmed in a pomegranate shell or rind, and dropped into the ears, helps the pain of them."

Caution: Rue needs to be treated with respect; juice from the plant can cause photosensitivity and skin irritation and it should never be used during pregnancy.

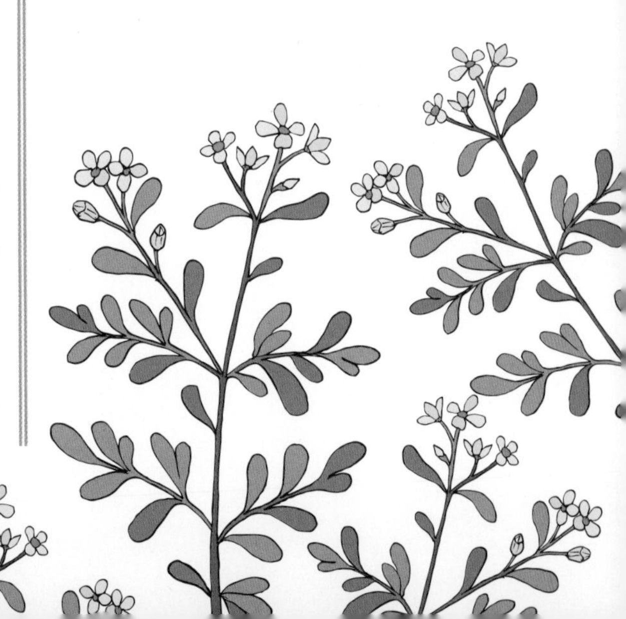

BUG REPELLENT LOTION BAR

Rue is a proven insect deterrent, however due to its many contraindications I have chosen not to use it in this recipe. These lotion bars are easy to carry, quick to apply and will keep most biting bugs away.

Makes approximately 120ml

INGREDIENTS

35g organic shea butter

35ml carrier oil

45g unrefined beeswax (I source mine from a local beekeeper)

10 drops citronella essential oil (insect repelling and wound healing)

10 drops lemongrass essential oil (gnats hate it)

5 drops tea tree essential oil (repels mosquitoes and soothes the skin)

5 drops cedarwood essential oil (repels ticks)

Equipment needed

Heatproof bowl

Silicone moulds

METHOD

Melt the beeswax, shea butter and carrier oil in a heatproof bowl placed over a pan of boiling water.

Once melted, take the mixture off the heat, combine and stir in the essential oil.

Pour into silicone moulds if you have them or you can use cupcake cases or any small flexible containers that you have around the kitchen.

Allow to cool completely before popping out of the mould.

The lotion bar will melt when rubbed over your skin before going outside and will remain solid at room temperature.

Always do a patch test before using.

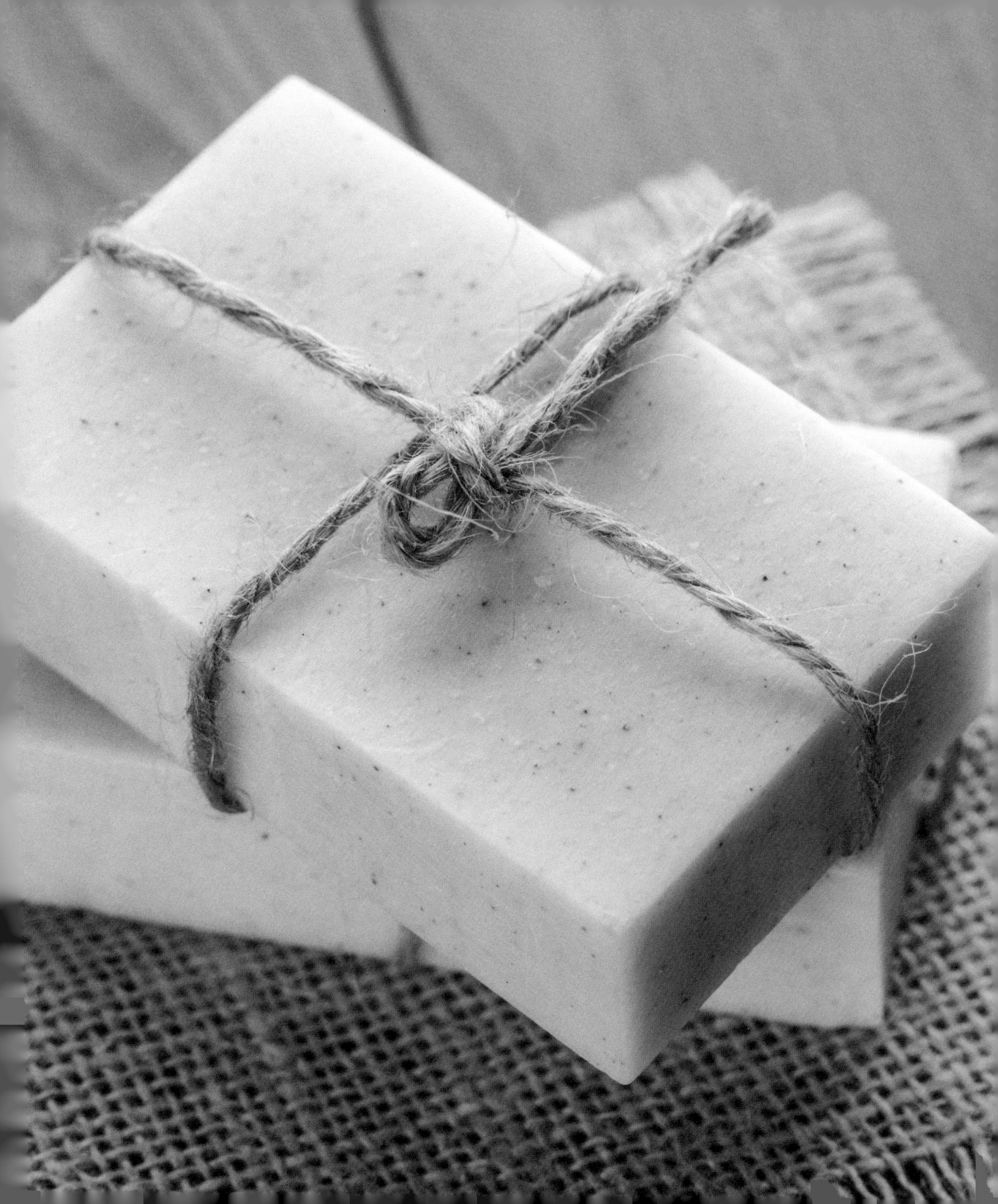

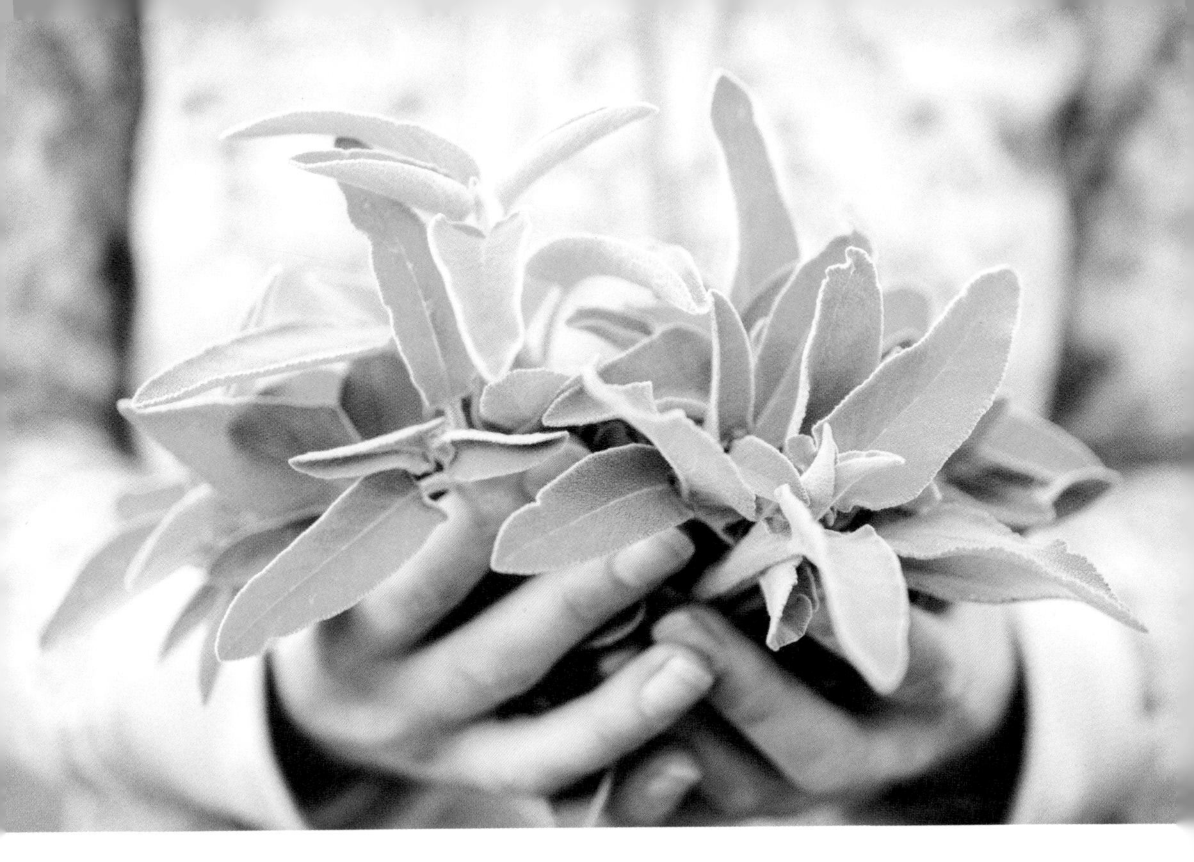

SAGE

Alternative names: Garden sage, Salvia officinalis, culinary sage, clairvoyant sage

HOW TO IDENTIFY: With soft, greyish green hairy leaves this square stemmed herb can grow up to 1.5 metres (5 feet) tall and can be identified by its distinctive strong earthy, musky smell.

HISTORY: Sage tea was drunk by Egyptian and Roman women to aid fertility and as a cure for sore throats. The Romans also used it to help them digest the fatty foods that were a big part of their diet. Like so many herbs that we rely on today, sage was introduced by the Romans for its medicinal and culinary properties. By the Middle Ages its use was well established in apothecary gardens and monasteries around the country.

FOLKLORE: In the Middle Ages it was wise to look after the sage growing in your garden as if it grew well the fortunes and health of the household would prosper, too. Similar to rosemary it was believed that sage would grow well in the garden of a dominant woman – some men would cut the sage down rather than suffer the ridicule of friends and neighbours.

"If the sage tree thrives and grows, the master's not the master, and he knows."
J. A. Langford, Warwickshire
Folk-Lore and Superstitions 1875

To manifest a wish, write it on a sage leaf and sleep with it under your pillow for three days then bury it in your garden.

Carrying sage can make you wise (hence the name) and by eating it every day in May you will enjoy a long and healthy life.

The burning of different herbs has long been used in many different cultures to cleanse, protect and purify houses, cattle and people. Smudging, involving burning dry bundles of white sage to create a cleansing smoke, is used during exorcisms to drive out negative influences, bad spirits and to protect from evil.

FOLK MEDICINE: Many cures use sage for healthy teeth and gums; a traditional Romany toothpaste recipe from the 1940s consisted of equal parts chopped sage and salt mixed together to be rubbed onto the teeth using Irish linen. A sage leaf with the vein removed can be put underneath dentures to relieve sore gums.

Sage was also used by dark-haired Romanies as a rinse to banish dandruff and keep their beautiful black hair from showing grey.

Regarded as a cure-all by many, Culpeper recommended that:

"The juice of sage in warm water helps the hoarseness or the cough. The leaves sodden in wine and laid upon the place affected with the palsy helps much, if the decoction be drank... helps the stinging and biting of serpents, and kills the worms that breed in the ear and in sores. The juice of sage drank in vinegar, hath been of good use in time of plague."

OTHER COMMON USES: Sage and onion stuffing not only tastes great but will help you digest your Sunday lunch, too!

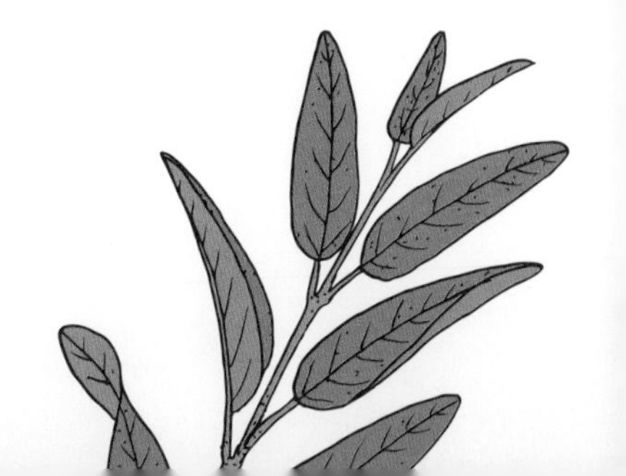

SAGE AND OREGANO FOOT POWDER

Sage is cooling and drying as well as being anti-fungal and antibacterial. Oregano also has natural anti-fungal and antibacterial properties, making it perfect for treating athlete's foot. Lemon essential oil is antibacterial and has a wonderful uplifting scent. Allow the leaves to dry completely on kitchen paper before using them, or use dried herbs instead for this recipe.

Makes 50g

INGREDIENTS

2 tbsp dried sage

4 tbsp dried oregano

20g cornflour

10 drops of lemon essential oil

Equipment needed

Herb grinder or pestle and mortar

Empty talc bottle or flour shaker

METHOD

Using a herb grinder or pestle and mortar crush the herbs to a fine powder.

Add in the cornflour and mix together thoroughly.

Add the lemon essential oil and combine.

Spread the powder onto a sheet of baking paper and allow to dry overnight.

Sift the powder to remove any lumps.

Store in an old talc container or flour shaker.

Sprinkle on clean dry feet, especially between the toes, daily and rub into the skin.

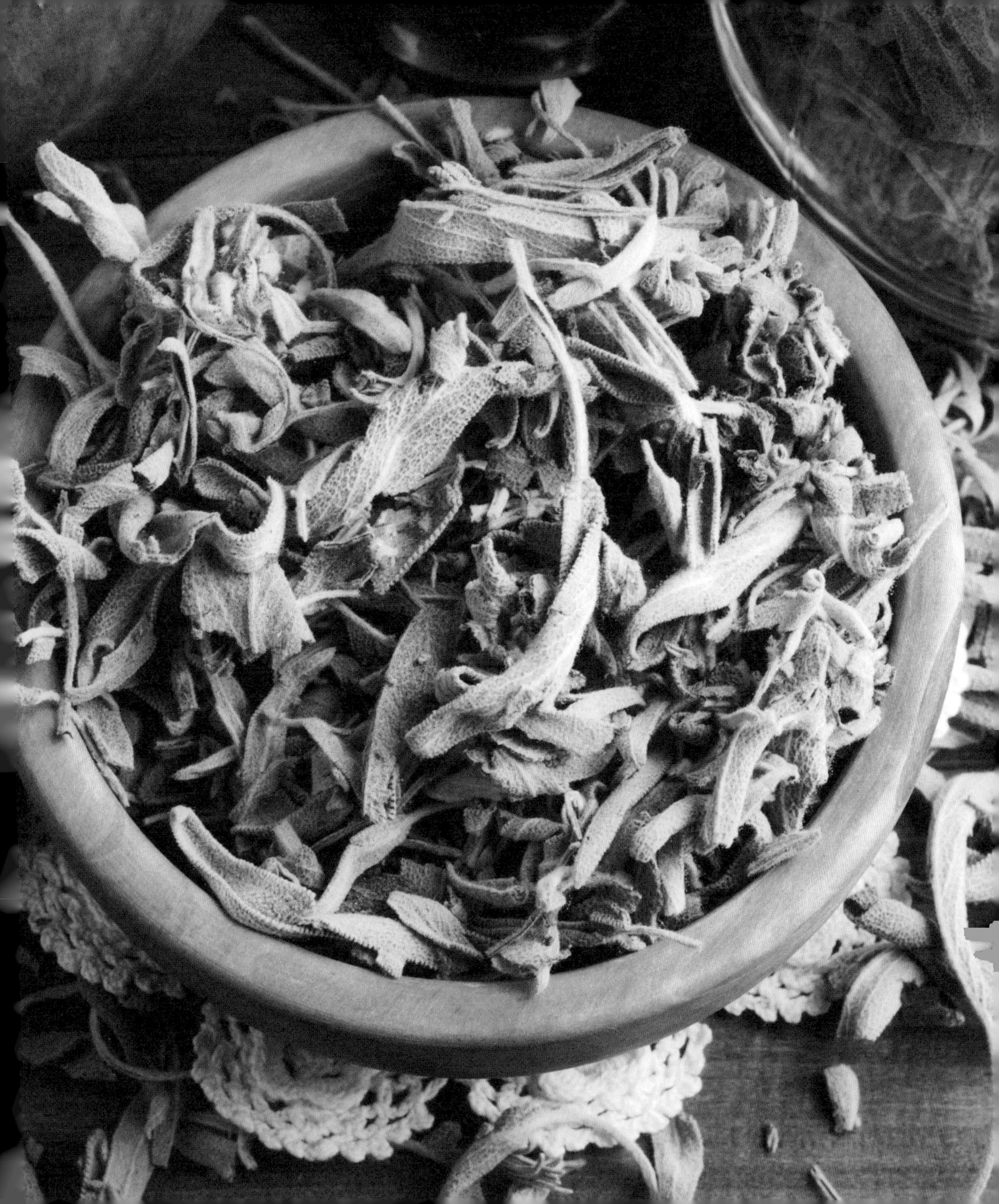

SAGE AND HONEY LINCTUS

Sage is anti-inflammatory and antibacterial, making it the perfect herb to help with this easy-to-make remedy. Raw honey, a traditional remedy for sore throats, is antioxidant, anti-inflammatory, anti-viral and anti-fungal. Supermarket honey has often been pasteurized, removing a lot of its health-giving properties; always try to source local raw honey if possible. Maple syrup or agave syrup can be substituted for honey if desired.

Makes 250ml

INGREDIENTS

Handful of fresh pesticide-free sage leaves

250ml raw runny honey

Equipment needed

Clean glass jar

METHOD

Wash and thoroughly dry the sage leaves, remove the stems. Pack the sage leaves into the jar.

Slowly drizzle in the honey allowing it to ooze between the leaves.

Stir well to cover all the leaves.

Leave for one to two weeks, stirring daily.

Take spoonfuls of the honey as needed or dilute with hot water and lemon for a soothing drink – the leaves can be added in, too.

Store in the fridge. Honey is a good preservative so it should keep for at least 6 months.

Sage is not recommended during pregnancy.

Raw honey is not to be given to children under 12 months old.

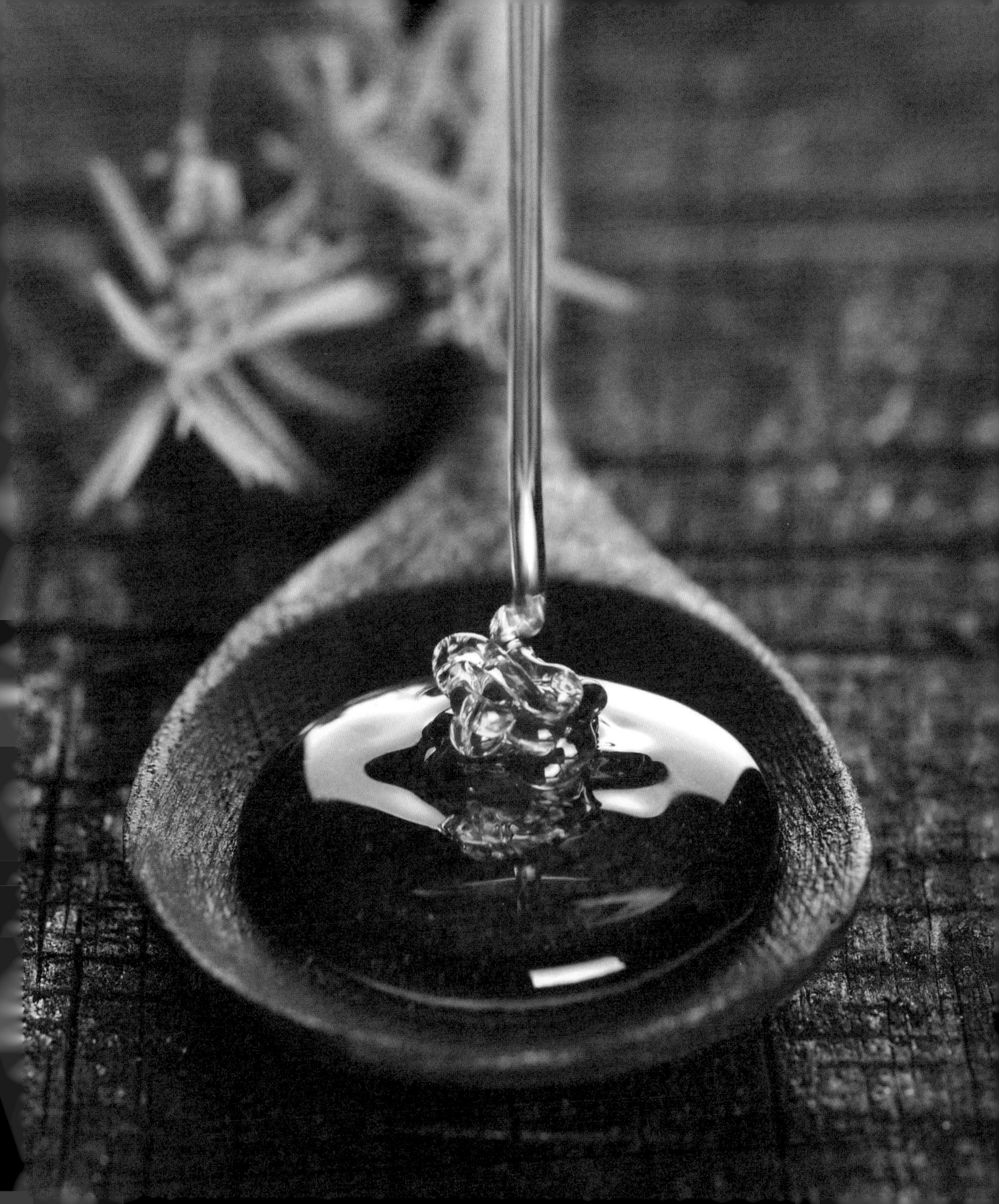

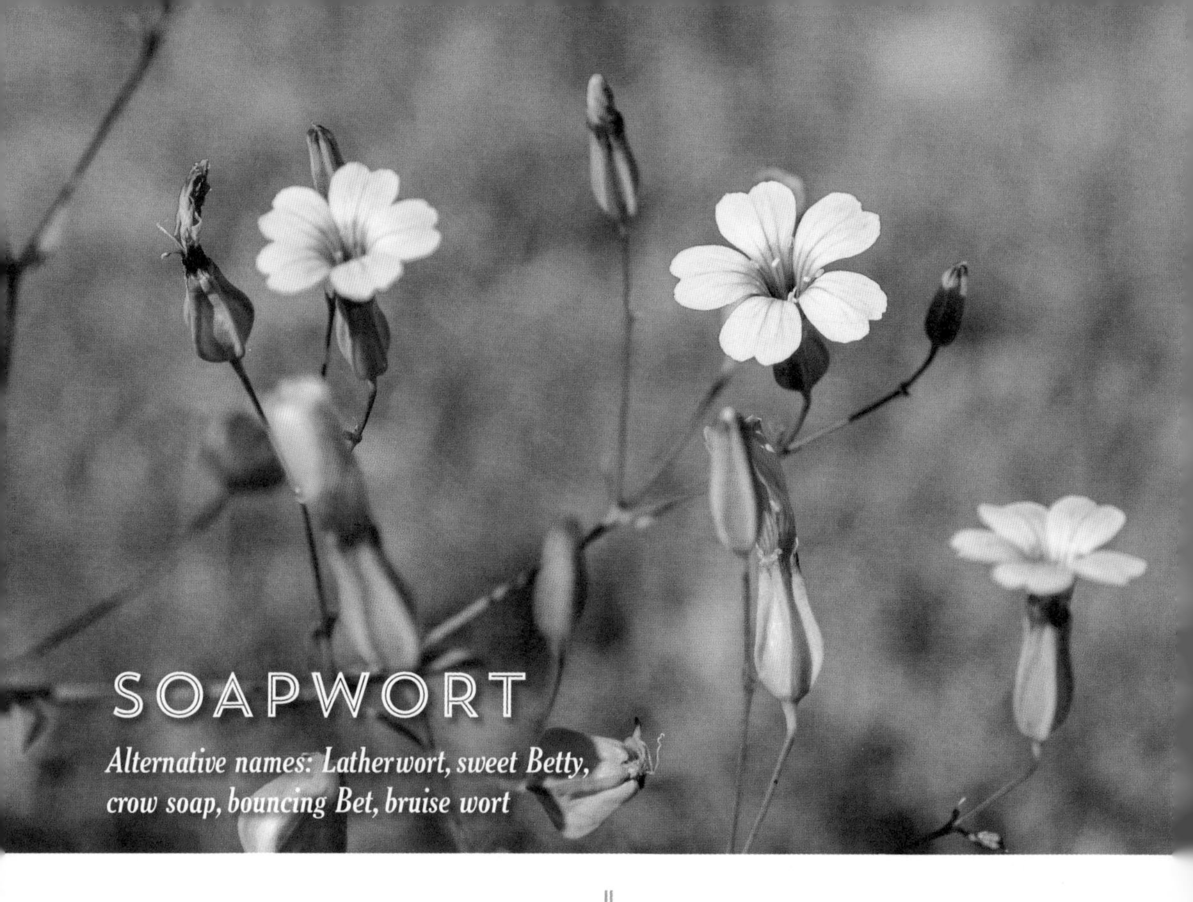

SOAPWORT

Alternative names: *Latherwort, sweet Betty, crow soap, bouncing Bet, bruise wort*

HOW TO IDENTIFY: This attractive plant grows up to 80cm (31 inches) tall, and in clumps, and is topped with dense clusters of pale pink sweet-smelling flowers.

HISTORY: Soapwort has been found growing around the remains of Roman bath houses and was, and I believe still is, used to gently clean the Turin shroud and other delicate textiles with its gentle foaming properties.

The early settlers took soapwort to America to use in sheep dips and for everyday washing tasks on the farm and in the bathroom.

By the end of the sixteenth century the use of soapwort for laundry and washing dishes had become widespread.

Soapwort was once grown commercially in the north of England so that it would be handily close to woollen mills and textile manufacturers.

Soapwort root is poisonous to fish and amphibians; don't grow it around ponds.

FOLKLORE: This useful little plant is used in purification spells – "*may the soapwort that fills the earth cleanse me*" – and is considered to be a gift from God.

FOLK MEDICINE: An old folk remedy for ringworm recommends a poultice made from soapwort, borage, onions or garlic, treacle, rue and wormwood.

Romanies boiled up soapwort root to speed up the healing of bruises. American settlers washed with it to soothe the itching from poison ivy and in the Netherlands it was prescribed as a treatment for jaundice.

The twentieth-century herbalist Maud Grieve used soapwort for the treatment of venereal disease "*especially where the use of mercury has failed*" and as a remedy for the skin eruptions associated with syphilis. Culpeper continues the theme: "*...a decoction of it externally cured the itch. The Germans make use of it, instead of sarsaparilla, for the cure of venereal disorders. In fact it cures virulent gonorrhoeas.*"

OTHER COMMON USES: Soapwort doesn't strip the lanolin from fleece and is used when crafters want to keep some of the water-repellent properties of wool.

Museum conservators still use soapwort to clean delicate historical fabrics and tapestries.

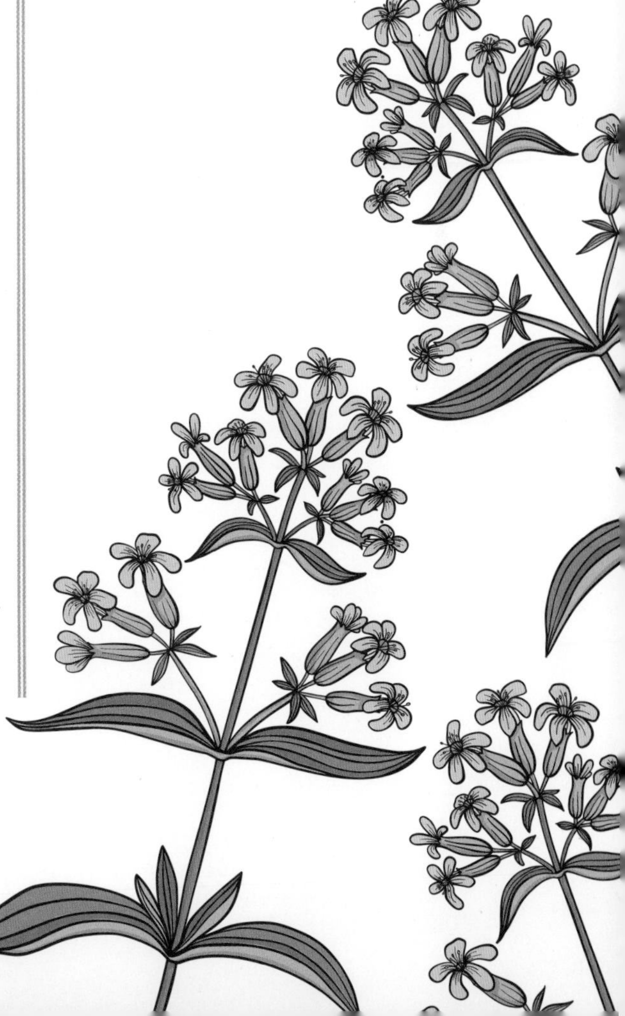

SOAPWORT SHAMPOO

Soapwort extracts are very gentle which makes them perfect if you have sensitive skin; always do a skin test to check for any reaction before use.

Makes 500ml

INGREDIENTS

500ml water

6 tbsp fresh soapwort leaves, chopped (or 2 tbsp of dried)

A handful of herbs of choice – camomile for blonde hair, rosemary or sage for dark hair, mint to combat dandruff, lavender to stimulate growth, nettle to strengthen, calendula for sensitive scalps

5 drops lavender or rose essential oil

Equipment needed

Muslin or fine sieve

Screw top bottle

METHOD

Bring the water to the boil in a saucepan.

Add the soapwort leaves and herbs of choice. Turn down to a simmer for 20 minutes with the lid on.

Allow to cool completely.

Strain through a muslin and squeeze as much liquid out as possible.

Stir in the essential oil.

Pour into a clean bottle with a screw top, an old squash bottle would work well.

Before use shake the bottle to activate the bubbles and use as normal – it won't have as much lather as you're used to but will make your hair squeaky clean.

Use within a month.

Not recommended for use during pregnancy.

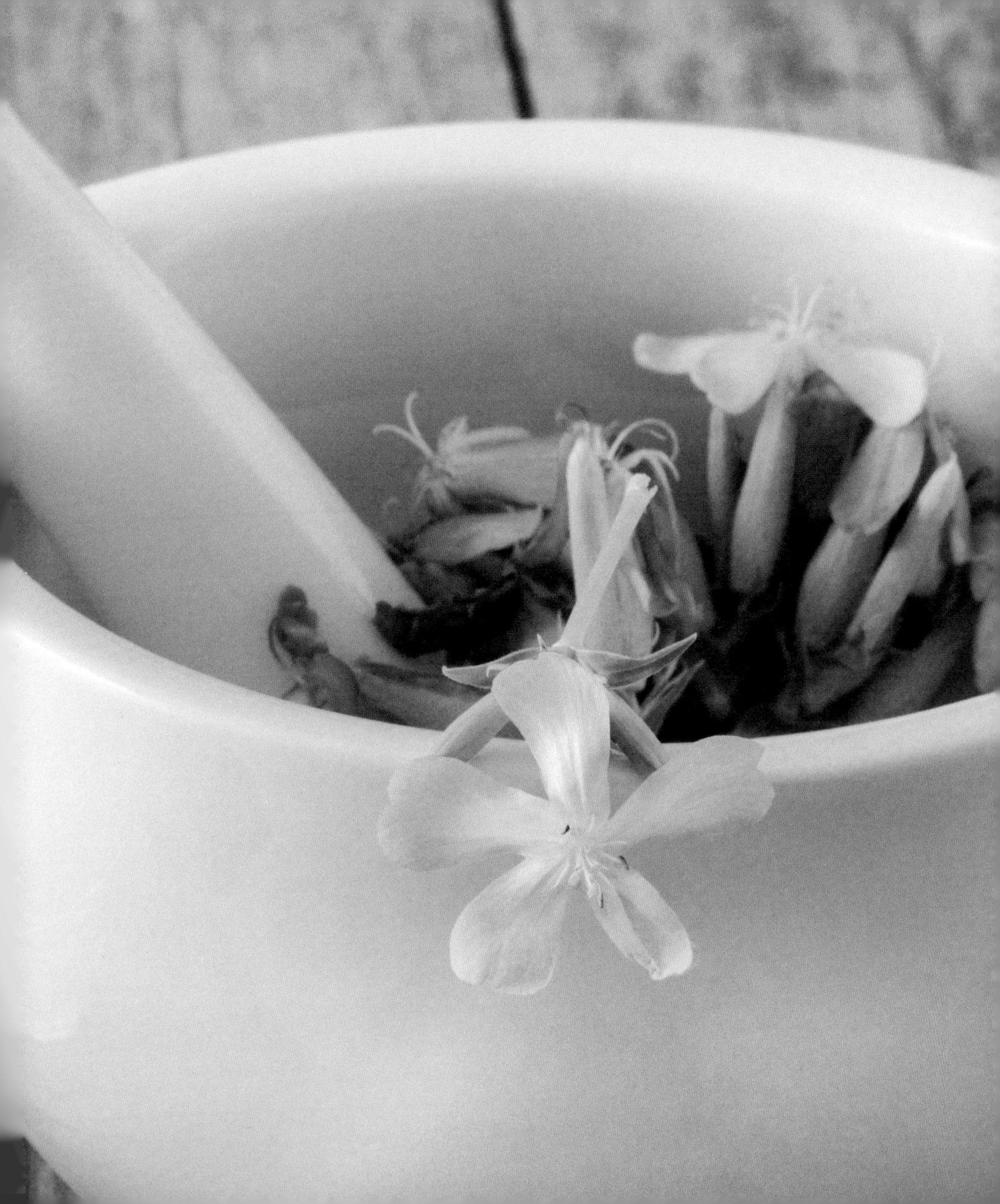

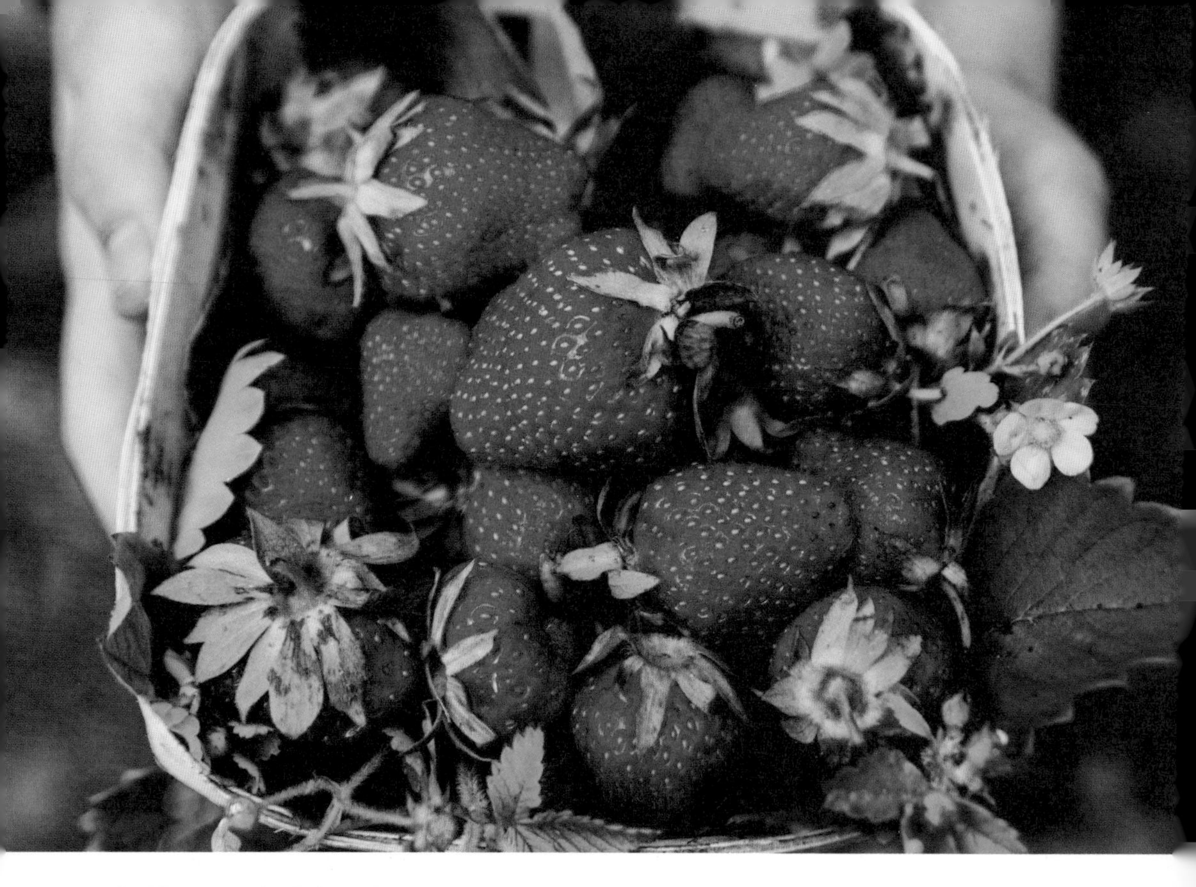

STRAWBERRY

Alternative names: Wild strawberry, alpine strawberry

HOW TO IDENTIFY: Wild strawberries grow to about 30cm (12 inches) with trefoil leaves and small white flowers. These give way to delicious miniature scarlet red fruits in early summer. The fruits of cultivated strawberries have been purposely grown to be much larger and juicier and are easier to harvest.

HISTORY: Native wild strawberries were foraged by our ancestors as long ago as 3000 BC throughout the British Isles.

The large fruited cultivated strawberry that we all know and love is a hybrid and came to our shores from France around the eighteenth century.

By the nineteenth century, England had gained a reputation for strawberry growing and these fruits could be found in most Victorian kitchen gardens.

Strawberries and cream appeared at the very first Wimbledon tennis tournament in 1877; Victorian railways ensured that the fruit would arrive the same day that it had been picked.

FOLKLORE: The German abbess Saint Hildegard Von Bingen announced that strawberries were unfit for human consumption as they grew along the ground where snakes and toads most likely crawled upon them. This had a huge effect among Europeans and discouraged people from eating strawberries for several years.

Clearly the food of lust according to the fifteenth-century paintings of Hieronymus Bosch, wild strawberries were threaded onto grasses to create bracelets to be exchanged by lovers. Carrying the leaves in your pocket while pregnant will relieve the pain of childbirth; strawberry plants were often associated with fertility.

For Christians the three leaves of the strawberry represented the Trinity and were associated with the Virgin Mary and John the Baptist.

If you are lucky enough to have a double strawberry, break it in half and share it with the person who you wish to fall in love with you.

Queen Anne Boleyn, second wife of Henry VIII, had a strawberry-shaped birthmark on her neck, proving to her enemies that she was a witch.

FOLK MEDICINE: Strawberry leaf tea was used as a laxative, diuretic and for digestive upsets while Cornish maidens rubbed leaves on their skin to improve their complexion.

Whitening toothpaste can be made by mashing a strawberry with baking soda, the malic acid in the strawberry acting as a whitening agent.

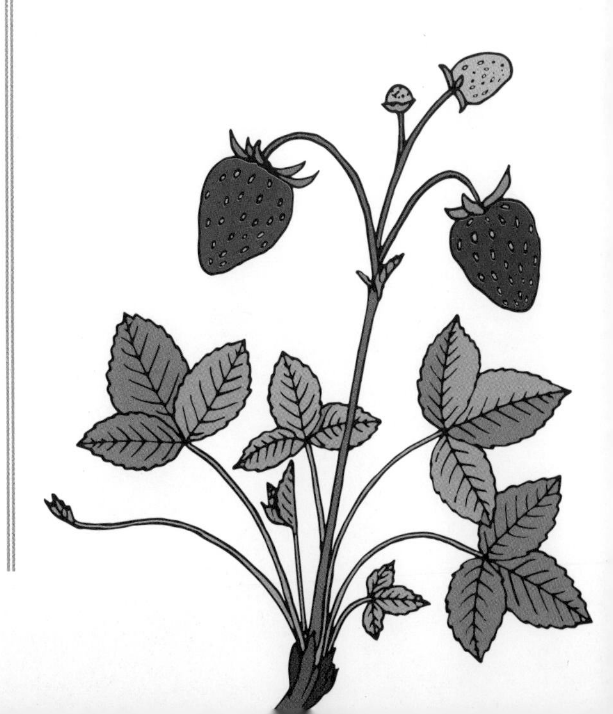

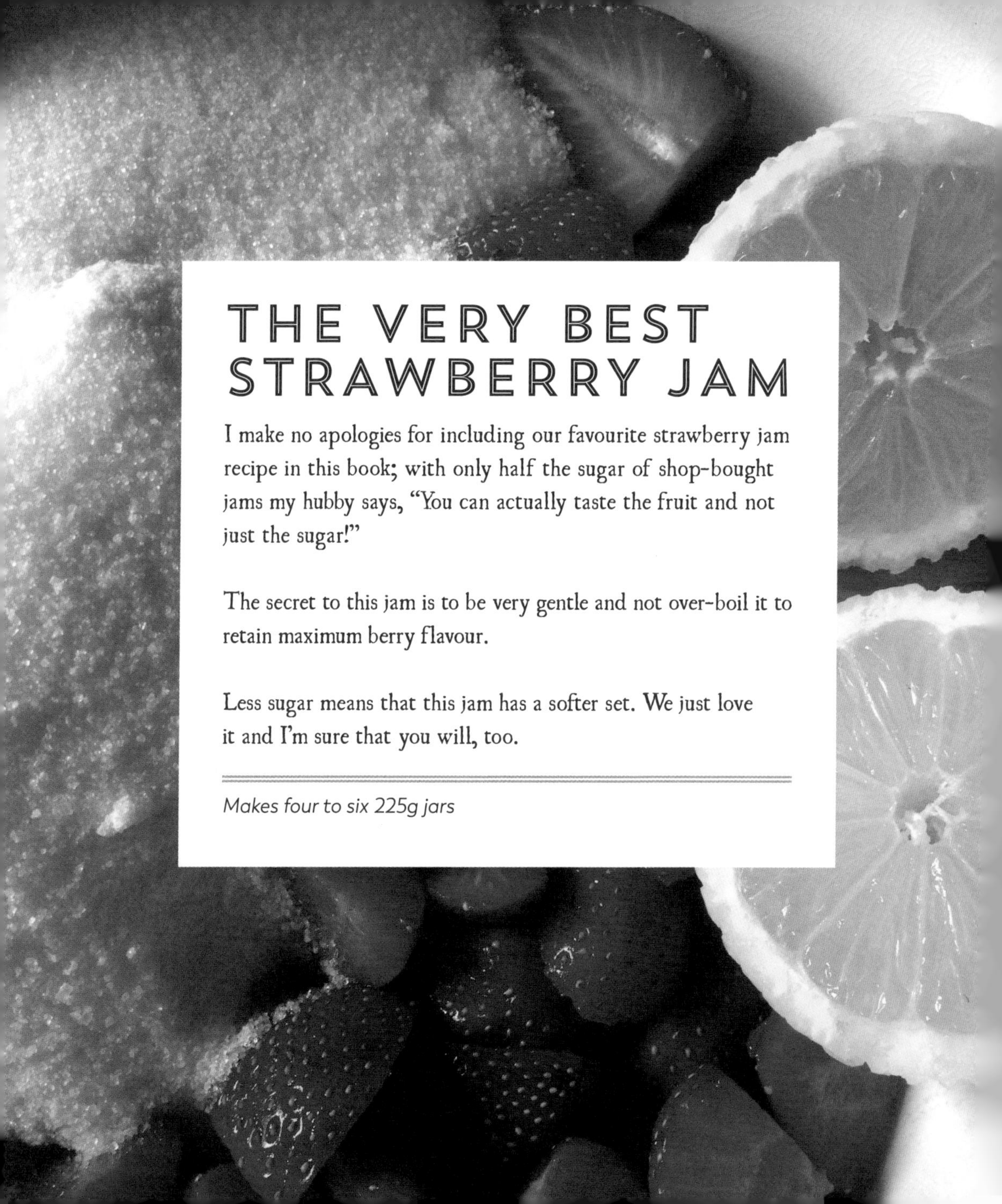

THE VERY BEST STRAWBERRY JAM

I make no apologies for including our favourite strawberry jam recipe in this book; with only half the sugar of shop-bought jams my hubby says, "You can actually taste the fruit and not just the sugar!"

The secret to this jam is to be very gentle and not over-boil it to retain maximum berry flavour.

Less sugar means that this jam has a softer set. We just love it and I'm sure that you will, too.

Makes four to six 225g jars

INGREDIENTS

1kg pesticide-free strawberries, halved

500g jam sugar (this has added pectin to help the jam set)

Juice of 1 organic lemon

Equipment needed

4–6 x 225g jam jars

METHOD

The night before you wish to make the jam put the strawberries, sugar and lemon juice into a large bowl. Stir and cover with a tea towel.

Pop a couple of saucers in the fridge to test for jam setting point.

Sterilize your jam jars (see page 16).

Stir the fruit; you'll notice that lots of liquid has appeared overnight where the sugar has dissolved.

Pour the mixture into a jam pan and start with a gentle heat, stirring all the time to dissolve the remaining sugar.

With a potato masher gently crush about half of the strawberries in the pan.

Bring up to a rolling boil, don't stir.

Boil for 5 minutes then remove from heat.

Check for "setting point" of your jam (see page 16).

If setting point hasn't been reached boil it for another two minutes and retest, be gentle and don't walk away.

Allow the jam to cool for 10 minutes before carefully pouring it into the hot jars.

Dry the lids thoroughly with kitchen paper and screw on tightly.

Refrigerate once open and use within six months, although I doubt it will last that long!

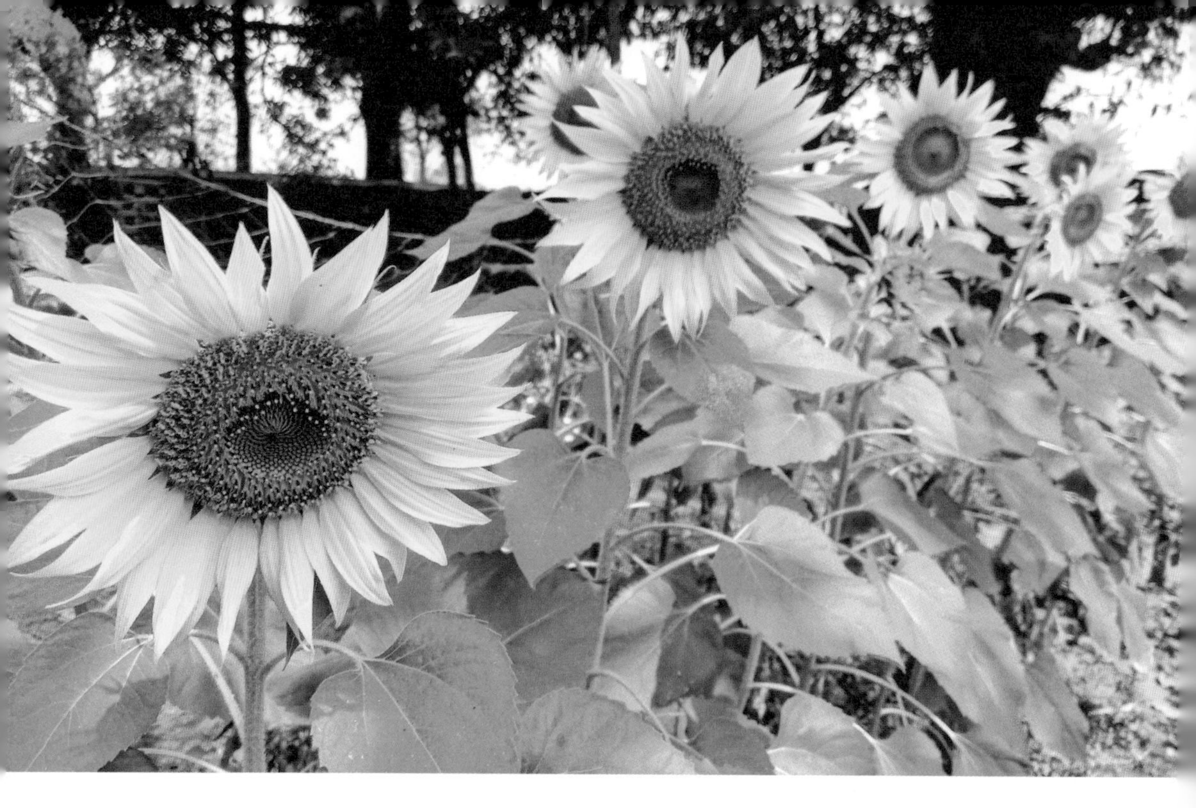

SUNFLOWER

Alternative names: Helianthus annuus, common sunflower

HOW TO IDENTIFY: The straight hairy stems of a sunflower can grow to 3.5 metres (11½ feet) in height. It's topped with an orange coloured central disc from which its yellow or even purple or brown petals radiate.

HISTORY: The wild sunflower is native to the Americas, first cultivated by the indigenous tribes who grew the single-headed plants in a variety of seed colours for culinary and medicinal use.

The ancient Inca tribes worshipped the sunflower. Images of sunflowers can be found drawn in the Inca temples in the Andes, priestesses wore golden sunflower discs on their robes and bowls of sunflower seeds were given as offerings to the dead.

Brought to Europe in the sixteenth century by Spanish explorers, sunflowers were once only seen as an ornamental plant. The herbalist John Gerard was disappointed that his sunflowers didn't grow as tall as expected and he noted that some of his contemporaries "have reported [sunflowers] to turn to the sun, which I could never observe, although I have endeavoured to find the truth of it."

The eighteenth-century physician Erasmus Darwin (grandfather to Charles) was inspired to write that the sunflower:

"Climbs the upland lawn,
And bows in homage to the rising dawn,
Imbibes with eagle eye the golden ray,
And watches as it moves, the orb of day."

FOLKLORE: Sunflowers are associated with truth, loyalty and honesty; sleep with a sunflower under your bed and the following day, before sunset, the truth about a situation that is troubling you will be revealed to you.

The sunflower is faithful to the sun, following it across the sky day after day – feeding your spouse or friends with sunflower oil or seeds will keep them faithful to you.

A crown or necklace of the blooms worn during the summer solstice will help to increase your fertility, as will taking a ritual bath in sunflower petals and eating sunflower seeds.

Planting sunflowers around your garden will bring you good fortune – pick a sunflower at sunset, make a wish and wear the flower the following day and before sunset your wish will come true.

In the seventeenth century "magic sunflower oil" was often made by infusing sunflowers and other summer blooms for three days in the sunshine. This was then turned into an ointment and applied to the body to enable faery folk to be seen more easily.

FOLK MEDICINE: Eating sunflower seeds is believed to be an aphrodisiac and also increase your chances of conception, containing magnesium, potassium, zinc, calcium, vitamins E and B, folic acid and selenium – all beneficial nutrients to aid fertility.

The anti-inflammatory properties of the leaves led to them being used as a poultice for snakebites and spider bites, and a tea made with the leaves can help to soothe tonsillitis and sore throats.

OTHER COMMON USES: Wild birds, particularly of the finch family, adore sunflower seeds so it's a great way to persuade them into your garden.

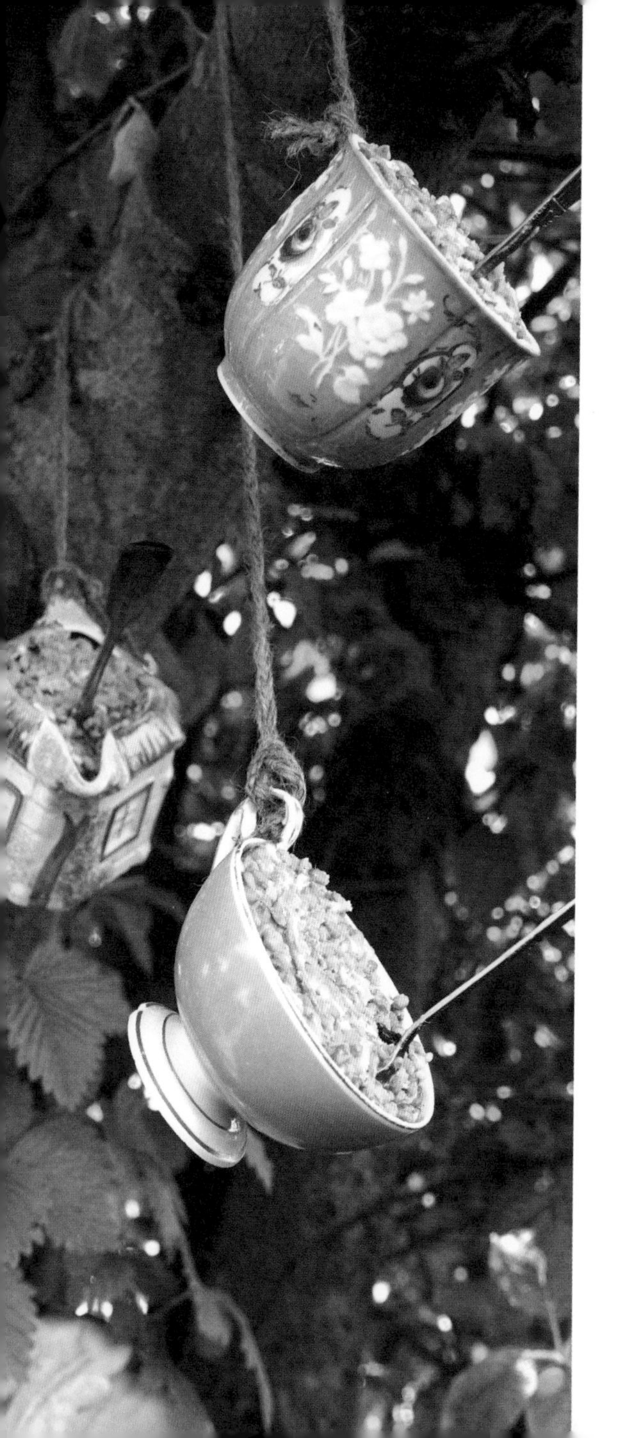

VINTAGE TEACUP BIRD FEEDERS

I try to encourage wildlife into my garden as much as possible. As a "lazy" gardener it's the perfect excuse for cultivating nettle patches and allowing some parts of the garden to become overgrown. This encourages more insects to inhabit the garden, which will in turn bring in more native birds to feed and nest.

During winter months when food is in short supply, it's even more important to feed our feathered friends with high-energy foods. Bird feeders don't have to be boring and the combination of dripping and a mix of seeds in a handy teacup will ensure that they make it through the winter in good health.

Makes four or five teacups depending on their size

INGREDIENTS

250g dripping (lard is too soft and likely to melt)

500g sunflower seeds and mixed birdseed

Equipment needed

4–5 vintage teacups (I get mine from boot fairs really cheaply)

4–5 teaspoons (also from a boot fair)

Strong twine

METHOD

In a saucepan carefully melt the dripping – don't walk away as you do this.

Once melted stir in the birdseed. You can also add any other bird-friendly scraps such as dried fruit or cooked bacon rind.

Allow to cool slightly until it begins to set.

Pack the mixture into the teacups.

Push a spoon into the seed mix to create a perch, pack the mix around it to hold it firm.

Pop into the fridge until solid.

Create a secure loop using the twine through the teacup handle.

Hang onto a tree branch and wait for the birds to discover it.

Once empty, wash out the teacup and refill.

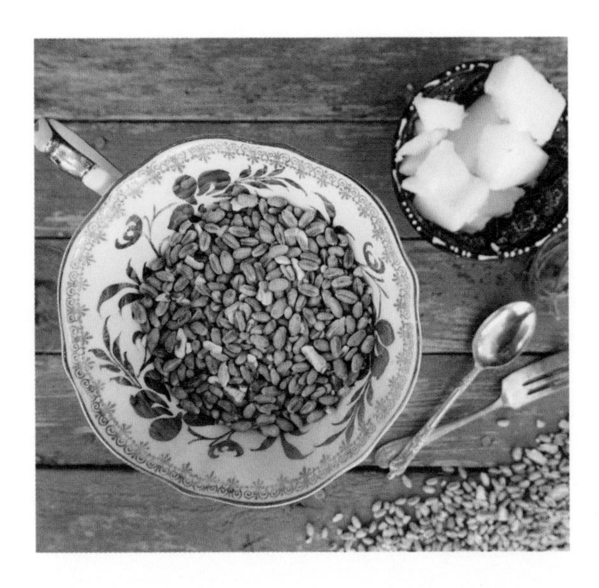

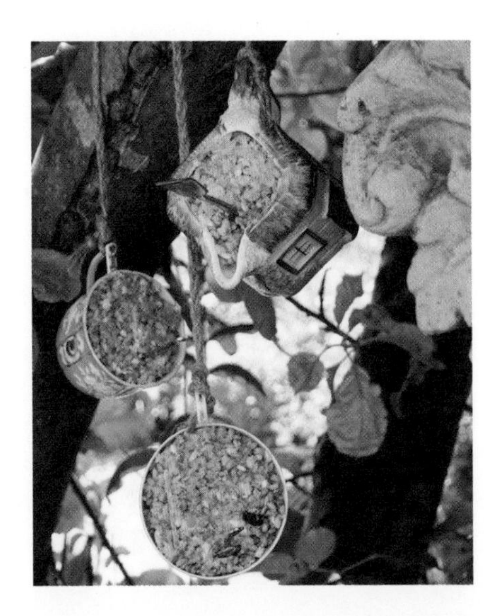

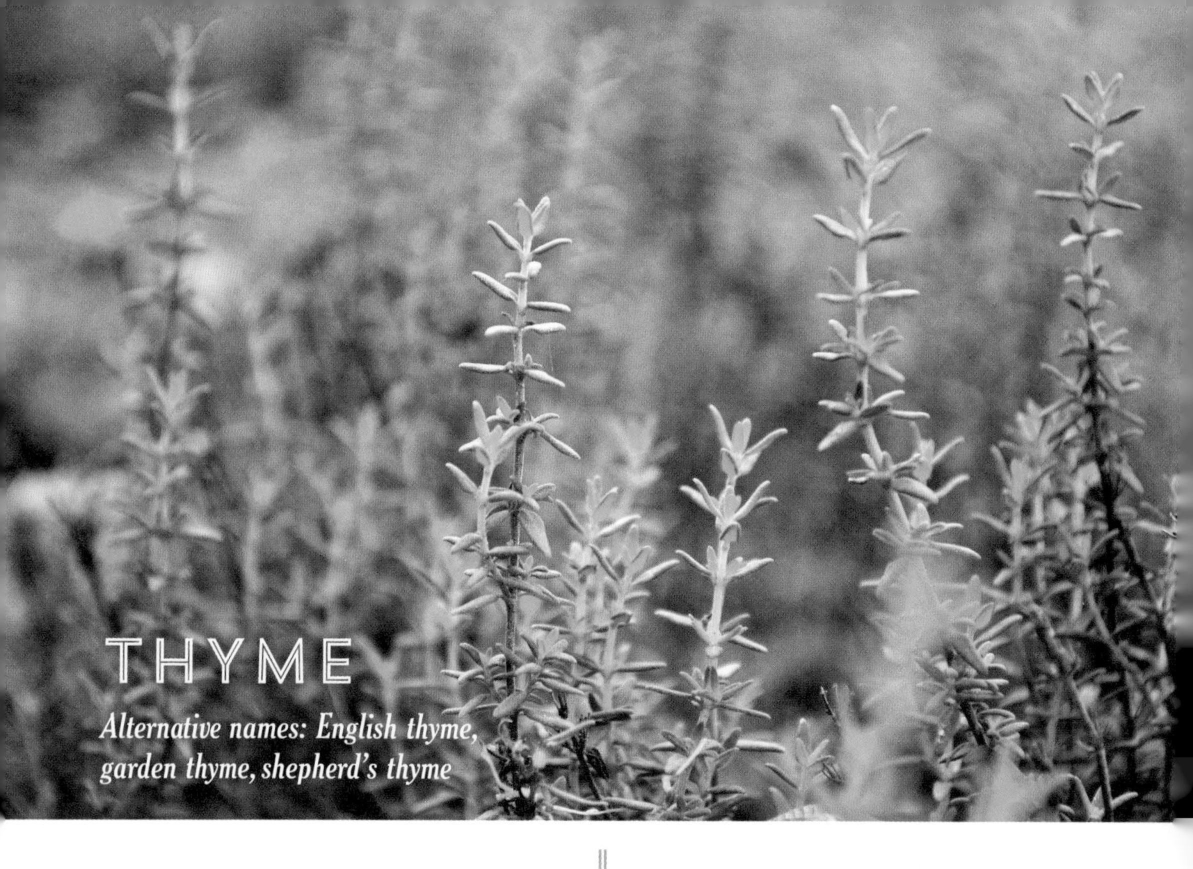

THYME

Alternative names: English thyme, garden thyme, shepherd's thyme

HOW TO IDENTIFY: Thyme is a low-growing woody plant with small aromatic leaves all the way up the stems. Wild thyme is one of the UK's native species and can still be found growing on heathland and meadows.

HISTORY: The many other varieties of thyme, such as lemon thyme and creeping thyme, originated in Mediterranean regions and were spread far and wide by the Romans. It was believed that eating thyme and even bathing in thyme would give them protection from poisoning; this made it especially popular with nervous Roman emperors.

Thyme was burned in both Roman and Greek temples for purification and inhaling the smoke gave courage to soldiers going into battle.

Thyme, along with other fragrant herbs, was rubbed onto the bodies of pharaohs as part of the mummification process; it was also believed to ease the passage of the spirit into the afterlife.

FOLKLORE: Faeries love to inhabit the twisted and knotted branches of wild thyme making it unlucky to bring into the house for fear of upsetting the fae. Thyme can be sprinkled on windowsills and doorsteps should you wish to invite the faery folk to visit; bathing your eyes in the dew from thyme leaves before dawn on the first day of May will enable you to see your special visitors. Patches of wild thyme were evidence that faeries had partied the night away on that very spot – this led to generations of young girls camping out in the hope of glimpsing faeries.

To find a lost object, leave an offering of thyme and honey in the woods on the night of a full moon and the faeries will do their best to find it for you. Romanies will never bring wild thyme into their wagons, regarding it as very unlucky; they will however drink thyme tea outdoors with a little vinegar and honey to cure a cough.

Plant thyme at the beginning of the waxing moon with several coins tucked into the root ball, look after it well and as the thyme grows so will your bank balance.

FOLK MEDICINE: Plague doctors in fourteenth-century England believed that diseases were carried by "miasma" (bad air) so they wore long beak-like masks stuffed with many herbs including thyme, peppermint and rosemary to avoid becoming infected by their patients.

To quote Culpeper:

> *"It purges the body of phlegm, and is an excellent remedy for shortness of breath. It kills worms in the belly... gives safe and speedy delivery to women in travail [labour]*
>
> *and brings away the afterbirth... An ointment of it takes away hot swellings and warts."*

Thyme is a natural antiseptic and antibiotic and has been used to treat a myriad of ailments including coughs and colds, warts, sciatica, headaches, hay fever and hangovers. Even before bacteria and infection were properly understood, nurses in the nineteenth century were soaking bandages in a solution of thyme water.

OTHER COMMON USES: Thymol is the powerful natural antiseptic contained in thyme and this can be found in mouthwash, hand sanitizer and acne medication. Bees love flowering thyme and the resulting honey takes on a delicious herby flavour that is much sought after by honey lovers.

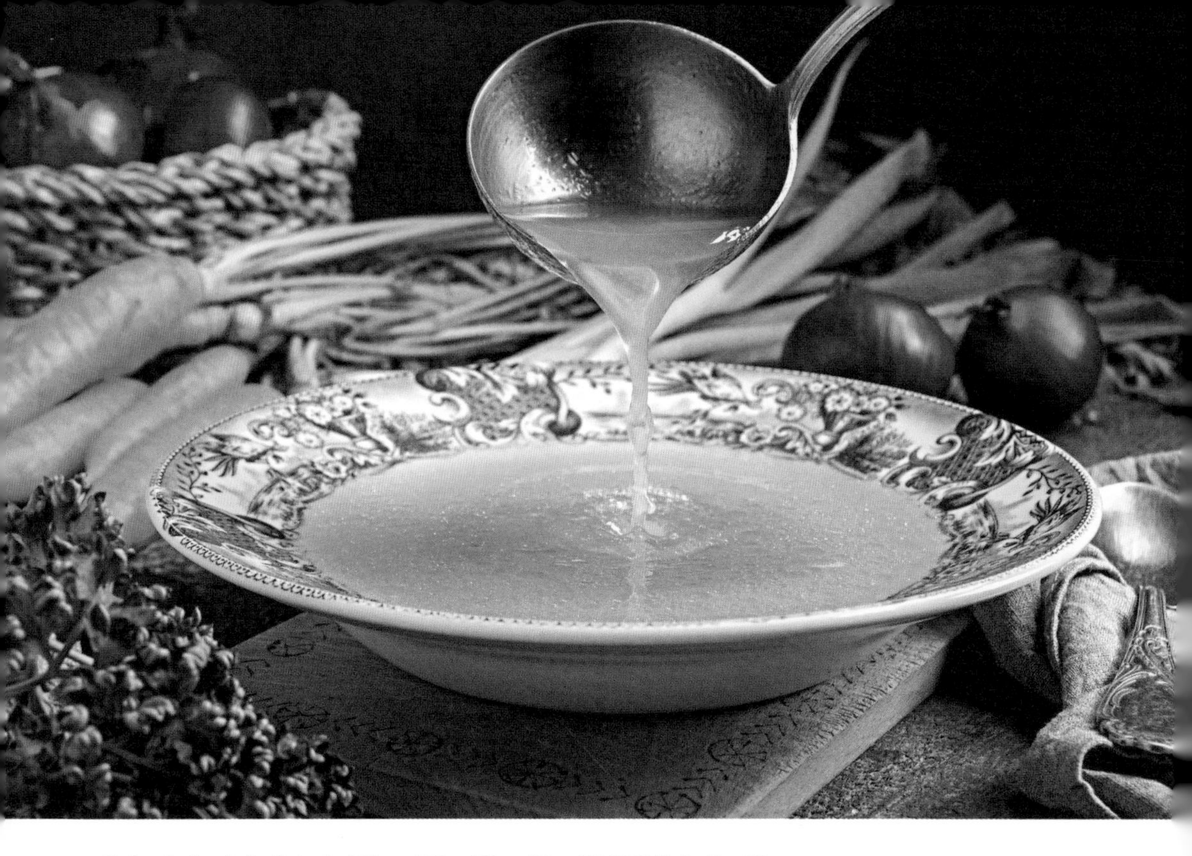

IMMUNE-BOOSTING CHICKEN AND THYME BROTH

When anyone in our household is recovering from illness or feels that a cough or cold is about to take hold, we like to make a batch of this hearty homemade soup that is full of immune-boosting ingredients.

Buy the best chicken that you can afford – there'll be plenty of meat left over to turn into risotto or chicken salad, making it well worth the extra money.

Makes 2–3 litres

INGREDIENTS

1 medium organic or free-range chicken

Bunch of thyme

2 celery sticks, chopped

1 large onion, chopped

2 garlic cloves

2 bay leaves

Thumb-sized piece of turmeric root, sliced (or 1 tsp dried)

Thumb-sized piece of root ginger, sliced

3 carrots, chopped

2 tbsp raw apple cider vinegar (see page 34)

2 tbsp coconut oil

Sea salt

Black peppercorns

2 tbsp miso paste

1 organic chicken stock cube

Equipment needed

Large stock pot or saucepan

METHOD:

Place all the ingredients except for the miso and stock cube in a large stock pot with just enough water to cover the chicken.

Bring to the boil, put on a lid and reduce to a simmer for at least 6 hours, topping up the water as needed.

Remove the cooked chicken and vegetables from the broth; sieve the liquid into a clean saucepan to remove any bones.

Stir some of the chicken, the miso paste and stock cube into the broth and check for seasoning.

I like to freeze this soup into individual portions to be used as required.

Keeps in the fridge for 2 days or freeze into handy portions to use as needed.

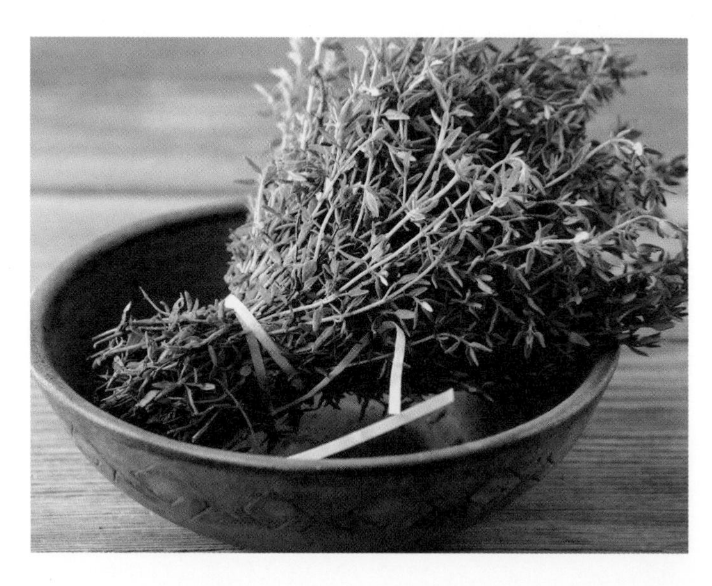

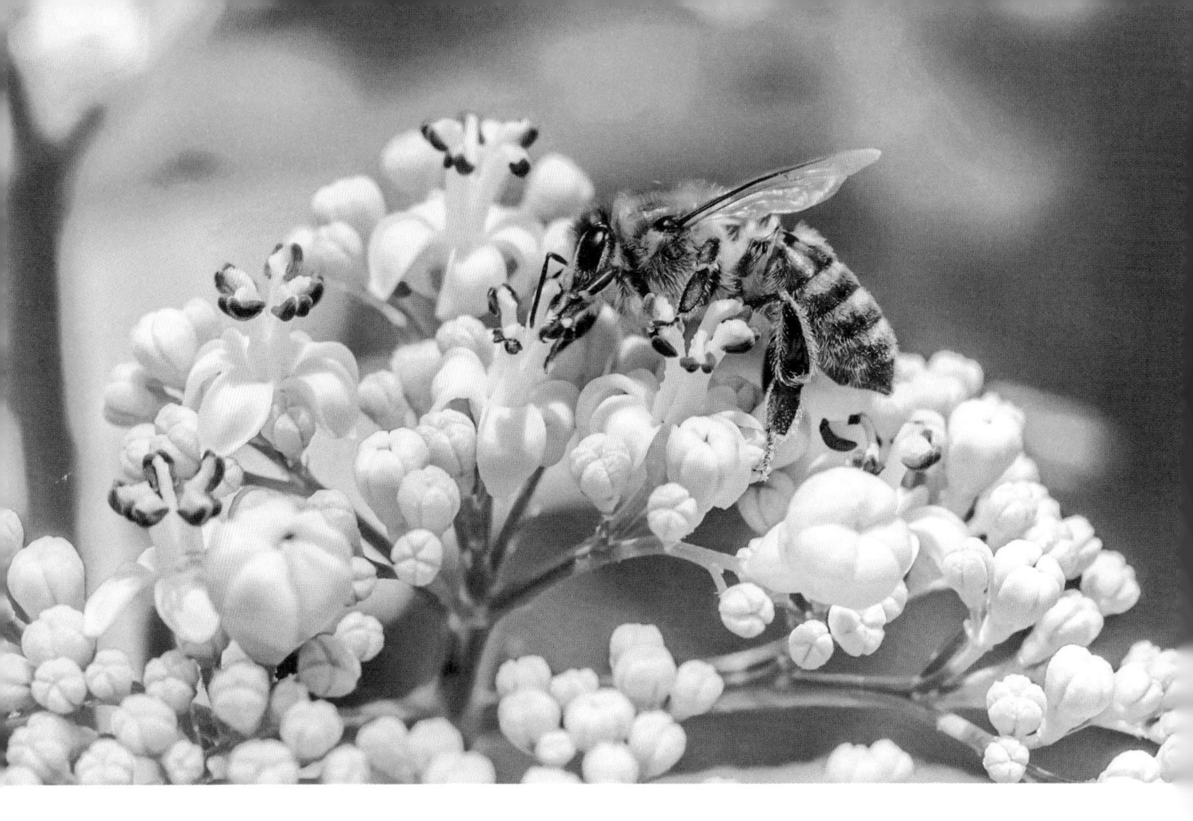

VALERIAN

Alternative names: All heal, cut finger, God's hand leaf, St George's herb, Valeriana officinalis

HOW TO IDENTIFY: Valerian can grow up to 2 metres (6½ feet) tall topped with clusters of pale pink five-petalled flowers.

HISTORY: Valerian is native to Europe and has been used medicinally since the eleventh century as records written by the Anglo Saxon leeches (healers) show.

Known as "the valium of the nineteenth century", valerian root was given to shell-shocked soldiers in the Great War and later prescribed to treat insomnia and nervous exhaustion in civilians during the Blitz of World War Two. Valerian was cultivated for medicinal use in parts of England but demand completely outstripped supply and the cost soared from 30 shillings (£1.50) per hundredweight to 120 shillings per hundredweight (£6) in 1915.

FOLKLORE: Cats, rats and other animals find the scent of valerian very attractive and it is believed that the Pied Piper of Hamelin carried valerian root in his pocket to lure the rats to their death in the river Weser.

The Celts hung bundles of valerian in their houses to protect from lightning strikes; placed under the pillow it not only cured insomnia and stopped nightmares but also acted as an aphrodisiac.

Love sachets containing valerian pinned to young ladies' clothing would cause men to follow them like children, or maybe rats?

FOLK MEDICINE: Culpeper wrote of how:

> *"The root boiled with liquorice, raisins and aniseed is good for those troubled with cough. Also, it is of special value against the plague, the decoction thereof being drunk and the root smelled. The green herb being bruised and applied to the head taketh away pain and pricking thereof."*

In the Middle Ages valerian was widely used in the treatment of epilepsy and St Vitas' Dance, now known as Sydenham's chorea; a disorder associated with rheumatic fever causing the body to jerk uncontrollably.

The sixteenth-century herbalist John Gerard wrote that "*no broth or medicine be worth anything if it did not contain valerian*" and recommended its use for "*chest congestion, convulsions, bruises and falls.*"

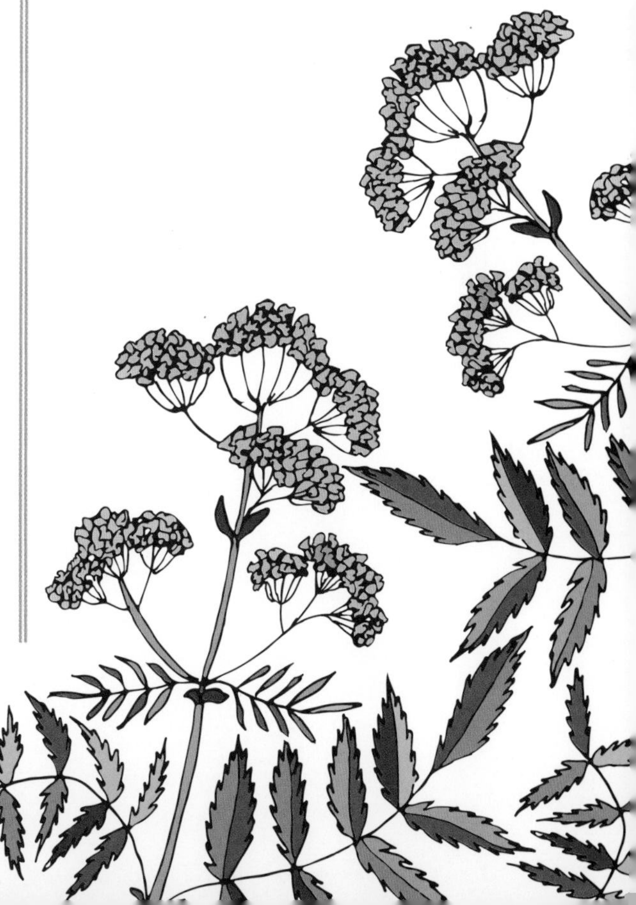

SLEEPY VALERIAN TEA

I've used dried herbs in this tea mixture mainly because you can make up a batch and it will keep for longer. Try to source organic herbs from a reputable supplier; the quality can sometimes be lacking if you go for the cheapest option.

INGREDIENTS

25g dried valerian root (sedative)

50g dried lemon balm (eases stress)

25g dried passion flower (helps the brain to switch off)

25g dried rose petals (sedative)

25g dried hop flowers (for insomnia)

25g dried lemongrass (for restful sleep)

Equipment needed

Small teapot or tea infuser ball

METHOD

Mix all the herbs together well. Store in an airtight jar in a cool, dry place.

Use one heaped tablespoon to a cup of boiling water. Place the herbs in a tea infuser ball or small teapot.

Allow to steep for 5 minutes. Discard the herbs.

Sweeten to taste with honey or a vegan alternative and drink 30 minutes before bedtime.

Keeps for 1 year.

This can be quite soporific; don't use before driving or operating machinery.

Valerian should not be consumed during pregnancy or breastfeeding.

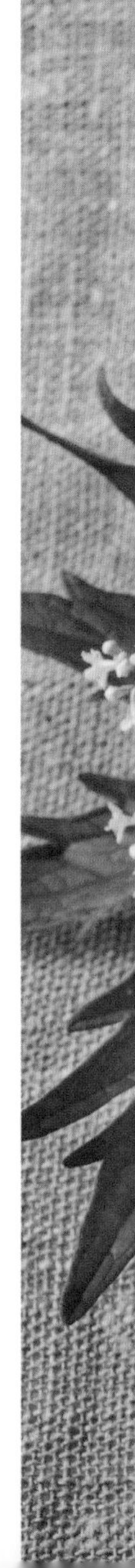

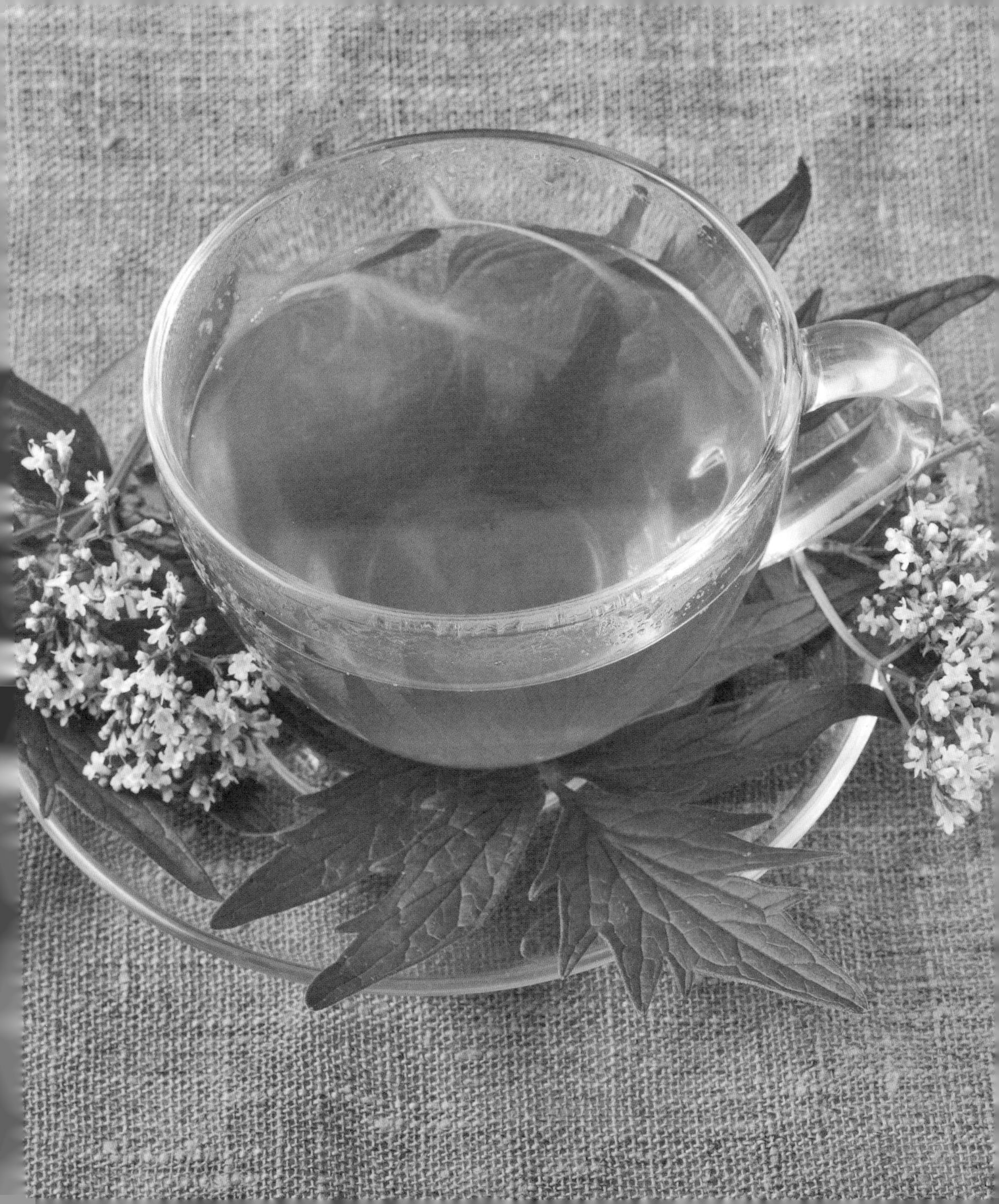

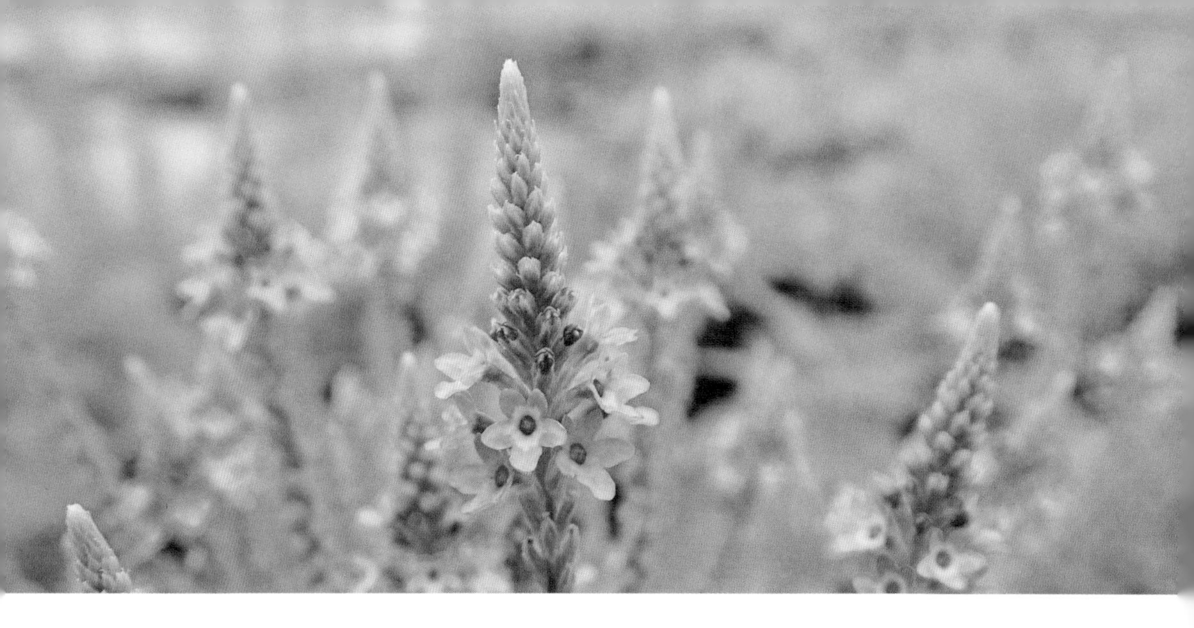

VERVAIN

Alternative names: Enchanter's plant, simpler's joy, wizard's herb, herb of the cross

HOW TO IDENTIFY: Small pale lilac flowers are carried on long slender spikes growing to around 1 metre (3 feet) tall.

HISTORY: It was said that vervain was used to halt the flow of blood from the wounds of Christ at Calvary and consequently it obtained its religious, magical and healing powers.

Vervain is native to southern Europe. From as long ago as 300 BC the ancient Druids believed vervain to be sacred and used it as a magical "altar plant", included it in their "lustral" (holy) water and tied it into bundles to cleanse the altar.

FOLKLORE: So sacred was vervain that it was only gathered by the Druids at the time of a dark (new) moon under the rising Dog Star (Sirius), otherwise its magical powers would be lost. Honey or honeycomb was poured onto the ground as an offering in exchange for this most magical of plants.

An old Elizabethan manuscript kept in a library in Manchester records that vervain was gathered before it flowered while saying these distinctly Christian words:

"All hele, thou holy herb vervain,
Growing on the ground,
In the mount of Calvary,
There was thou found,
Thou helpest many a grief,
And staunchest many a wound,
In the name of sweet Jesus,
I take thee from the ground,
O Lord, do effect the same,
That I go about,
In the name of god on mount Olivet,
First I found thee,
In the name of Jesus,
I pull thee from the ground."

In New Orleans Hoodoo folk magic, VanVan Oil, made from vervain, citronella, ginger and patchouli, is used to banish negativity, change bad luck into good, attract love, and recharge amulets and lucky charms.

The scent of vervain is believed to be an aphrodisiac. In Germany the bride was presented with a wreath containing vervain to ensure fertility and good luck.

Pouches of vervain were given to babies to make them more intelligent, vervain tea helped with insomnia and soothed nervous excitement, burying it in the garden brings good luck and rubbing vervain on your hand will ensure that anyone you touch will fall in love with you.

FOLK MEDICINE: Culpeper wrote of vervain:

"It consolidates and heals also all wounds, both inward and outward, stays bleeding, and if used with some honey heals all old ulcers and fistulas in the legs or other parts of the body...or used with hogs' grease, it helps the swellings and pains in the secret parts in man or woman, also for the piles and haemorrhoids."

The advice for treating throat tumours from the physician to Emperor Theodosius was: "*cut vervain root into two pieces, tie one around the throat and hang the other over a fire. As the root in the fire shrivels the tumour will shrivel too.*"

During the Middle Ages vervain became a popular treatment for minor skin conditions such as acne and spots, Culpepper claimed that "*The leaves bruised, or the juice mixed with vinegar, does wonderfully cleanse the skin, and take away morphew, [lesions or blisters caused by scurvy].*"

OTHER COMMON USES: Vervain incense is still burned in the home for protection against evil spirits.

PEACEFUL SLEEP BATH SOAK

Nothing relaxes the body before bedtime more than a warm herbal bath; this remedy includes vervain to calm the nerves, camomile and lavender for their soporific qualities, rosemary to ease stress, mugwort for pleasant dreams and spearmint to improve sleep. If you wish to use fresh herbs just double the quantities.

INGREDIENTS

2 tbsp dried vervain

1 tbsp dried camomile

1½ tbsp dried lavender flowers

½ tbsp dried rosemary

½ tbsp dried mugwort

½ tbsp dried peppermint

Equipment needed

Small cotton or muslin drawstring bag

METHOD

Place all the herbs into the cotton bag and tie securely.

Tie the cotton bag underneath the hot tap as you run your bath, ensuring that the water flows through it. Alternatively, just pop it into the tub squeezing it out into the water occasionally.

Maybe place a couple of cornflower compresses (see page 72) onto your eyes for extra luxury.

Lie back and relax.

Not to be used if pregnant or breastfeeding.

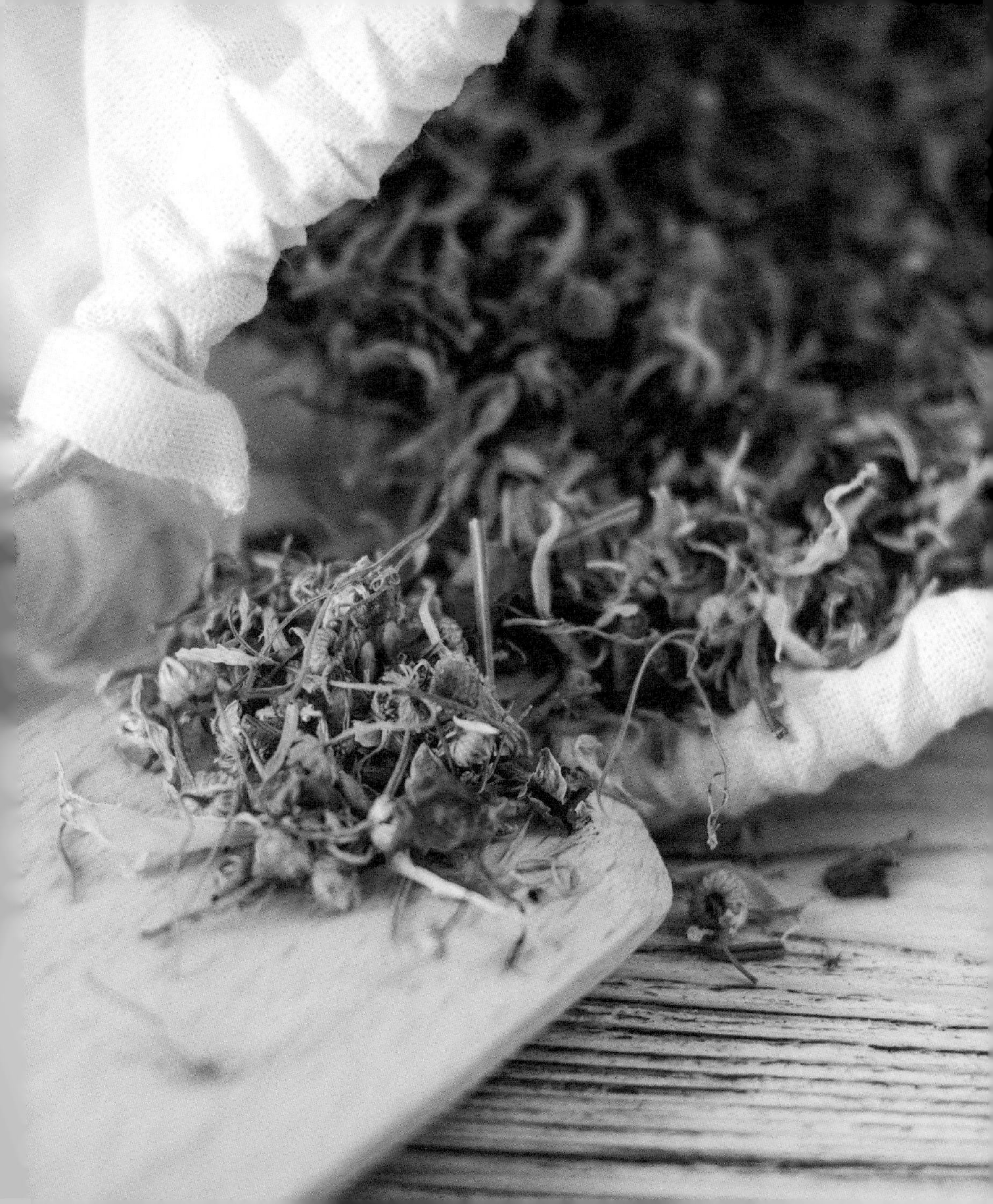

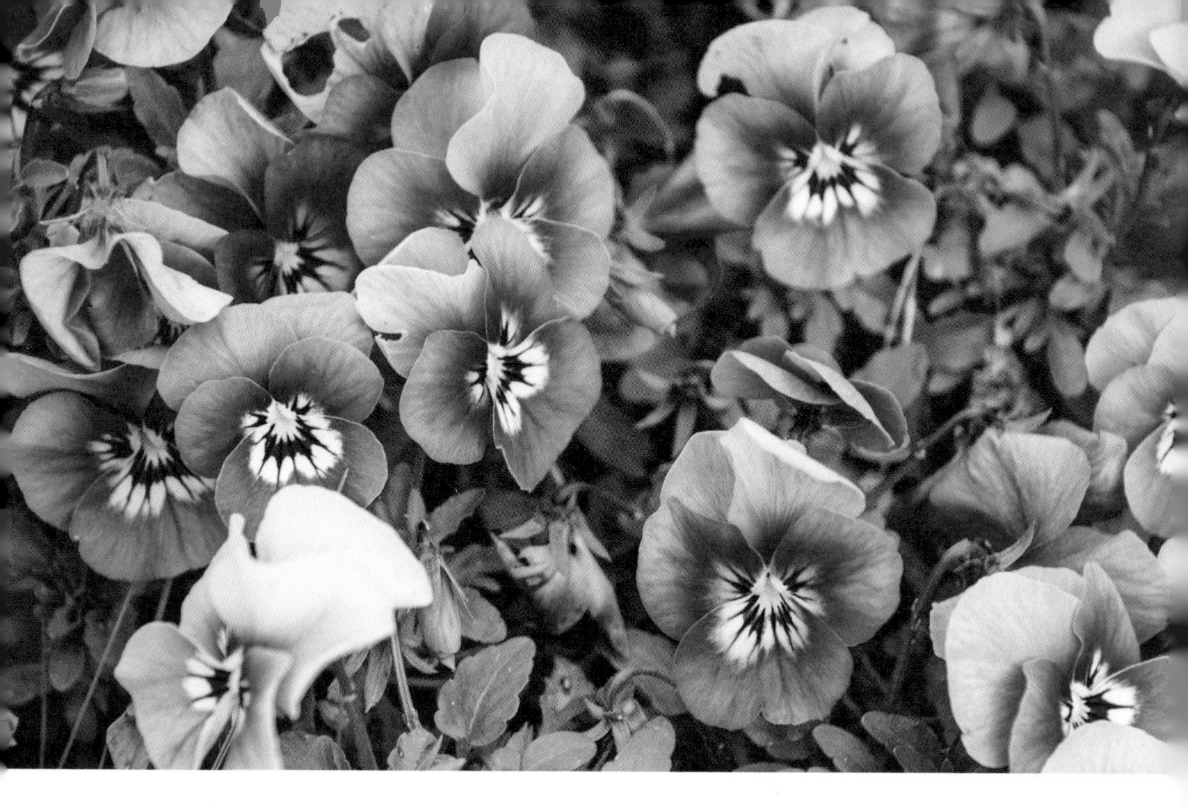

VIOLA

Alternative names: Love lies bleeding, heartsease, Jack-jump-up-and-kiss-me, kiss behind the garden door, wild pansy, love-in-idleness

HOW TO IDENTIFY: Viola has pansy-like cream, white and violet flowers, grows to 12cm (5 inches) tall and flourishes in partial shade.

HISTORY: Representing chastity, viola was the favourite flower of Elizabeth I and she had them embroidered onto her clothing and linens. Also linked to the Virgin Mary, the three colours of heartsease flowers are used to symbolize purity, joy and mourning.

FOLKLORE: Very much associated with love, viola was originally pure white but it became tricolour after being struck by one of Cupid's arrows.

Lovesick Oberon in *A Midsummer Night's Dream* sends Puck to gather "*...love in idleness. Fetch me that flower; the juice of it on sleeping eyelids laid will make man or woman dote on the next live creature that it sees.*" Unfortunately, that first creature seen by Titania didn't turn out to be Oberon!

Plant your viola in a heart-shaped pot to keep your relationship alive or sleep with them under your pillow if you'd like to attract a new partner.

Picking the flowers when the morning dew is on them will bring about a death to someone in the family.

Pick some viola, pluck off a petal and count the streaks on the petals to predict your future:

Four lines – signify hope
Five lines – there could be trouble coming
Six lines – a surprise is coming to you
Seven lines – your love will be true
Eight lines – indecisiveness
Nine lines – a change of heart
Ten lines – you will be rich
Eleven lines – many children

If the central line is the longest then you should choose a Sunday as your wedding day.

FOLK MEDICINE: As well as being used as a love potion, Culpeper, rather ironically, recommended that: "*A strong decoction of the herbs and flowers, if you will, you may make it into a syrup, is an excellent cure for the French pox [syphilis]*" and that '*...it is excellently good for the convulsions in children, as also for the falling sickness [epilepsy] and a gallant remedy for the inflammation of the lungs and breasts, pleurisy, scabs, itch etc.*"

An infusion of viola is also suggested as a treatment to mend a broken heart, for bronchitis, asthma and the common cold.

OTHER COMMON USES: The flowers are edible and look beautiful in salads, frozen into ice cubes, or on top of cakes and have also been used to make green, blue and yellow dyes.

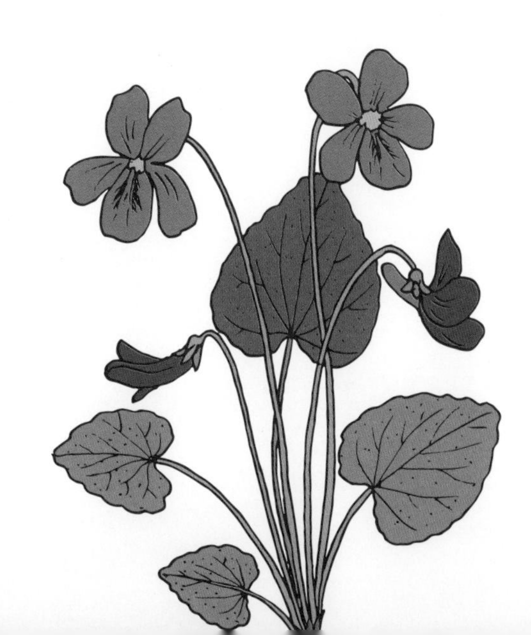

BLUEBERRY LEMON MOUSSE CAKE WITH VIOLA

I am extremely grateful to my dear friend Charlotte of Frog Hollow Catering for coming up with this amazing recipe decorated with viola flowers especially for this book. Blueberry lemon mousse cakes are not only incredibly tasty but also vegan and gluten-free and made without the use of any refined sugar.

Charlotte doesn't share her recipes with many people so we are very lucky indeed.

Makes six

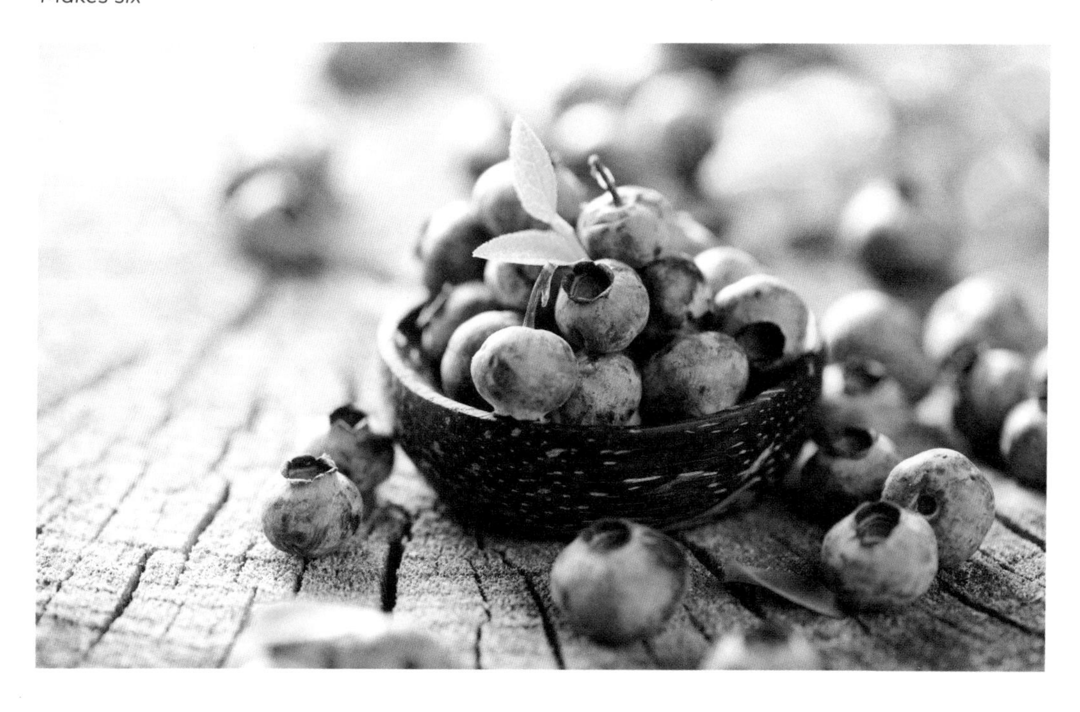

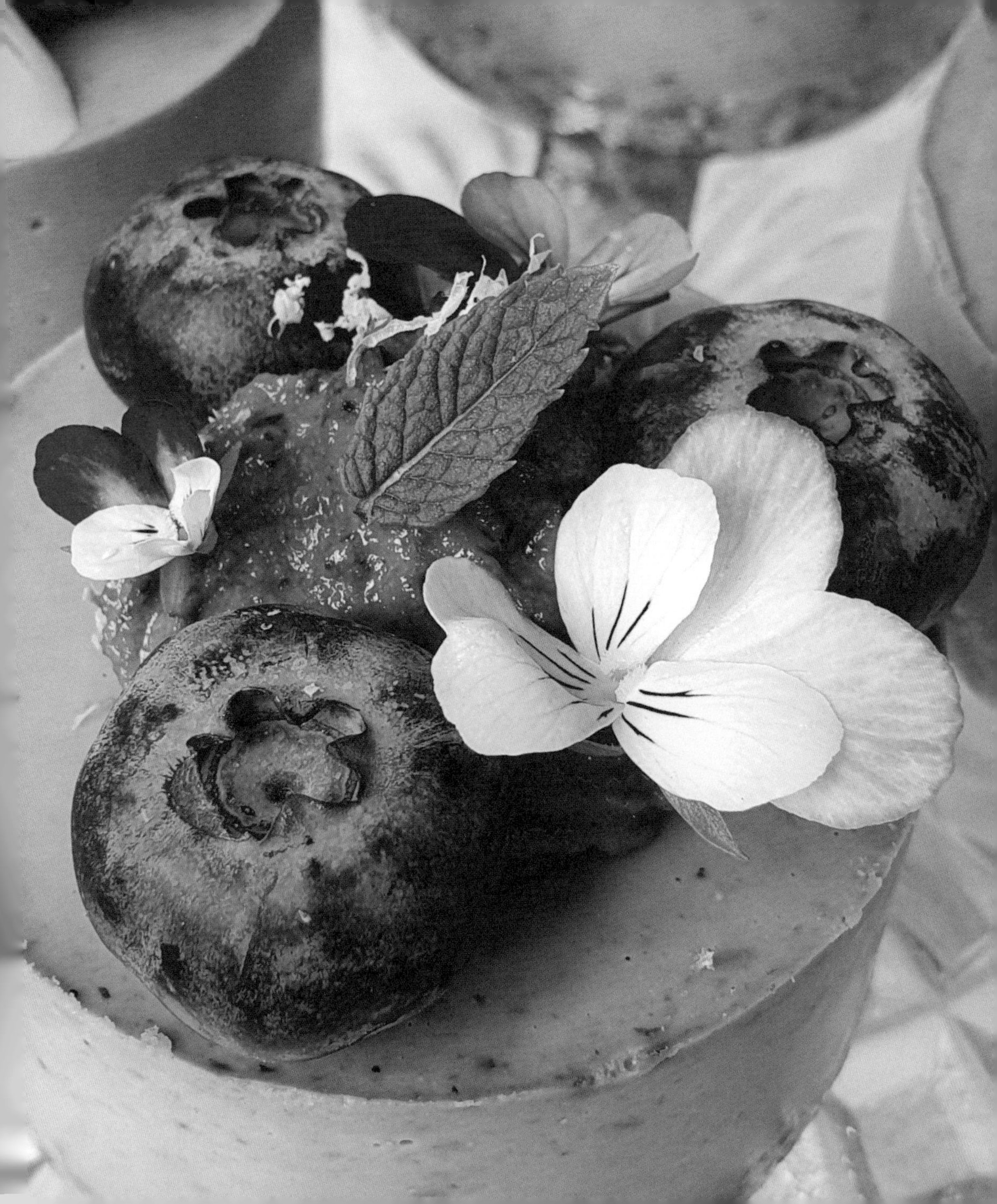

INGREDIENTS

For the filling:

100g cashew nuts

100g blueberries fresh or frozen (defrosted)

25g coconut milk powder

75ml water

1 lemon, grated zest

50ml lemon juice

5g maple syrup

Pinch of Himalayan pink rock salt

100g coconut oil, melted

For the vanilla base:

50g pitted Medjool dates

Pinch of Himalayan pink rock salt

¼ tsp vanilla extract

35g desiccated coconut

18g hulled hemp seeds

15g coconut oil, melted

METHOD

Blitz all of the blueberry filling ingredients except the coconut oil in a high-powered liquidizer and let the cashew nuts soak in the blitzed blueberry juice while you make the bases.

To make the bases:

Chop up the pitted dates with the salt and vanilla in a food processor to form a stiff paste. Add the desiccated coconut and the hemp seeds and blitz to combine.

Melt the base coconut oil, and add to the food processor. Chop until everything is combined.

Measure and press 20g of base mix between six silicone portion moulds. Chill in the refrigerator to set.

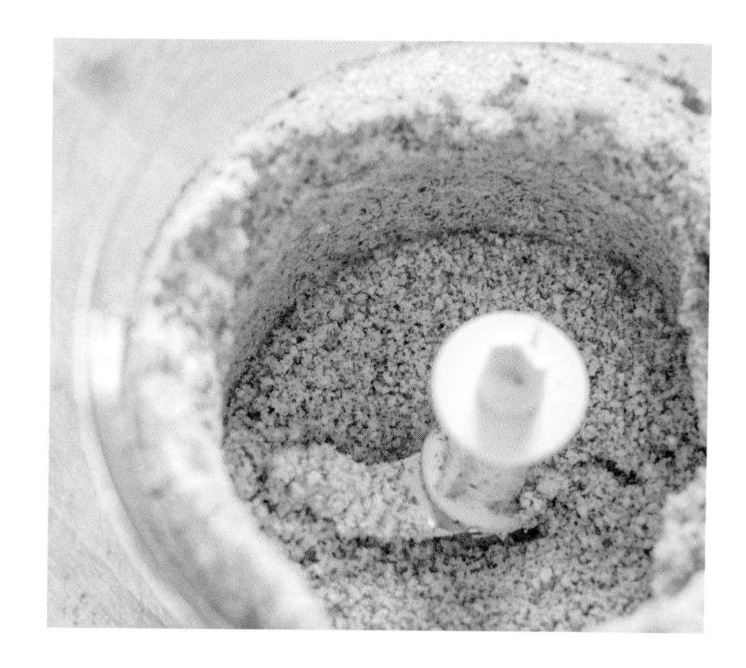

Blueberry cream to decorate:

50g cashews, soaked in ½ tbsp water and a pinch of salt

50g blueberries fresh or frozen (defrosted)

6g coconut milk powder

8g maple syrup

12g coconut oil, melted

¼ tsp vanilla extract

Decoration:

½ a lemon, grated zest

100g fresh blueberries

A few viola flowers

Mint leaves

Equipment needed

Liquidizer

Food processor

Six silicone moulds

Piping bag with star nozzle

To finish the filling:

Whizz the blueberry mix again in the liquidizer until it is completely smooth, then add the melted coconut oil and whizz again until fully incorporated.

Pour the blueberry mousse filling over the bases and tap the trays to level. Cover and freeze overnight or for at least 6 hours until solid.

To make the blueberry decorating cream:

Whizz all the ingredients together in a liquidizer until smooth.

Chill in the refrigerator until almost set, but still soft enough to pipe.

To serve:

Un-mould the frozen mousses onto a serving plate.

Prepare a piping bag with a star nozzle and fill with the soft blueberry cream. Pipe swirls of cream over the top of each one.

Press three whole blueberries into the cream and arrange the viola flowers and mint leaves over the top and sprinkle with grated lemon zest to finish.

Delicious with a cup of tea in the garden or serve as a dessert.

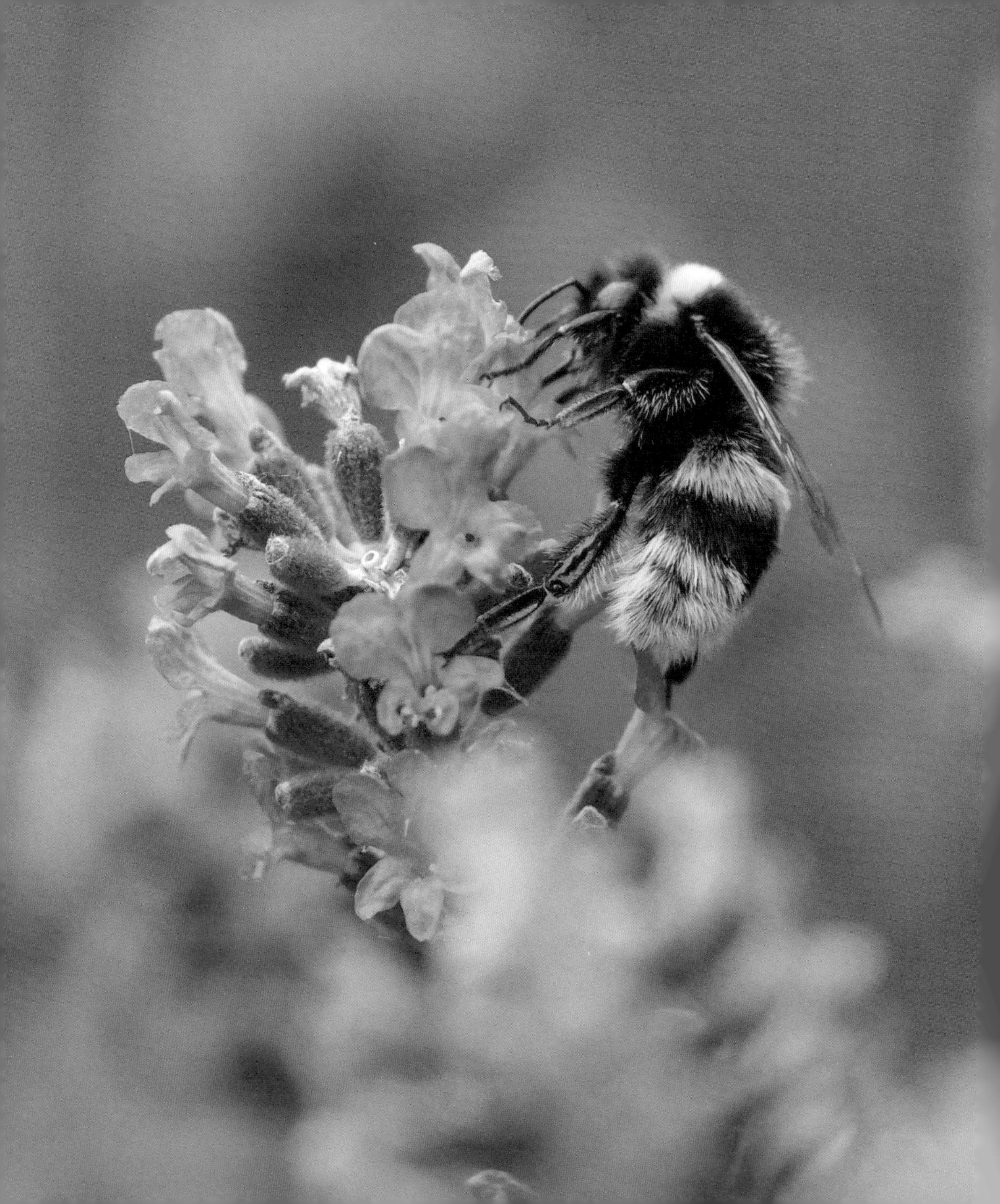

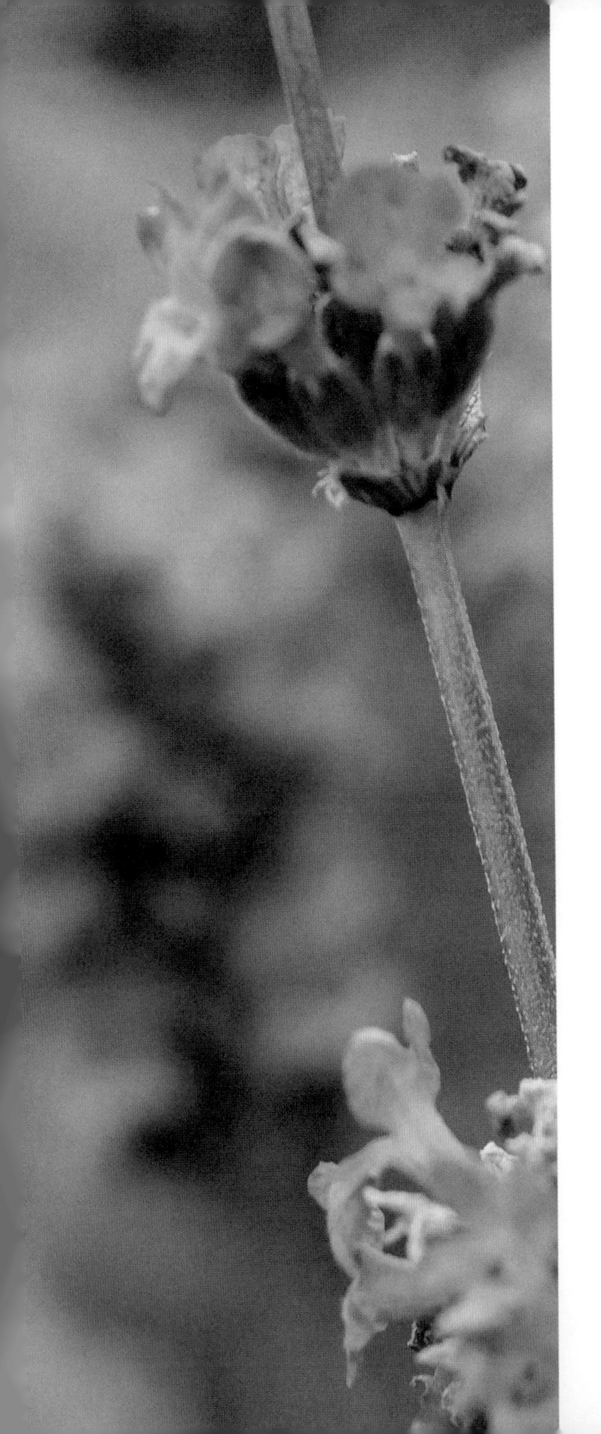

FINAL THOUGHTS

I've had such fun writing my second apothecary book; it has opened my eyes to the many wonders to be found just outside in my own back garden. Without doubt I will be looking to my own plot to grow lots more native plants to make use of – even better if they have some fascinating folklore attached.

I hope that this book will inspire you to gather some goodies from your own back gardens and turn them into straightforward home-grown remedies and treats.

Friends and family will love the fact that you have taken the time to create something just for them that is both natural and homemade.

Believe me you will have fun doing it, too!

THE HEALING PROPERTIES OF PLANTS

	Antibacterial	Anti-fungal	Anti- inflammatory	Anti-viral	Antioxidant	Antiseptic	Antihistamine	Soporific	Pain relieving
Agrimony								✓	
Aloe Vera	✓	✓	✓	✓					
Angelica			✓		✓				✓
Apple					✓				
Basil	✓	✓	✓						✓
Bay			✓		✓				
Borage			✓		✓				
Calendula	✓	✓	✓			✓			
Camomile			✓		✓		✓	✓	
Cherry			✓		✓			✓	
Cornflower			✓						
Daisy			✓						✓
Dandelion	✓		✓	✓	✓				
Dill			✓		✓				
Fennel	✓	✓	✓						

Hollyhock			✓						
Lady's Mantle			✓						
Lavender	✓	✓	✓	✓	✓	✓	✓	✓	✓
Lemon Balm	✓		✓		✓				
Lemon Verbena	✓		✓		✓			✓	
Lilac	✓		✓	✓	✓				
Mint	✓		✓		✓				
Nettle			✓		✓		✓		
Parsley	✓		✓						
Passion Flower								✓	
Pear			✓		✓				
Red Clover			✓		✓				
Rose			✓		✓	✓			
Rosemary	✓	✓	✓	✓	✓	✓			
Sage	✓	✓	✓						
Soapwort			✓						
Strawberry			✓		✓				
Sunflower			✓		✓				
Thyme	✓	✓	✓	✓		✓			
Valerian								✓	✓
Vervain									✓

ONLINE SUPPLIERS

G. Baldwins & Co – the oldest herbalist suppliers in London carrying a wide variety of dried herbs and pages of advice.
www.baldwins.co.uk

Naturally Thinking – organic carrier oils, natural beeswax, butters and essential oils and also a variety of eco-friendly packaging options for creams and balms.
www.naturallythinking.com

Wares of Knutsford – a wonderful range of decorative bottles, jars and kitchen equipment.
www.waresofknutsford.co.uk

Herbal Haven – grow over 150 varieties of medicinal, culinary and aromatic herbs (UK only).
www.herbalhaven.com

The Soap Kitchen – silicone moulds and lotion and soap-making supplies.
www.thesoapkitchen.co.uk

Lordington Lavender – West Sussex lavender growers and producers of pesticide-free lavender essential oil.
www.lordingtonlavender.co.uk

Image credits

Front cover – illustration © 4clover/Shutterstock.com; background texture © Art_Textures/Shutterstock.com

Back cover – top and bottom image © Christine Iverson; middle image © Ksenija Toyechkina/Shutterstock.com; illustrations © 4clover/Shutterstock.com; background texture © Art_Textures/Shutterstock.com

pp.11, 12, 13, 16, 17, 25, 36, 54, 55, 56, 88, 102, 104, 105, 171, 172 © Christine Iverson

p.4 – top row: © Christine Iverson; © TGTGTG/Shutterstock.com; middle row: © Frog Hollow Catering; © Christine Iverson; bottom row: © Christine Iverson; pp.6–7 – © STEVENSON/Shutterstock.com; pp.8–9, 208 and endpapers – © galsand/Shutterstock.com; p.15 © Seija/Shutterstock.com; p.18 – © Conrad Barrington/Shutterstock.com; pp.20–1 © KAN.Y/Shutterstock.com; p.22 – © thipjang/Shutterstock.com; p.23 – © Alenka Karabanova/Shutterstock.com; p.26 – © riet bloemen/Shutterstock.com; p.27 – © Anastasia Panfilova/Shutterstock.com; p.29 – © mirzamlk/Shutterstock.com; pp.30–1 © Mark Heighes/Shutterstock.com; p.32 – © Yana Peneva/Shutterstock.com; p.33 – © EngravingFactory/Shutterstock.com; p.34 – © Madeleine Steinbach/Shutterstock.com; p.38 – © Nadya So/Shutterstock.com; p.39 – © Cat_arch_angel/Shutterstock.com; pp.40–1 – © Billion Photos/Shutterstock.com; p.42 – © Formatoriginal/Shutterstock.com; p.43 – © Cat_arch_angel/Shutterstock.com; pp.44–5 – © Halil Ibrahim mescioglu/Shutterstock.com; p.46 – © Michael gromov/Shutterstock.com p.47 – © Cat_arch_angel/Shutterstock.com; pp.48–9 – © Madeleine Steinbach/Shutterstock.com; p.51 – © Magdanatka/Shutterstock.com; p.52 – © LutsenkoLarissa/Shutterstock.com; p.53 – © Foxyliam/Shutterstock.com; p.58 – © irink/Shutterstock.com; p.59 – © lucky strokes/Shutterstock.com; p.61 – © Alina Kruk/Shutterstock.com; p.63 – © kazmulka/Shutterstock.com; p.64 – © Serhii Brovko/Shutterstock.com; p.65 – © Melniklena/Shutterstock.com; p.67 – © iuliia_n/Shutterstock.com; p.68 – © john mobbs/Shutterstock.com; p.69 – © cuttlefish84/Shutterstock.com; p.71 – © TGTGTG/Shutterstock.com; pp.72–3 – © Ariene Studio/Shutterstock.com; p.74 – © Flower_Garden/Shutterstock.com; p.75 – © Cat_arch_angel/Shutterstock.com; pp.76–7 – © TGTGTG/Shutterstock.com; p.78 – © Vitaly Slavinsky/Shutterstock.com; p.81 – © Madeleine Steinbach/Shutterstock.com; p.82 – © Scharfsinn/Shutterstock.com; p.83 – © Foxyliam/Shutterstock.com pp.84–5 – © manulito/Shutterstock.com; p.86 – © nnattalli/Shutterstock.com; p.87 – © Irina Vaneeva/Shutterstock.com; p.91 – © Oksana Shufrych/Shutterstock.com; p.92 – © Ole Schoener/Shutterstock.com; p.93 – © Cat_arch_angel/Shutterstock.com; p.95 – © Ole Schoener/Shutterstock.com; p.96 – © sasimoto/Shutterstock.com; p.97 – © Foxyliam/Shutterstock.com; p.98 – © neroli/Shutterstock.com; p.100 – © ESstock/Shutterstock.com; p.101 – © Foxyliam/Shutterstock.com; p.106 – © S.O.E/Shutterstock.com; p.107 – © Foxyliam/Shutterstock.com; p.109 – © Scharfsinn/Shutterstock.com; p.110 – © Julie Clopper/Shutterstock.com; p.111 – © Foxyliam/Shutterstock.com; p.112 – © Julie Clopper/Shutterstock.com; p.113 – © Lida Reviako/Shutterstock.com; p.114 – © Maya Kruchankova/Shutterstock.com; p.115 – © Bubnova Natalia/Shutterstock.com; p.117 – © Vlada Tikhonova/Shutterstock.com; p.118 – © IAM PRAWIT/Shutterstock.com; p.121 – © New Africa/Shutterstock.com; p.122 – © Sunrise Hunter/Shutterstock.com; p.123 – © Cat_arch_angel/Shutterstock.com; p.124 – © zoryanchik/Shutterstock.com; p.126 – © Andrey Venhlovskyi/Shutterstock.com; p.129 – © Liudmyla Yaremenko/Shutterstock.com; p.130 – © Flower_Garden/Shutterstock.com; p.133 – © Julija Ogrodowski/Shutterstock.com; p.134 – © docstockmedia/Shutterstock.com; p.135 – © EngravingFactory/Shutterstock.com; pp.136–7 – © Tatiana Vorona/Shutterstock.com; p.138–9 – © robertsre/Shutterstock.com; p.140 – © vvoe/Shutterstock.com; p.141 – © Cat_arch_angel/Shutterstock.com; p.143 – © Ekaterina Kondratova/Shutterstock.com; p.144 – © Bobyleva Kseniya/Shutterstock.com; p.147 – © iva/Shutterstock.com; p.148 – © Alexander Raths/Shutterstock.com; p.151 – © kostrez/Shutterstock.com; p.152 – © Karen Kaspar/Shutterstock.com; p.153 – © Cat_arch_angel/Shutterstock.com; p.155 – © HUIZENG/Shutterstock.com; p.156 – © Olesya Baron/Shutterstock.com; p.157 – © Foxyliam/Shutterstock.com; p.159 – © MoDaVi Art/Shutterstock.com; p.161 – © Justyna Kaminska/Shutterstock.com; p.162 – © DVY/Shutterstock.com; p.163 – © Nina Fedorova/Shutterstock.com; pp.164–5 – © Gaston Cerliani/Shutterstock.com; p.166 – © ElenaVah/Shutterstock.com; p.167 – © Foxyliam/Shutterstock.com; p.168 – © 4mai/Shutterstock.com; p.170 – © Mr. Arun/Shutterstock.com; p.174 – © Barbara Bekei/Shutterstock.com; p.176 – © Madeleine Steinbach/Shutterstock.com; p.177 – © Afanesieva/Shutterstock.com; p.178 – © Lipatova Maryna/Shutterstock.com; p.179 – © Foxyliam/Shutterstock.com; p.181 – © Snowbelle/Shutterstock.com; p.182 – © Dan4Earth/Shutterstock.com; p.185 – © AlexSamDnDz/Shutterstock.com; p.186 – © Brita Seifert/Shutterstock.com; p.187 – © Foxyliam/Shutterstock.com; p.188–190 – © Frog Hollow Catering; p.192–3 – © muroPhotographer/Shutterstock.com

NOTES

ALSO BY CHRISTINE IVERSON

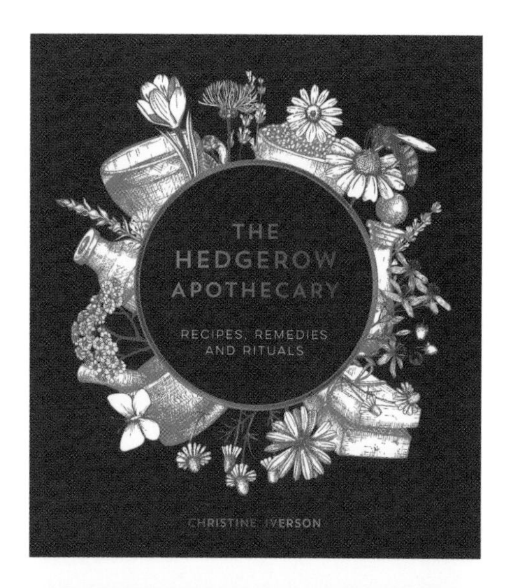

THE HEDGEROW APOTHECARY

Recipes, Remedies and Rituals

Hardback
ISBN: 978-1-78783-029-5

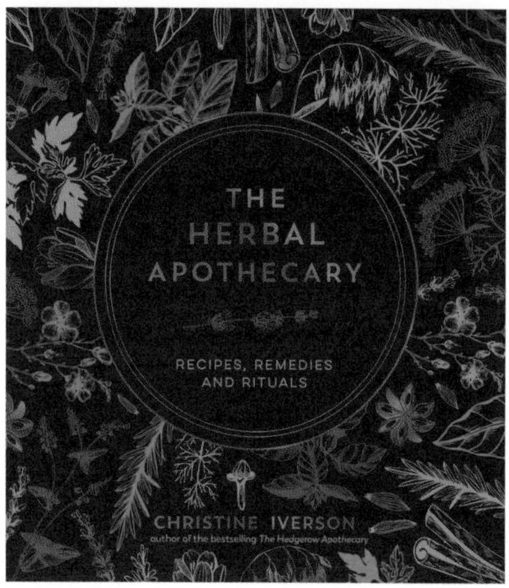

THE HERBAL APOTHECARY

Recipes, Remedies and Rituals

Hardback
ISBN: 978-1-80007-985-4

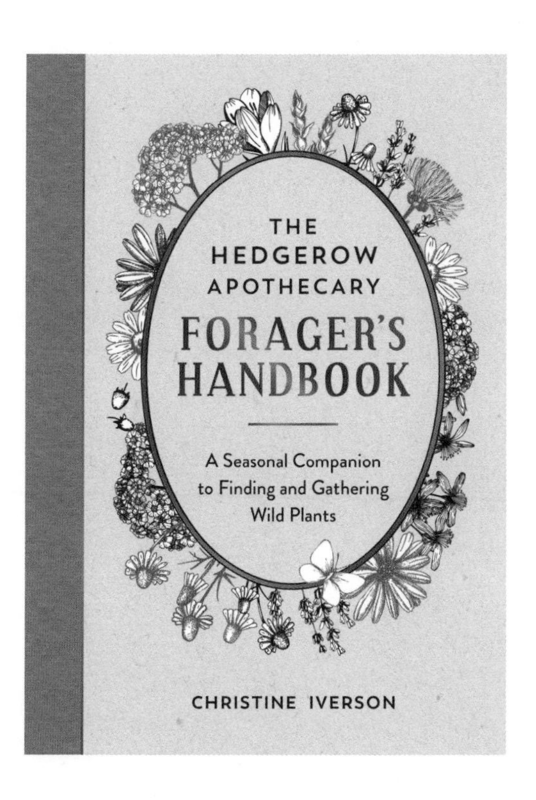

THE HEDGEROW APOTHECARY FORAGER'S HANDBOOK

A Seasonal Companion to Finding and Gathering Wild Plants

Paperback
ISBN: 978-1-80007-181-0

Learn to forage in the hedgerows like the herbalists of the past

As many of us look for ways to live a more planet-friendly lifestyle, the sustainable and ethical art of foraging offers us a way to connect with the world around us. It is a practice rich in tradition and steeped in history, and one that links us to our past and our future.

This foraging companion is designed to be taken with you on your adventures into the hedgerows, forests and woodland all year round. Helpfully arranged by season, this book includes clear photographs to aid plant identification, ideas on how best to prepare and preserve your finds, fascinating foraging and plant folklore, and handy pages to make your own notes and drawings.

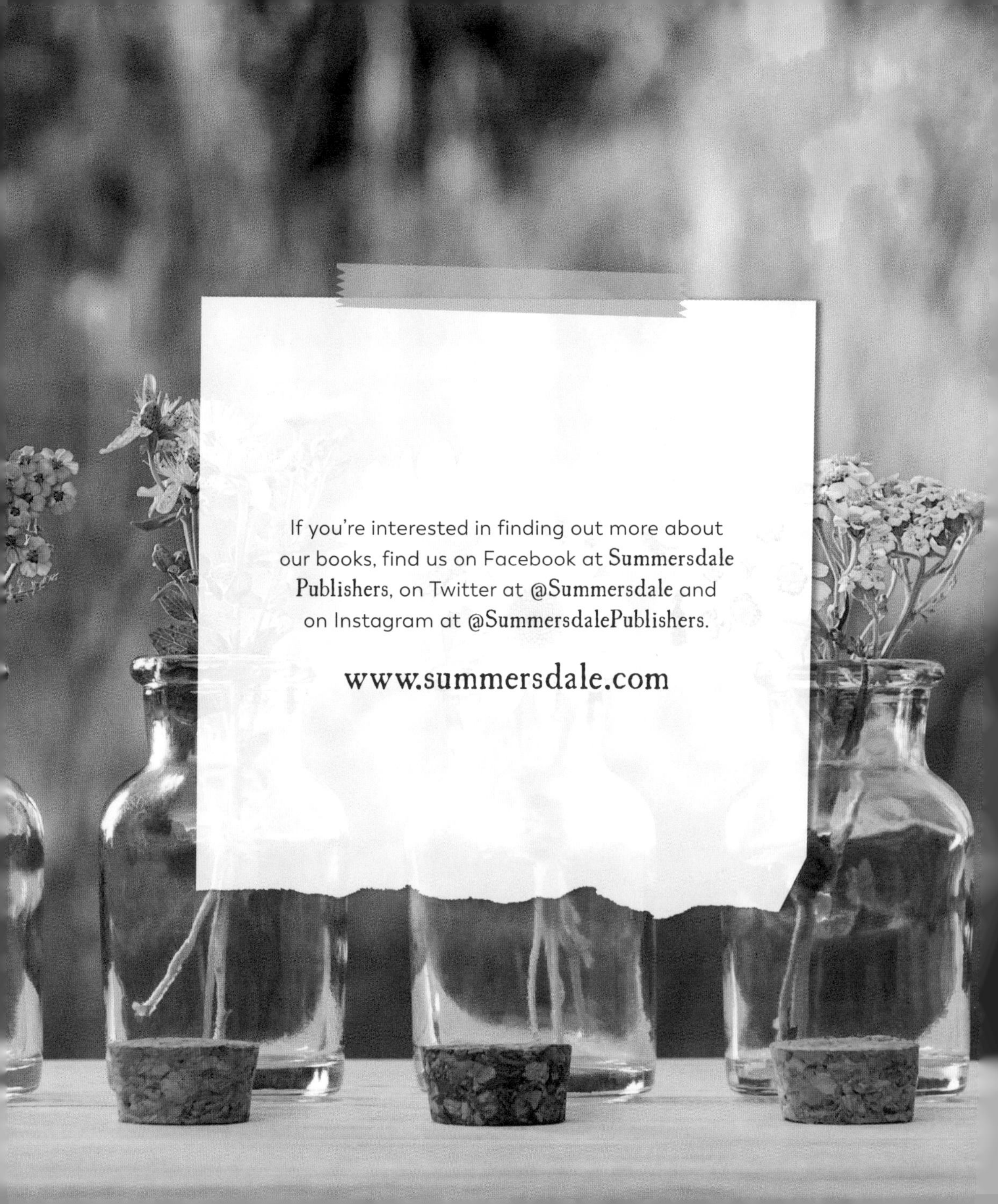

If you're interested in finding out more about our books, find us on Facebook at Summersdale Publishers, on Twitter at @Summersdale and on Instagram at @SummersdalePublishers.

www.summersdale.com

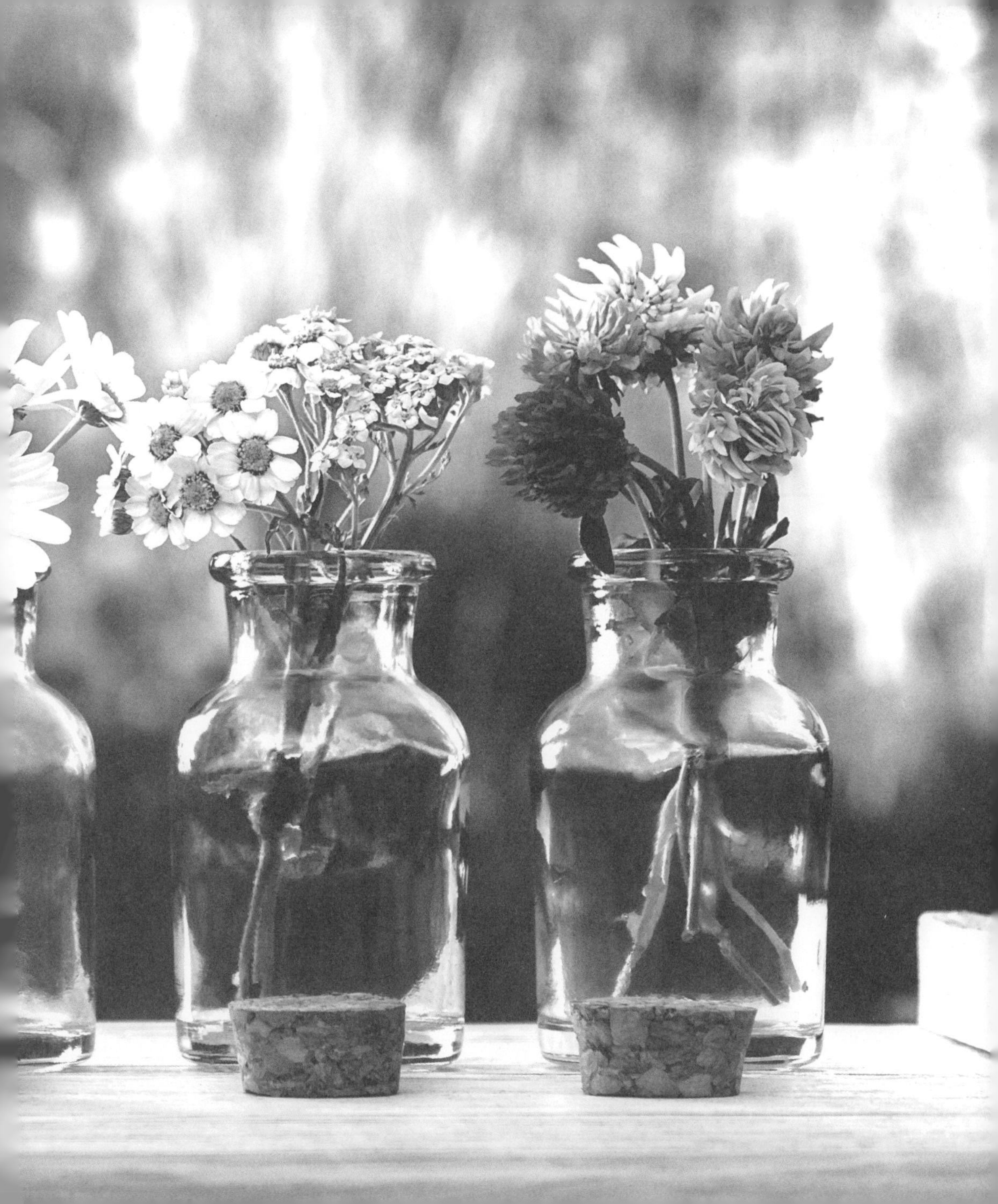

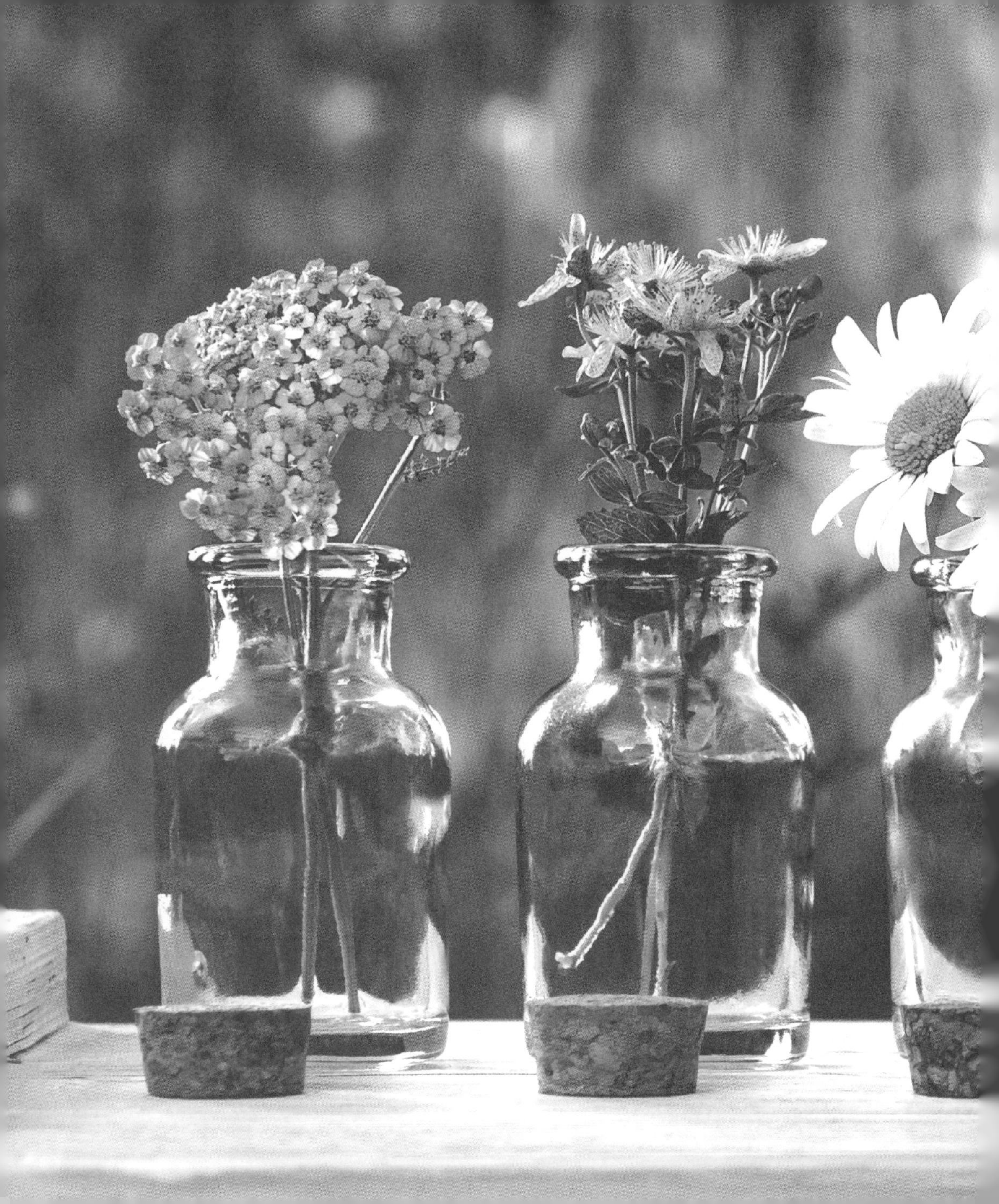